Mechanisms in Respiratory Toxicology

Volume I

Editors

Hanspeter Witschi, M.D.
Senior Research Staff Member
Biology Division
Oak Ridge National Laboratory
Oak Ridge, Tennessee

Paul Nettesheim, M.D.
Chief
Laboratory of Pulmonary Function and Toxicology
National Institute of Environmental Health Sciences
Research Triangle Park, North Carolina

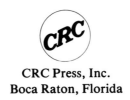

CRC Press, Inc.
Boca Raton, Florida

Library of Congress Cataloging in Publication Data

Main entry under title:

Mechanisms in respiratory toxicology.

  Includes bibliographies and indexes.
  1. Lungs--Diseases. 2. Respiratory organs--Diseases.
3. Toxicology. I. Witschi, Hanspeter.
II. Nettesheim, P. [DNLM: 1. Lung--Pathology. 2. Lung
diseases--Chemically induced. WF 600 M486]
RC732.M43   616.2'4   81-2135
                                    AACR2

Direct all inquiries to CRC Press, Inc., 2000 N.W. 24th Street, Boca Raton, Florida 33431.

© 1982 by CRC Press, Inc.

International Standard Book Number 0-8493-5689-X

Library of Congress Card Number 81-2135
Printed in the United States

PREFACE

Over the last decade, pulmonary toxicology has become an exciting and fast moving field. A main reason for this is the realization by many investigators, which occurred about 10 years ago, that the lung is not simply a gas-exchanging organ. At the same time there was an increasing awareness that lung tissue may not become damaged by airborne agents alone, but also by chemicals carried by the bloodstream. Among these are naturally and manmade agents, some of which have considerable economic or medical value. It was also realized that the main problem in environmentally induced pulmonary disease is not so much acute, but rather long-term low-level toxicity and it became clear that very little information is available on chronic injury.

It seemed an appropriate undertaking to review some of the current knowledge on the pathobiology of toxic lung damage. This could have been done by describing the toxicology of individual agents. However, such an analysis might not provide an in-depth insight into underlying general pathogenetic principles and might also become overly repetitious, since many of the more thoroughly studied toxic agents produce similar end results. We therefore chose to focus on the cellular and biochemical mechanisms of lung tissue responses to chemical injury.

In the first volume of *Mechanisms in Respiratory Toxicology* an overview is presented on the access toxic agents have to the lung. This includes description of the anatomical features of the lung as well as a discussion of the kinetics of the delivery of chemicals either by the airways or the bloodstream. Once toxic agents reach their target, they set in motion a sequence of events such as cell death, development of edema, and changes in the activity of the mucociliary escalator.

In the second volume pulmonary defense mechanisms and endogenous factors modulating the biological response are discussed. Equally important for understanding the diversity of toxic reactions is the knowledge of biotransformation of chemicals in their target cells. Finally, two clinically important conditions resulting from chronic lung damage are discussed, namely fibrosis and emphysema.

Throughout the two volumes emphasis is placed on cellular and biochemical mechanisms. It is hoped that a discussion of general pathogenetic principles will interest all who are concerned with the action of toxic chemicals on the lung.

It is a pleasure to acknowledge the dedicated and highly competent work of all contributors to this book. Our thanks also go to the staff of CRC Press for skillfully editing the two volumes.

THE EDITORS

Hanspeter Witschi, M.D., is a Senior Research Staff Member at the Biology Division, Oak Ridge National Laboratory. Dr. Witschi received his M.D. degree from the University of Bern, Switzerland, in 1960. He worked as a research fellow in the MRC Toxicology Research Unit in Carshalton/England, the Kettering Laboratory at the University of Cincinnati, and in the Department of Pathology, University of Pittsburgh. From 1969 to 1977 he was at the Department of Pharmacology, Faculty of Medicine, University of Montreal before moving to Oak Ridge National Laboratory. His present research concerns mechanisms of acute and chronic lung damage.

Paul Nettesheim, M.D., is Chief of the Laboratory of Pulmonary Function and Toxicology at the National Institute of Environmental Health Sciences, National Institutes of Health, Department of Health and Human Services. Dr. Nettesheim received his M.D. degree from the University of Boun Medical School in 1959. His professional experience includes training in Pathology at the University of Freiburg i Br. and the University of Pennsylvania between the years 1960 to 1963. He was a member of the research staff at the Biology Division of Oak Ridge National Laboratory from 1963 to 1978. In 1978 he became a member of the National Institute of Environmental Health Sciences. His present research concerns pulmonary cell biology and respiratory tract carcinogenesis.

CONTRIBUTORS

Michael R. Boyd, M.D., Ph.D.
Chief, Molecular Toxicology Section
Clinical Pharmacology Branch
National Cancer Institute
Bethesda, Maryland

Kathryn H. Bradley
Chemist
Pulmonary Branch
National Heart, Lung, and Blood
  Institute
National Institutes of Health
Bethesda, Maryland

Arnold R. Brody, Ph.D.
Head, Pulmonary Pathology Group
Laboratory of Pulmonary Function and
  Toxicology
National Institute of Environmental
  Health Sciences
Research Triangle Park, North
  Carolina

Carroll E. Cross, M.D.
Professor
School of Medicine
Departments of Physiology and
  Medicine
University of California
Davis, California

Ronald G. Crystal, Ph.D.
Chief, Pulmonary Branch
National Heart, Lung, and Blood
  Institute
National Institutes of Health
Bethesda, Maryland

Gerald S. Davis, M.D.
Chief
Division of Pulmonary Medicine
University of Vermont
Burlington, Vermont

Michael J. Evans, Ph.D.
Associate Director
Medical Sciences Department
SRI International
Menlo Park, California

Victor J. Ferrans, M.D.
Chief, Ultrastructure Section
Pathology Branch
National Heart, Lung, and Blood
  Institute
National Institutes of Health
Bethesda, Maryland

Joan Gil, M.D.
Associate Professor of Medicine and
  Anatomy
Cardiovascular-Pulmonary Division
Department of Medicine
University of Pennsylvania
Philadelphia, Pennsylvania

Arnold B. Gorin
Assistant Professor in Medicine
School of Medicine
University of California
Davis, California

Kaye H. Kilburn, M.D.
Ralph Edgington Professor of Medicine
Director
Environmental Sciences Laboratory
University of Southern California
  School of Medicine
Los Angeles, California

Charles Kuhn, M.D.
Professor of Pathology
Washington University School of
  Medicine
Associate Pathologist
Barnes Hospital
St. Louis, Missouri

Jerold A. Last, Ph.D.
Associate Professor of Internal
  Medicine and Biological Chemistry
University of California
Davis, California

Lee V. Leak, Ph.D.
Professor of Anatomy
Director
Ernest E. Just Laboratory of Cellular
  Biology
College of Medicine
Howard University
Washington, D.C.

Marvin Lesser, M.D.
Chief of Pulmonary Medicine
Bronx Veterans Administration Medical
  Center
Assistant Professor of Medicine
Mount Sinai Hospital
Bronx, New York

Gibbe H. Parsons, M.D.
Director
Medical and Respiratory Intensive Care
  Unit
University of California Davis Medical
  Center
Sacramento, California

John A. Pierce, M.D.
Director, Pulmonary Disease Division
Professor of Medicine
Washington University
St. Louis, Missouri

Otto G. Raabe, Ph.D.
Associate Adjunct Professor
Department of Radiological Sciences
School of Veterinary Medicine
University of California
Davis, California

Stephen I. Rennard, M.D.
Senior Staff Fellow
Pulmonary Branch
National Heart, Lung, and Blood
  Institute
National Institutes of Health
Bethesda, Maryland

Sami I. Said, M.D.
Chief, Pulmonary Disease Section
Veterans Administration Medical
  Center
Professor of Internal Medicine and
  Pharmacology
University of Texas Health Science
  Center
Dallas, Texas

Robert M. Senior, M.D.
Associate Professor of Medicine
Washington University School of
  Medicine
Co-Director, Pulmonary Disease and
  Respiratory Division
The Jewish Hospital
St. Louis, Missouri

Alan G. E. Wilson, Ph.D.
Senior Research Toxicologist
Metabolism Section
Environmental Health Laboratory
Monsanto Company
St. Louis, Missouri

TABLE OF CONTENTS

Volume I

Volume II

Delivery of Toxic Agents to the Lung

Chapter 1

COMPARATIVE MORPHOLOGY AND ULTRASTRUCTURE OF THE AIRWAYS

Joan Gil

TABLE OF CONTENTS

I. INTRODUCTION

The purpose of this chapter is to describe the anatomy of the mammalian lung with emphasis on those structures and features that are apt to be involved in early toxicologic reactions. In this context, boundaries seem particularly important, e.g., those between air and tissue or between inspired and alveolar air. The air spaces of the lung are comprised of conducting airways (trachea, bronchi, and bronchioles) and terminal airways (ducts and alveoli) where the gas exchange takes place. Both of them are lined, at least in part, by extracellular fluids of relatively unclear composition and uncommon physicochemical properties: the seromucous secretions in the conducting airways and the extracellular lining layer ("surfactant") in the alveoli. The boundary between blood and endothelium is also to some extent unique because the capillary bed seems to be subjected to frequent changes in shape, size, and level of perfusion, depending on a variety of factors. This presentation is limited to the morphological aspects of lung function. In keeping with current research trends, it includes data on morphometry of different parts of the lung.

II. CONDUCTING AIRWAYS

Conducting airways are a system of branching tubes of regular, cylindrical, or somewhat irregular cross section that extend from the trachea down to the last respiratory bronchioles. From the point of view of particle penetration and deposition and airborne environmental injury, dimensions and geometry of the bronchial tree are of outermost significance, but other important features include the cellular composition and the nature of the fluid lining of the lumen of the airways. These aspects have been the object of very intensive research in recent times.

A. Airway Morphometry

The significance of the airway geometry in connection with different problems of pulmonary physiology or environmental aggression was recognized early. First attempts at casting airways with diverse materials were already reported in the 19th century, and advanced morphometric studies on airway casts are still being published. Although not primarily anatomical in nature, the work of Rohrer[1] in 1915 deserves mention because it pioneered a mathematical approach to the basis of airflow resistance in the respiratory system. A solution to the problems raised by Rohrer's and subsequent studies on lung mechanics required a realistic knowledge of the airways both in qualitative and quantitative terms (for review see Pedley et al.[2]).

Weibel offered the first comprehensive quantitative treatment of airway branching in his book.[3] Division of an airway takes place by irregular dichotomy, i.e., a mother branch divides into two daughter airways of different diameter which, in turn, become parent branches. As we shall see below, irregularity of the branching pattern is one of the major problems encountered in morphometry of the conducting airways. Information needed for the study of important items, such as dead space, type of airflow (turbulent or laminar), airflow resistance, and pattern of particle deposition, includes the following anatomic features: number of dichotomic divisions, length-to-diameter ratios of the simple branches, number of units in each generation, particularly number of units in the last generation, and changes in airway diameter after each division. For special purposes, knowledge of branch angles and inclination to gravity may also be necessary. Weibel studied detailed casts of the more proximal generations of airways beginning with the trachea, and additionally he performed measurements on the total amount of peripheral airways visible in histologic specimens. From this he established that after assigning to the trachea the generation number 0, the average number of generations down to the last airways (alveolar sac) was 23, with the terminal bronchioles, the last purely conducting airways, being on the average generation 16.

Most airflow studies are based on the above-described Model A of Weibel which, without ignoring the branching irregularity, imposes a workable pattern by simply taking the mean values of length and diameter for each generation. The effective length of individual paths could be anywhere between 15 and 30 generations. Tables listing data for individual airway generation (number, diameter, length, and total cross section and volume)[3] and airflow data (Reynolds number at different airflow rates) have been published.[2] Plotting the progressive reduction of diameter d of conducting airways against the generation number, Weibel derived the relationship

$$d_z = d_0 \cdot 2^{-\frac{z}{3}} \qquad\qquad (1)$$

(where d_0 is the diameter of the trachea (1.8 cm), and d_z is the average diameter of the branches in generation Z) which is favorable from the point of view of hydrodynamics. This relationship holds only until Z = 16 (terminal bronchioles, d_z = 0.06 cm). Subsequent branchings, from Z = 17 to 23 show much larger diameters. In this model, the total number of branches (n) of a generation is evidently n = 2^z which explains why in this system the trachea must be assigned the generation number 0. Useful as this model was, certain relevant parameters were missing from this model. These have been listed by Phalen et al.[4] as follows:

1.   The model did not provide branching angles.
2.   It did not consider the effects of asymmetry in daughter segments.
3.   It did not describe local differences in anatomy among lobes.

Irregular dichotomy was to become the major concern of many workers. According to Horsfield and Cumming,[5] an asymmetrical dichotomously branching system is one with variation in the diameters or lengths of the branches in a given generation or a variation in the number of divisions down the end branches. These authors stressed that in an irregular system, it is an unjustified restraint to count generations from the trachea (generation 0) down to end branches because any intermediate generation number embodies branches different in size and possibly in function. They proposed to number the branches upward starting with branches of a diameter equal to 0.07 cm ("lobular branches") to which the order number 1 was arbitrarily assigned. Thinner branches were designated 0. Horsfield and Cumming[5] performed a painstaking counting of the amount and individual measurements of all the airways between the above-indicated 0.07-cm bronchioles and the trachea (a total of 8298). The shortest path length was reached after 8 branchings, and the longest was found after 25 divisions, with the mean being 14.6. Additionally these authors measured samples of the last distal airways between the 0.07-cm branches and the end. They found the number of distal divisions to range from two to seven.

This careful study in fact showed that Weibel's model was reasonably accurate in spite of the assumptions made. Additionally it has proven very difficult to use asymmetrical systems in modeling for flow dynamics.[2] In a comprehensive, careful study of compared airway morphometry in humans and three other mammals, Phalen et al.[5] point out that asymmetry and its effects are more pronounced in larger than in smaller airways. The most common branching angle appears to be 37.5°.[4,6]

B. Airway Organization

1. Histology of Airway Epithelium

The conducting airways are lined by a pseudostratified ciliated epithelium on a thick basement membrane. Its extraordinary complexity has only recently been recognized: it is an epithelial lining, a mechanical and an immunological defense organ, and an exocrine and an endocrine gland. At the onset, one must point out at the existence of numerous species differences and the variability of the quantitative relationship between cell types.

a. Cells

Several detailed reviews on the structure of epitheliel cells have been recently published by Kuhn,[7] Breeze and Wheeldon,[8] and Jeffery and Reid.[9] The enumeration of the cell types is surprisingly long.

The ciliated cells account for the bulk of cells (see Figures 1 to 4) and are responsible for moving the mucous secretions. They are columnar, electron lucent with abundant mitochondria, secondary lysosomes, rough endoplasmic reticulum, multivesicular bodies, smooth vesicles, and well-developed Golgi. Their lumenal surface is covered with long, slender microvilli and approximately 250 cilia per cell, each 6-μm long and 0.3-μm wide (see Figure 2). The cilia contain an axoneme, a system of nine peripheral double tubules with dynein arms arranged forming a ring around two single central microtubules. Each cilium is anchored to basal bodies, identical with the centrioles active in cell mitosis, and these are fixed by a dense system of "root" microtubules, believed to be a cytoskeletal feature. The tip of the ciliar shaft is provided with claw-like projections which may adhere to the underface of the mucous blanket. The molecular organization and physiology of ciliar beat have been extensively discussed.[7,10]

The goblet cells (see Figure 1) are tall columnar, with slender basis and broad apex. Their cytoplasm is dark; it contains extensive rough endoplasmic reticulum and a supranuclear large Golgi. The apical portion contains variable amounts of secretion granules, sometimes fusing with each other. These granules which often show a dense core by electron microscopy contain some form of mucus, and their histochemical characteristics are well known.[9] Accounts of the normal amount of goblet cells vary greatly; an often-repeated figure for humans is 6800 cells per square millimeter. At the root of the problem, we face the fact that they undergo hyperplasia as unspecific response to irritation (together with increase of the epithelial mitotic index and hypertrophy of the seromucous glands).[9] It has been claimed by several workers that goblet cells are rare in specific pathogen-free adult animals. These cells evidently secrete mucus, but it is dubious at what extent they contribute to the movable blanket of bronchial mucus. In the intestinal epithelium, similar cells perform a general protective function.

The small, pyramidal *basal cells* are generally regarded as the progenitors of the other cell types.

Brush cells are columnar, with a broad basis. They are characterized by the presence of a brush border of very thick microvilli (200 μm in diameter and 800 μm in length) with conspicuous tonofilaments.

Intermediate cells seem to represent stages between young basal cells and fully differentiated cells.

Special type cells occur only in some species. They usually do not reach the lumenal surface; they interdigitate heavily with neighboring cells and contain specific, membrane-bound granules of moderate electron density placed peripherally.

Epithelial serous cells were recently described in the rat trachea. They are thought to be similar to the serous secretory cells of the seromucous glands and contain homogeneous, ovoidal, large inclusions.

Endocrine cells include Kultschitsky, amine uptake and decarboxylation (APUD) or

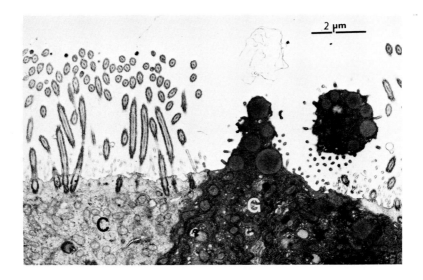

FIGURE 1.   Trachea of rat lung fixed by filling the airspaces with glutaraldehyde; C, ciliated cell; G, goblet cell. Note that tips of cilia and of goblet cell reach similar height.

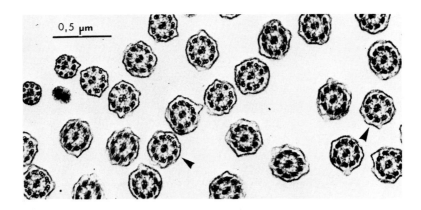

FIGURE 2.   Same material as Figure 1, cross sectional views of cilia. Arrows point at cilia where the subcellular arrangement of tubules is well visible. (See complete description in the reviews by Kuhn[7] and Sleigh.[10])

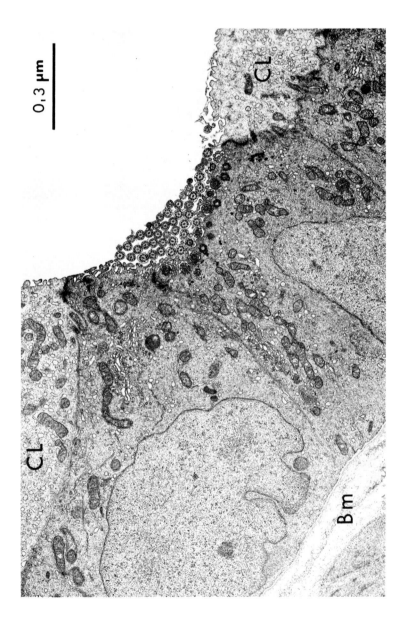

FIGURE 3.   Bronchiole of rat lung fixed by perfusion of the pulmonary artery. Two cuboidal, moderately dark ciliated cells rest on a basement membrane (Bm) and are flanked by two Clara cells (CL) with smooth vesicles. On left, lower corner, is a smooth muscle cell.

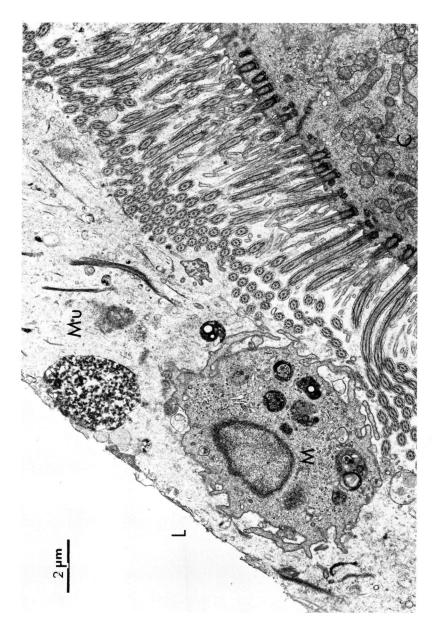

FIGURE 4. Electron micrograph of large bronchus in rabbit lung fixed by vascular perfusion of OsO₄, through the pulmonary artery. C is the top of a ciliated cell with many small mitochondria. Numerous cilia cut in different directions originate from kinetosomes and are embedded in electron lucent fluid (sol phase), covered by a mucus layer Mu (gel phase). Inside the mucus, a small macrophage profile (M) is visible, as well as other impurities of uncertain nature. Floating on top of the mucus are some tubular myelin of alveolar origin. L is bronchial lumen.

small granules cells, either individually interspersed or clustered in neuroepithelial bodies.[11] Their characteristic feature is the existence of small basal granules with a dense core. Their secretion products are unknown, but they are thought to be the source of vasoactive substances. One of the problems involved in their study is that they are sparse and difficult to stain. Some progress in the development of suitable stains has been recently reported.[12]

Clara cells (see Figure 4) are present mainly in the peripheral airways such as bronchioles. Owing to species differences, there are many conflicting descriptions in the literature. A constant finding is the existence of large amounts of smooth endoplasmic reticulum (which in other cells is related to functions such as steroid synthesis, detoxification, or phospholipid synthesis). It has been shown that Clara cells are a cellular site of cytochrome P-450 dependent mixed function oxidase activity in the lung,[47] which is localized in the apices of the cells. Clara cells are frequent targets of injury in chemical poisoning. In certain species, large mitochondria with few cristae have been described. One usually sees apical granules of small size, sometimes crystalline in nature.[7]

Rare cell types include the oncocytes, cells literally stuffed with mitochondria (for instance, like the parathyroideal chief cells), which are particularly notorious after oxygen exposure: the globule leukocytes which seem to be immigrant cells stuffed with very large granules, and are, to some extent, similar to the mast cells, but with larger globules; and also lymphocytes, as in many other epithelial membranes.

Finally, one should mention the intraepithelial axons, believed to be afferent, unmyelinated nerve endings.[13] The search for lung receptors, and their identification — irritant, stretch, and J-receptors — has been generally frustrating. These naked intraepithelial axons, associated with different cell types, are regarded as irritant receptors responsible for reflex hyperpnea and bronchconstriction on inhalation of irritant substances.

b. Glands

The submucosal seromucous glands are thought to be the main source of tracheobronchial secretions. Human glands have been the object of a three dimensional reconstruction.[14] They consist of a ciliated duct continuous with the surface epithelium, a collecting duct lined by tall, nonciliated cells, and of mucous and serous secretory end pieces. The precise nature of the serous secretions is not known. If it is permissible to compare the serous cells with similar cells of the salivary or pancreatic glands, one would expect them to secrete enzymes for the purpose of modulating the final composition of the mucus produced by mucous cells of the glands.

c. Mucous Layer

Back in 1934, Lucas and Douglas[15] proposed a biphasic fluid layer consisting of a viscous gel layer (the mucus in the usual sense) continuously cleared toward the trachea by ciliary motion and a thin sol layer underneath, between the gel and the cell surface, in which the cilia beat. Fixation by vascular perfusion or by rapid freezing permits preservation of some mucous material *in situ* (see Figure 3). There is, however, widespread disagreement about whether or not the layer is biphasic, continuous, or of constant thickness.[16] Much of this disagreement may be related to species differences. This mucous layer is not to be confused with the lining described over the bronchiolar epithelium by Gil and Weibel[17] because mucus is not supposed to be present in the small bronchioles.

2. Major Conducting Airways
a. Trachea

The human trachea has in the average a length of some 12 cm and contains in its walls U-shaped cartilages. The dorsal aspect of the trachea is spanned between the ends of the cartilage plates, contains smooth muscle, and is called *Paries membranaceus*. As a hollow tube, the trachea is comparatively rigid, but allows for modest changes in both width and length. Most textbooks describe a mucous, a submucous and a fibrocartilagineous layer, although the boundaries between them are diffuse. The epithelium of the mucosa has been described above. In the trachea, it is very tall and clearly pseudostratified; as one progresses toward the periphery, the epithelium progressively loses height until in the bronchioles it clearly becomes cuboidal (see Figures 3 and 4). There appear to be also some changes in the relative frequency of cell types, although this is not clear for all cell types.

b. Bronchi

These are characterized by the loss of the U-shaped cartilage rings which are replaced by more irregular plates interconnected by bundles of smooth muscle cells. The arrangement of the muscle is such that the airway shortens as it narrows. As they penetrate into the lungs, bronchi become embedded in a sheath of loose connective tissue which contains structures, such as lymphatics, nerves, bronchial blood vessels, and pulmonary arteries. In smaller airways, the pulmonary artery runs alongside the sheath embedded in a connective tissue layer of its own which is interconnected with the peribronchial tissue by a thin lamella. Von Hayek[18] already showed that these sheaths and their contents (essentially conducting airways and arteries) form a compartment separated from the gas exchanging parenchyma. Sheaths are relevant as sites of fluid accumulation during edema development (peribronchial and perivascular "cuffs").

The histology of the epithelium is nearly identical to that of the trachea, as discussed above.

c. Bronchioles

There is no universally accepted definition of a bronchiole. They are small in diameter, devoid of cartilage in their walls, devoid of glands, and the goblet cells are gradually replaced by Clara cells, described above which are among the most interesting features of the bronchioles. The function of Clara cells has never been clear; in connection with carcinogenic studies, increasing attention is paid to these cells which under the effect of nitrosamines develop lamellar bodies similar to those normally seen in Type II cells.[19] Additionally, they seem to be progenitors of ciliated cells.[20] The bronchioles possess a double, but incomplete layer of smooth muscle cells; the two layers are helicoidal and cut each other in an oblique angle. The epithelial cells here are cuboidal; their short cilia are embedded in an extracellular fluid as shown by Gil and Weibel[17] in rat lungs fixed by vascular perfusion.

3. Bronchus Associated Lymphatic Tissue (BALT)

In keeping with the increasing significance of immunologic studies in pulmonary research, growing attention is being paid to the recently described BALT.[21] Localized infiltrations of the lamina propria of the mucosa with lymphocytes have always been known to exist. What the notion of BALT implies is that there are permanent lymphatic structures immediately under the epithelium, comparable to those which constitute the gut associated lymphatic tissue (GALT). The description of BALT includes an attenuated, thin squamous epithelium in place of the usual pseudostratified epithelium of the conducting airways. Under this epithelium typical lymphatic tissue is found (lymphocyte infiltrations in a framework of reticular cells). BALT areas have been reported to occupy regions of up to several square millimeters and to protrude above the surfaces of neighboring cilia, but in view of the universal exposure of airways to infection, it will be difficult to decide what is their normal size.

III. GAS-EXCHANGING PARENCHYMA

Gas-exchanging parenchyma is the area where air and blood come close enough for gas exchange to take place. Blood and air remain separated at all times by at least an endothelium and a thin epithelial lining (air-blood barrier).

A. Organization

The alveolar region is best understood as a peripheral extension of the conducting airways, which continue undergoing dichotomic division four more times past the last respiratory bronchioles (generation 19). These airways, three generations of ducts and the final, blind airway, the alveolar sac, lack a wall of their own in the ordinary sense; they are wide spaces surrounded by lateral, wide open air chambers, the alveoli. The reinforced entrance rings of the alveoli form a kind of chicken wire fence around the lumen of the duct. Alveoli are outpocketings of the last airways, beginning in the respiratory bronchioles. When fully inflated they can be regarded as polygonal structures. A random section of the alveolar region, however, is bound to produce confusion because of the difficulty in distinguishing between duct and alveolar spaces and because of the continuous changes of direction of the ducts which usually stay in the plane of the section for only a short distance. Alveolar geometry is a topic of significance in connection with specific problems of pulmonary mechanics. Evidently alveoli undergo distortion during most routine fixation procedures, mainly because geometry is dependent on large extent on intraalveolar forces generated at the air tissue interfaces which are often altered during fixation (This can be avoided by using vascular fixation or freezing procedures.).[22] In the air-filled lungs, alveolar walls tend to be straight and form angles to each other. In these angles, where interfacial forces are strongest, one occasionally sees pleatings of the alveolar wall and pools of an intraalveolar fluid (see Figure 5).[23-25] These pools moderate the intraalveolar recoil forces by evening out the final alveolar surface and are relevant to alveolar mechanics and to fluid exchange.

From the point of view of gas exchange or of inhalation studies, a notable property of the final airways is that they are blind. Therefore a complete replacement of the air during ventilation is impossible. The boundary between alveolar and inspired air is set up relatively high, probably at the end of the respiratory bronchioles, although this matter is controversial.[2,26,27] The gas-exchange regions are reached only by the way of gas mixing. This is relevant not only to gas exchange physiology; it also bears significance to inhalation problems. Accordingly, most environmental-related acute lesions have been reported to be centroacinar (i.e., close to the bronchioles).

B. Histology

The alveolar septum (see Figure 6) or wall between neighboring alveoli is a structure of a notable homogeneity throughout the whole lung in most mammals. In a totally stretched septum, one would see an incomplete connective tissue midplane, formed by bundles of collagen or reticular fibrils and elastic fibers. As it has been pointed out recently,[24] for specific purposes it is practical to distinguish between primary septa (those partitions placed between and common to two different ducts) and secondary septa (those placed between and separating two alveoli open to the same duct). The tip of the secondary septa is thickened, forming the above-mentioned reinforced entrance rings of the alveoli which in many species contain muscle. The over-all arrangement of the connective tissue inside the septal midplane and its connections with the subpleural and the axial connective tissue to form a fibrous continum is important in both normal pulmonary mechanics and experimental lung pathology. It has been extensively reviewed.[29] It must be pointed out here, for its potential significance, that a number of resident interstitial cells of the kind usually regarded as fibrocytes are be-

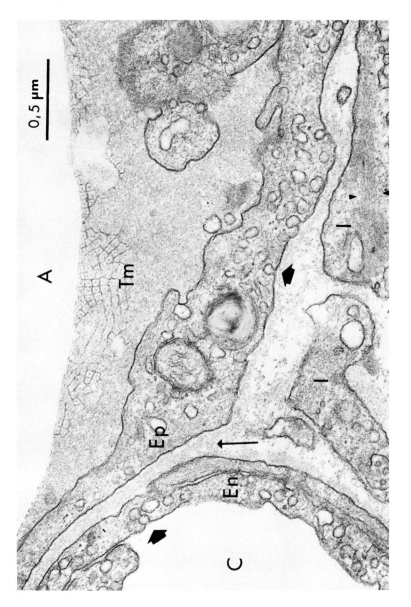

FIGURE 5. Rabbit lung fixed by perfusing osmium through the pulmonary artery. Ep is a squamous alveolar epithelial cell Type I. A pool of fluid is located in this depression of the alveolar wall. Some of this fluid is in the form of tubular myelin (Tm), a fluid crystal; C is an empty capillary. In the bottom are profiles of two interstitial cells labeled I. In one of them a bundle of (contractile?) filaments between thin arrowheads. Thick arrowheads point at pinocytotic vesicles. Long arrow points at fusion between the epithelial and endothelial basal laminae. En is endothelial cell.

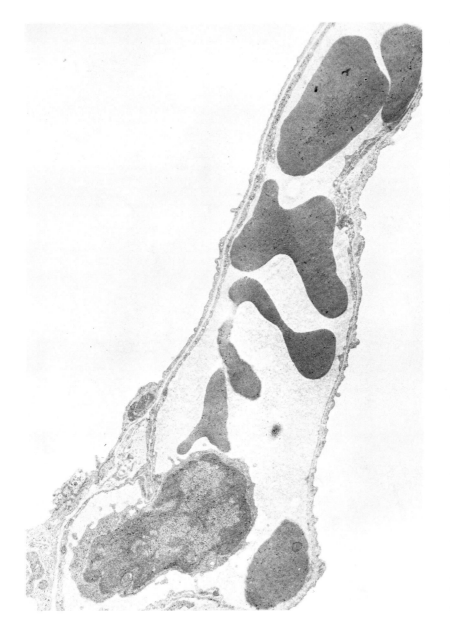

FIGURE 6.   Septum of rat lung fixed by filling the airspaces with glutaraldehyde. Thick black line shows the connective tissue midplane. In the circle is air-blood barrier.

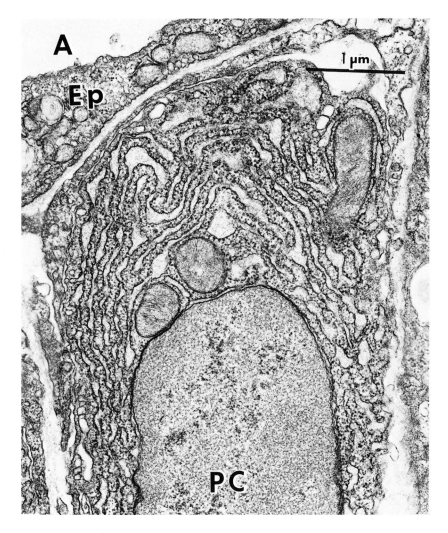

FIGURE 7. Plasma cell (PC) in the interstitial space of rabbit lung. Ep is an epithelial Type I cell. A is alveolar space.

lieved to be contractile and contain bundles of filaments (see Figure 5, bottom right).[30] Immigrant interstitial cells, mainly plasma or mast cells, (see Figure 7) are rarely found in the gas-exchanging area; they appear to be more frequent around small blood vessels or in the peribronchial connective tissue sheaths. We recently described that alveolar connective tissue cells spread out as they reach the points of insertion of the septa into extra-alveolar connective tissue sheaths forming an apparent boundary between alveolar and extra-alveolar interstitial compartments.[51] Collagen types are different in both compartments; lymphatics are confined to extra-alveolar interstitium.

Large portions of the alveolar wall (see next section) are occupied by a very dense capillary network. As Weibel[3] recognized, these capillary segments form on face views roughly hexagonal networks. Capillary segments are alternatively placed on both sides of the connective tissue midplane (see Figure 6). The result of this arrangement will be that each capillary is asymmetrically placed and that the capillary network continuously crosses the midplane in both directions. Each capillary will have a thin and a thick side (see Figures 6 and 8). The capillaries are of the closed type without openings or fenestrations; the intercellular junctions are zonulae occludentes (see Figure 7), but less tight than the epithelial functional complexes. Endothelial (as well as epithelial)

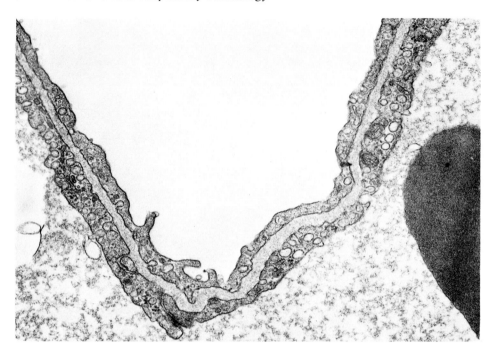

FIGURE 8.   "Thin" part of the air-blood barrier of the rabbit lung. A is alveolar space, C is capillary space, and E is an erythrocyte. Arrowhead points at intercellular junction of the endothelium which, under circumstances, could become leaky.

cells contain extremely high amounts of pinocytotic vesicles. Pinocytotic vesicles are supposed to be primarily a shuttle system for the transcellular transport of macromolecules; it has been claimed that certain of these vesicles ("caveolae") morphologically undistinguishable from the rest, contain enzymes important in the metabolism of vasoactive peptides.[28] The recent notion of "receptor-mediated endocytosis" is linked to coated pits and vesicles surrounded by a geodesic basketwork of a unique protein called "chlathrin" which is supposed to possess specific receptors for certain chemical compounds such as low density lipoproteins.[44] The ultrastructure of the air-blood barrier has been reviewed in detail several times.[29,31] The alveolar wall is continuously lined by two cell types, alveolar epithelial cell Type I (squamous) and alveolar epithelial cell Type II (cuboidal and granular pneumocyte). A third pneumocyte, similar to the brush cell of the conducting airways, is more rare. Opinions about their frequency differ widely; in this author's experience with common laboratory rodents (rats and rabbits) it is very tedious to find one. The Type I cells line in excess of 95% of the alveolar surface. The nucleus with some pericaryon is placed in a pit between two capillaries; it sends out very long, thin cytoplasmic extensions which sometimes line several alveoli. These cells are not capable of division. It is said that Type I cells are poor in organelles, but they contain sizable amounts of smooth endoplasmic reticulum which appear to proliferate under the effect of toxic agents; one also sees some dark, irregularly shaped mitochondria and extremely large amounts of pinocytotic vesicles; these cells form tight functional complexes between themselves and with type II cells. It is generally accepted that the alveolar epithelium forms the real permeability barrier of the lung, opposite to the endothelium which under certain circumstances is more capable of leaking.

Alveolar epithelial cells Type II (see Figures 9 and 10) are cuboidal, placed also in niches between capillaries, and are notorious for their wealth in organelles, particularly

17

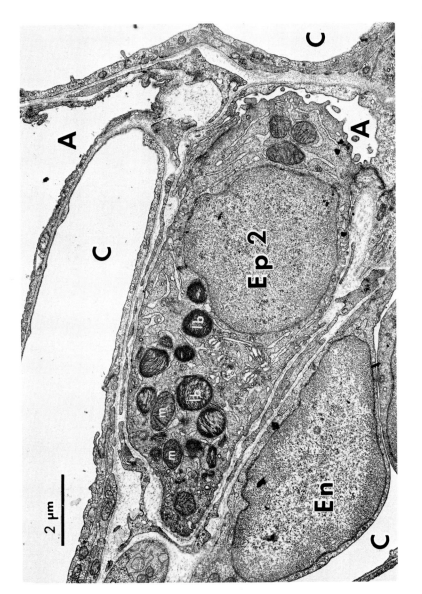

FIGURE 9. Rabbit lung fixed by vascular perfusion with osmium. Ep 2 is an epithelial cell Type II with lamellar bodies (lb) and mitochondria (m); C is capillary space (flushed out by the fixative), and A are airspaces. This area shows septal pleating.

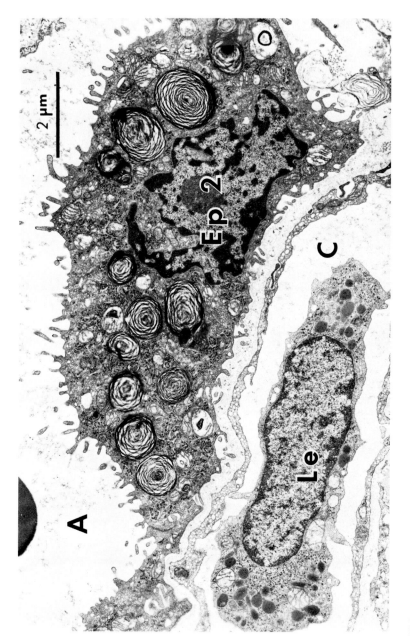

FIGURE 10.   Human epithelial cell Type II. Surgical biopsy of a female patient affected by Goodpasture syndrome (erythrocytes and edema in alveolar space A); capillary C contains a leukocyte Le.

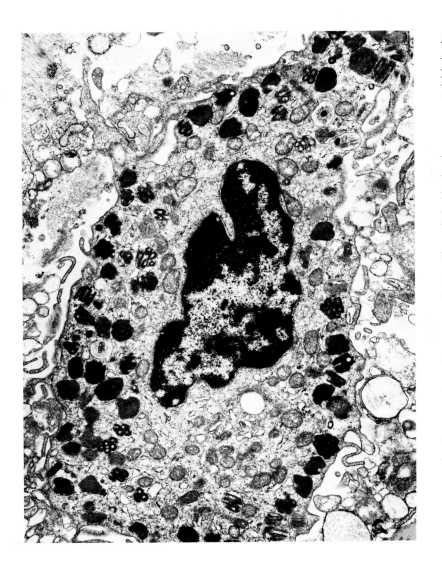

FIGURE 11. Alveolar macrophage from same patient as Figure 9. Inside alveolar space material is in the process of being organized.

the osmiophilic lamellar bodies which represent intracellular storage sites of surfactant. They have some irregular microvilli; they can undergo mitotic division and are supposed to be the progenitor cells of the squamous Type I cells. If a denudation of the alveolar epithelium occurs (as it is known to occur in early stages of the respiratory distress syndrome), this denudation is immediately covered by a proliferation of Type II cells.

Epithelial cells rest on a continuous basal lamina, as endothelial cells do. In thin parts of the air-blood barrier, both laminae are fused; on the thicker side, they stay separated. Interstitium is the part of the septum between the basal laminae of the epithelium and the endothelium. It contains the connective tissue backbone described above.

Inside the alveolus, the macrophage (see Figure 10) deserves special mention because of the increasing recognition of its immunological significance and the role that it plays in lung pathology.[45] Very conspicuous are the large amounts of primary and secondary lysosomes, but surprisingly one rarely recognizes ingested foreign material. Macrophages have been thought to play a major role in the removal of the lipid-rich surfactant material; therefore most of its inclusions are heavily osmiophilic, similar to inclusions of the Type II cells, but without the same organization. In lungs fixed by instilling fixatives into the airways, macrophages are rounded-off; in preparations fixed by vascular perfusion, they are always stuck to the epithelial surface, have a smooth surface, and send out thin extensions mostly devoid of inclusions. They usually have no microvilli, although they seem to be immersed in the fluid lining layer. Morphologists tend to regard as macrophages all the cells of the intraalveolar and intrabronchial space. This is not so. It has been shown by Gorenberg and Daniele[32] that in the guinea pig lung, where a tracheobronchial lavage will contain on the average 14×10^6 cells, some 68% of them seem to be macrophages, 20% are eosinophils, and some 12% are lymphocytes (with T cells predominating over B lymphocytes). The origin and life history of the bronchoalveolar lymphocyte is under study.[33]

Finally in adequately prepared lungs, one can find small pools of fluid adding to the smoothness of the alveoli (see Figure 5). This is closely related to alveolar surfactant, secreted by Type II cells. Inside the accumulations of fluid, one often sees a peculiar liquid crystal, tubular myelin, formed by a system of parallel tubes of osmiophilic wall with a periodicity of some 60 nm. Fluid pools are sometimes lined by an osmiophilic dark line which may be present over a certain length of the surface, but morphological examinations have never shown the existence of a continuous fluid lining layer which others have predicted. The material seen in our specimens (see Figure 5) gives the impression of being a free fluid which forms no appreciable contact angle with the tissue and therefore is likely to be able to spread easily.

C. Morphometry

The need for quantitative ("morphometric") assessment of histologic specimens of the lung has been widely recognized in recent years. This is particularly evident when trying to define slight pathological changes or to correlate a function with the structure that performs it. For a general description of the technique both at the light and electron microscopic level, the reviews by Weibel[34] can be consulted. We have base line data currently along two main lines of interest: (1) information on organ characteristics of the lung, such as alveolar and capillary volume and surface and arithmetic and harmonic mean thickness of the air-blood barrier, or (2) data on characteristics and number of specific cell types (i.e., what is the size of a Type I cell, are there more Type I than Type II, or vice versa). Alveolar surface is a very popular parameter, but one must keep in mind that it is always dependent on the magnification chosen, simply because higher magnification reveals more detail.[35] When describing surface measurements, the magnification at which they were made must always be indicated.

Table 1
SELECTED QUANTITATIVE DATA ON LUNGS OF COMMON LABORATORY ANIMALS[a]

	Small dog	Large dog	Monkey	Rabbit	Small rat	Mouse
W(kg)	11.2 ± 0.4	22.8 ± 0.6	3.71 ± 0.8	3.6 ± 0.5	0.14 ± 0.007	0.023 ± 0.002
V_L(ml)	736 ± 25	1501 ± 74	184 ± 3.6	79 ± 12	6.3 ± 0.2	0.74 ± 0.075
Sa(m²)	41 ± 4	90 ± 7	13 ± 0.5	5.9 ± 0.05	0.39 ± 0.02	0.068 ± 0.075
Sc(m²)	33 ± 1.6	72 ± 4.5	12 ± 0.6	4.7 ± 0.4	0.41 ± 0.02	0.059 ± 0.006
Vc(ml)	50 ± 5	119 ± 14	15 ± 1.1	7.2 ± 0.8	0.48 ± 0.02	0.084 ± 0.009
TAU(μm)	1.64 ± 0.01	1.42 ± 0.08	1.52 ± 0.05	1.51 ± 0.1	1.42 ± 0.07	1.25 ± 0.08
TAU_h(μm)	0.46 ± 0.01	0.48 ± 0.01	0.50 ± 0.01	0.48 ± 0.02	0.38 ± 0.02	0.32 ± 0.006
Sc/Sa	0.8	0.8	0.89	0.82	1.05	0.87

Note: All data from lungs fixed by inflating the airspaces with fixatives at pressure.

[a] Explanation of symbols: W = body weight, V_L = total lung volume, Sa = total alveolar surface, Sc = total capillary surface, Vc = total capillary volume, TAU = arithmetic mean thickness of air-blood barrier, TAU_h = harmonic mean thickness of barrier, Sc/Sa = capillary-to-alveolar surface ratio (which in part reflects the degree of capillary loading).[29,31,37,49]

Table 2
QUANTITATIVE DATA FROM EIGHT ADULT HUMAN LUNGS

	Highest	Lowest	Mean
W	—	—	74 ± 4
V_L(ml)	4680	3500	4341 ± 285
Sa(m²)	194	97	143 ± 12
Sc(m²)	189	74	126 ± 12
Vc(ml)	387	125	213 ± 31
TAU(μm)	3.28	1.35	2.22 ± 0.20
TAU_n (μm)	0.85	0.49	0.62 ± 0.04
Sc/Sa	—	—	0.88

Note: Symbols as in Table 1. Same fixation procedure. Data are from electron microscopic examination. Columns of highest and lowest values not necessarily from the same lungs.[35]

That quantitative data on the histology of terminal airspaces are needed for certain types of predominantly physiological studies have been recognized many years ago. Among others one must mention the influential paper by Tenney and Remmers[36] and the book by Weibel.[3] During the last years, a wealth of reliable comparative data in different animals and even humans has accumulated. Table 1 has been constructed with data on common laboratory animals taken from several publications.[29,31,37,49] Table 2 with human data contains results from a recent publication by Gehr et al.[35] The original publications should be consulted for more extensive data. Two values are offered for the mean thickness of the barrier (TAU): the arithmetic and harmonic means. The latter is the average of the reciprocal value of the thickness and is the one to be used when TAU is to be entered as a denominator, as is the case in formulas for diffusing capacity. Weibel[37] has shown by regression analysis that many morphometric parameters (Y) can be related to body weight W by a simple allometric function: Y =

Table 3

CYTOLOGICAL COMPOSITION OF THE GAS-
EXCHANGING PARENCHYMA OF PERFUSED RAT
LUNGS

	V_v*	N_N (%)	$\bar{v}(\mu m^3)$	$\bar{s}(\mu m^2)$
Epithelial cells I	0.13 ± 0.01	8	812	4003
Epithelial cells II	0.09 ± 0.01	14	336	69
Endothelial cells	0.27 ± 0.01	39	352	995
Interstitial cells	0.35 ± 0.01	39	472	—
Noncellular interstitium	0.12 ± 0.01	—	—	—
Macrophages	0.04 ± 0.00	—	—	—

Note: Data are from five rats.[40] V_v* is the volume density (fraction of volume taken up by each cell as related to the total tissue volume without
blood or air); N_N is the relative number of cells; $\bar{v}$ is the mean volume
of each cell, and $\bar{s}$ is the mean lumenal surface of each cell. The three
last parameters are final averages obtained by pooling together all
primary data; hence they have no SE. The interstitial cells are largely
fibrocytes.

$a \cdot W^b$. This is useful because it can be utilized for predictive purposes. A table listing values of a and b derived from plots, including most common laboratory animals for the most relevant parameters, can also be found in the original publications.[37,49]

Another area that can be greatly helped by organ morphometry is the study of volume-dependent changes in lung histology. Recent studies include a morphometric assessment at the light microscopic levels of rat lungs fixed at different inflation degrees[38] and of the same lungs at the electron microscopic levels.[39]

An additional study of rabbit lungs fixed at different levels of inflation in the physiological volume range[23] revealed comparatively small changes of alveolar dimensions. The presence of small areas of reversible pleatings of alveolar septa in corners was constant (see Figure 9). The observations seem to suggest that much of the volume changes take place in the duct space. It shall be noted that if the front between inspired and alveolar air is formed practically at the entrance of the acinus, it does not matter much where volume changes taken place, since in most airspaces this will be distal to the boundary. More data are needed before comprehensive quantitative information on this difficult but important subject can be offered.

Studies on cytologic morphometry of the lung are less numerous probably because of the technical difficulties involved. We[40,52] conducted a laborious study involving five rat lungs fixed by vascular perfusion. The tissue volume (i.e., tissue excluding air and blood volume) was used as a reference system. Data are summarized in Table 3. This type of work involves handling an extraordinary volume of primary point counting data. These studies have become possible as a result of the recent development of high-performance desktop calculators with large storage capacities. Crapo et al.[41] have recently published cytomorphometric data in normal rats and in rats tolerant to pure O_2 and partially cross tolerant to NO_2. Morphometry provides an effective tool of studying changes in cell population and individual cell reactions. Cell counting is, however, a most difficult endeavor. Normally the worker must count nuclear profiles because the electron microscopic cell profiles are of far-fetched shapes and too variable in size. The worker interested in this area is exposed to rather difficult theoretical problems.

D. Blood Vessels

The lung has in common with the liver the existence of two separate sets of vessels:

vasa privata or bronchial arteries which nourish and provide oxygen for the conducting airways and vasa publica or pulmonary arteries which exchange oxygen for the benefit of the whole organism. Bronchial arteries form plexuses in the bronchial wall; most of their blood is eventually drained into the pulmonary veins. It is generally believed that only 25% of the bronchial arterial flow is drained by the comparatively small bronchial veins, although probably there are species differences.

The pulmonary arteries enter the lung at the hilum and become associated with the airways. Essentially they branch dichotomously following the airways. However, Elliott and Reid[42] showed that the arteries branch too often which results in the formation of supernumerary arteries. These run isolated in the gas-exchanging parenchyma and supply the most peripheral parts of the acinus with blood. The axial pulmonary arteries run parallel to the airways, originally embedded in their connective tissue sheaths. Somewhere around the last bronchioles, the arteriole disappears and joins the capillary network of the alveolar walls.

The situation with the veins is less clear. The textbooks describe large veins surrounding the periphery of segments until they eventually join the airways and arteries in their way out of the lung. Smaller veins can be seen apparently isolated in the parenchyma. It is difficult to define a relationship of a small vein to any of the terminal airspaces (for instance, between ducts of different acini or parallel to a certain ducts). Their venular origin is also difficult to establish.

Relevant to gas exchange are above all the capillaries contained inside the alveolar wall which have already been described above. Most electron micrographs show fully open capillaries, but the situation in vivo in more complex as it has become evident that capillary segments can be recruited and derecruited. This has been shown in rapidly frozen lungs and in lungs fixed by vascular perfusion of the fixatives.[24,25] Fung and Sobin[43] developed the imaginative model of the sheet flow; these authors visualize the intraseptal vascular spaces as a sheet interrupted by "posts", the connective tissue structures placed in the center of the hexagonal network. Their usual analogy is with a low ceiling parking garage with pillars. The consequence of this model is that no parts of the network can be identified as individual tubes. A hydrodynamic analysis of blood flow will be different, depending on whether the vascular spaces are a network of tubes or a sheet with localized obstacles, the posts. Anatomically, these are simply two ways of interpreting the pictures, but whatever the situation is, one should keep in mind the existence of primary and secondary septa. Another difficult problem is the existence of bundles of capillaries in certain alveolar corners where the septum is reversibly pleated.[24] These topics will require additional studies.

ACKNOWLEDGMENT

Work of the author was supported by NHLBI grants HL 00389 and HL 00436.

REFERENCES

1. **Rohrer, F.,** Der Strömungswiderstand in den menschlichen Atemwegen und der Einfluss der unregelmässigen Verzweigung des Bronchialsystems auf den Atmungsverlauf in verschiedenen Lungenbezirken, *Arch. Ges. Physiol.,* 162, 225, 1915.
2. **Pedley, T. J., Schroter, R. C., and Sudlow, M. F.,** Gas flow and mixing in the airways, in *Bioengineering Aspects of the Lung,* West, J. B., Ed., Marcel Dekker, New York, 1977.
3. **Weibel, E. R.,** *Morphometry of the Human Lung,* Academic Press, New York, 1963.
4. **Phalen, R. F., Yeh, H. C., Schum, G. M., and Raabe, O. G.,** Application of an idealized model to morphometry of the mammalian tracheobronchial tree, *Anat. Rec.,* 190, 167, 1978.
5. **Horsfield, K. and Cumming G.,** Morphology of the bronchial tree in man, *J. Appl. Physiol.,* 24, 373, 1968.
6. **Horsfield, K., Relea, F. G., and Cumming, G.,** Diameter, length and branching ratios in the bronchial tree, *Respir. Physiol.,* 26, 351, 1976.
7. **Kuhn, Ch.,** The cells of the lung and their organelles, in *Biochemical Basis of Pulmonary Function,* Crystal, R. G., Ed., Marcel Dekker, New York, 1976.
8. **Breeze, R. G. and Wheeldon, E. B.,** The cells of the pulmonary airways, *Am. Rev. Respir. Dis.,* 116, 705, 1977.
9. **Jeffery, P. K. and Reid, L. M.,** The respiratory mucous membrane, in *Respiratory Defense Mechanisms,* Part I, Brain, J. D., Proctor, D. F., and Reid, L. M., Eds., Marcel Dekker, New York, 1977.
10. **Sleigh, M. A.,** The nature and action of respiratory tract cilia, in *Respiratory Defense Mechanisms,* Part I, Brain, J. D., Proctor, D. F., and Reid, L. M., Eds., Marcel Dekker, New York, 1977.
11. **Lauweryns, J. M., Cokelaere, M., and Theunynck, P.,** Neuro-epithelial bodies in the respiratory mucosa of various animals. A light optical, histochemical and ultrastructure investigation, *Z. Zellforsch. Mikrosk. Anat.,* 135, 569, 1972.
12. **Sorokin, S. P. and Hoyt, R. F.,** PAS-lead hematoxylin as a stain for small-granule endocrine cell populations in the lungs, other pharyngeal derivatives and the gut, *Anat. Rec.,* 192, 245, 1978.
13. **Das, R. M., Jeffery, P. K., and Widdicombe, J. G.,** The epithelial innervation of the lower respiratory tract of the cat, *J. Anat.,* 126, 123, 1978.
14. **Meyrick, B., Sturgess, J., and Reid, L.,** Reconstruction of the duct system and secretory tubules of the human bronchial submucosal gland, *Thorax,* 24, 729, 1969.
15. **Lucas, A. M. and Douglas, L. C.,** Principles underlying ciliary activity in the respiratory tract. II. A comparison of nasal clearance in man, monkey and other mammals, *Arch. Otolaryngol.,* 20, 518, 1934.
16. **Luchtel, D. L.,** The mucous layer of the trachea and major bronchi in the rat, in *Scanning Electron Microscopy,* Vol. 2, SEM Inc., O'Hare, Ill., 1978.
17. **Gil, J. and Weibel, E. R.,** Extracellular lining of bronchioles after perfusion-fixation of rat lungs for electron microscopy, *Anat. Rec.,* 169, 185, 1971.
18. **Von Hayek, H.,** *Die Menschliche Lunge,* Springer Verlag, Heidelberg, 1953.
19. **Reznik-Schüller, H.,** Sequential morphologic alterations in the bronchial epithelium of Syrian golden hamsters during N-nitrosomorpholine-induced pulmonary tumorigenesis, *Am. J. Pathol.,* 89, 59, 1977.
20. **Evans, M. J., Cabral-Anderson, L. J., and Freeman, G.,** Role of the Clara cell in renewal of the bronchiolar epithelium, *Lab. Invest.,* 38, 648, 1978.
21. **Bienenstock, J., Johnston, N., and Percy, D. Y. E.,** Bronchial lymphoid tissue. I. Morphologic characteristics, *Lab. Invest.,* 28, 686, 1973.
22. **Gil, J.,** Preservation of tissues for electron microscopy under physiological criteria, in *Techniques of Biochemical and Biophysical Morphology,* vol. 3, Glick, D. and Rosenbaum, R. M., Eds., Wiley-Interscience, New York, 1977.
23. **Gil, J., Bachofen, H., Gehr, P., and Weibel, E. R.,** Alveolar volume-surface area relation in air- and saline-filled lungs fixed by vascular perfusion, *J. Appl. Physiol.,* 47, 990, 1979.
24. **Gil, J.,** Morphologic aspects of alveolar microcirculation, *Fed. Proc. Fed. Am. Soc. Exp. Biol.,* 37, 2462, 1978.
25. **Gil, J.,** Influence of surface forces on pulmonary circulation, in *Pulmonary Edema,* Fishman, A. P. and Renkin, E., Eds., American Physiological Society, Bethesda, Md., 1979.
26. **Chang, H. K., Cheng, R. T., and Farhi, L. E.,** A model study of gas diffusion in alveolar sacs, *Respir. Physiol.,* 18, 386, 1973.
27. **Pack, A. I., Hooper, M., Nixon, W., and Taylor, J.,** A computational model of gas transport incorporating effective diffusion, *Respir. Physiol.,* 29, 101, 1977.
28. **Ryan, V. S. and Ryan, J. W.,** Correlations between the fine structure of the alveolar-capillary unit and its metabolic activities, in *Metabolic Functions of the Lung,* Bakhle, Y. S. and Vane, J. R., Eds., Marcel Dekker, New York, 1977.

29. Weibel, E. R. and Gil, J., Structure-function relationships at the alveolar level, in *Bioengineering Aspects of the Lung*, West, J. B. Ed., Marcel Dekker, New York, 1977.

30. Kapanci, Y., Assimacopoulos, A., Irle, C., Zwahlen, A., and Gabbiani, G., "Contractile interstitial cells" in pulmonary alveolar septa: a possible regulator of ventilation/perfusion ratio? Ultrastructural immunofluorescence and in vitro studies, *J. Cell. Biol.*, 60, 375, 1974.

31. Weibel, E. R., Morphological basis of alveolar-capillary gas exchange, *Physiol. Rev.*, 53, 419, 1973.

32. Gorenberg, D. J. and Daniele, R. P., Characterization of immunocompetent cells recovered from the respiratory tract and tracheobronchial lymph node of normal guinea pigs, *Am. Rev. Respir. Dis.*, 114, 1099, 1976.

33. Daniele, R. P., Beacham, C. H., and Gorenberg, D. J., The bronchoalveolar lymphocyte. Studies on the life history and lymphocyte traffic from blood to the lung, *Cell Immunol.*, 31, 48, 1977.

34. Weibel, E. R., *Practical Methods for Biological Morphometry*, Vol. 1, Academic Press, London, 1979.

35. Gehr, P., Bachofen, M., and Weibel, E. R., The normal human lung: ultrastructure and morphometric estimation of diffusion capacity, *Respir. Physiol.*, 32, 121, 1978.

36. Tenney, S. M. and Remmers, J. E., Comparative quantitative morphology of mammalian lungs; diffusing areas, *Nature (London)*, 197, 54, 1963.

37. Weibel, E. R., Morphometric estimation of pulmonary diffusion capacity, V. Comparative analysis of mammalian lungs, *Respir. Physiol.*, 14, 26, 1972.

38. Gil, J. and Weibel, E. R., Morphological study of pressure-volume hysteresis in rat lungs fixed by vascular perfusion, *Respir. Physiol.*, 15, 190, 1972.

39. Weibel, E. R., Untersee, P., Gil, J., and Zulauf, M., Morphometric estimation of pulmonary diffusion capacity, VI. Effect of varying positive pressure inflation of air spaces, *Respir. Physiol.*, 18, 285, 1973.

40. Haies, D., Gil, J., and Weibel, E. R., unpublished data.

41. Crapo, J. D., Marsh-Salin, J., Ingram, P., and Pratt, P. C., Tolerance and cross-tolerance using NO_2 and O_2. II. Pulmonary morphology and morphometry, *J. Appl. Physiol. Respir. Environ. Exercise Physiol.*, 44, 370, 1978.

42. Elliott, F. M. and Reid, L., Some new facts about the pulmonary artery and its branching pattern, *Clin. Radiol.*, 16, 193, 1965.

43. Fung, Y. C. and Sobin, S. S., Pulmonary alveolar blood flow, in *Bioengineering Aspects of the Lung*, West, J. B., Ed., Marcel Dekker, New York, 1977.

44. Goldstein, J. L., Anderson, R. G. W., and Brown, M. S., Coated pits, coated vesicles, and receptor-mediated endocytosis, *Nature (London)*, 279, 679, 1979.

45. Brain, J. D., Godleski, J. J., and Sorokin, S. S., Quantification, origin, and fate of pulmonary macrophages, in *Respiratory Defense Mechanisms*, Brain, J. D., Proctor, D. F., and Reid, L., Eds., Marcel Dekker, New York, 1977.

46. Gil, J., Organization of microcirculation in the lung, *Annu. Rev. Physiol.*, 42, 177, 1980.

47. Boyd, M. R. Evidence for the Clara cell as a site of cytochrome P-450-dependent mixed-function oxidase activity in lung, *Nature (London)*, 269, 713, 1977.

48. Weibel, E. R., *Practical Methods for Biological Morphometry*, Academic Press, London, 1979.

49. Gehr, P., Mwangi, D. K., Amman, A., Maloiy, G. M. O., Taylor, C. R., and Weibel, E. R., Design of the mammalian respiratory system. V. Scaling morphometric pulmonary diffusing capacity to body mass: wild and domestic mammals, *Respir. Physiol.*, 44, 61, 1981.

50. Gil, J., Silage, D. A., and McNiff, J. M., Distribution of resicles in cells of air-blood barrier in the rabbit, *J. Appl. Physiol. Respir. Environ. Exercise Physiol.*, 50, 334, 1981.

51. Gil, J. and McNiff, J. M., Interestitial cells at the boundary between alveolar and extra-alveolar connective tissue in the lung, *J. Ultrastr. Res.*, in press.

52. Gil, J., Alveolar wall relations, *Ann. N.Y. Acad. Sci.*, in press.

Chapter 2

DEPOSITION AND CLEARANCE OF INHALED AEROSOLS

Otto G. Raabe*

TABLE OF CONTENTS

*   Supported by the Office of Health and Environmental Research (OHER) of the U.S. Department of Energy (DOE) under contract with the University of California, Davis.

I. INTRODUCTION

When aerosols consisting of either liquid droplets or solid particles are inhaled by people, some of the particles are not exhaled, but are either directly deposited upon contact with airway surfaces in various regions of the respiratory tract or mixed with unexhaled air and subsequently deposited. The remainder is exhaled. This deposition of inhaled airborne particles has a probability that depends upon the aerodynamic properties of the particles, the anatomy of the respiratory tract, and the airflow and mixing behavior in the airways. The pattern of deposition of inhaled aerosols which may include toxic agents within the anatomical regions of the respiratory tract will influence the fate of the deposited material and the potential for injury.

In inhalation toxicology, the term deposition refers specifically to the quantity or fractions of inhaled airborne particles that are never exhaled, but are ultimately deposited on surfaces in the respiratory tract and to the initial regional pattern of these deposited particles. The term clearance refers to the subsequent translocation, transformation, and removal of deposited particles from the respiratory tract or from the body. The temporal distribution of uncleared deposited materials is called retention. Hence, both clearance and retention are described with respect to time after deposition. For a brief aerosol exposure, the relationship of these three concepts may be described by the equation: RETENTION (t) = DEPOSITION − CLEARANCE (t), where (t) refers to a function of time after deposition occurs. These are important dosimetric relationships that need to be evaluated if biological responses are to be fully understood.

The mechanisms involved in the deposition of inhaled aerosols are affected by the physical and chemical properties of the aerosols, including particle size or size distribution, density, shape, surface area, electrostatic charge, hygroscopicity or deliquescence, and chemical composition and related reactions. The geometry of the respiratory airway from nose and mouth to the lung parenchyma also influences aerosol deposition; the important morphometric parameters include the diameters, lengths, and branching angles of airway segments. Physiological factors that affect deposition include breathing patterns, air flow dynamics in the respiratory tract, and variations of relative humidity and temperature within the airways. With quantitative information concerning those elements, theoretical models of regional deposition can be developed to predict the fate of inhaled aerosols of various types. Carefully collected data from experiments with human volunteers provide a basis for testing these theoretical predictions.

Clearance from the respiratory tract depends on many factors, including site of deposition, chemical composition and properties of the deposited particles, and such biological functions as biochemical and cellular reactions, mucociliary transport in the tracheobronchial tree, macrophage phagocytosis in the deep lung, and pulmonary lymph and blood flow.

Translocation of materials from the lung to other organs can be an important aspect of inhalation toxicology, since the lung is frequently the portal of entry for toxic agents. Hence, multicompartment models of clearance from the respiratory tract to other organs can provide predictive information about the potential for injury to those other organs. Mathematical representations of lung retention and translocation require input about the various factors that affect deposition and clearance.

This chapter summarizes the essential features of the main factors affecting the mechanism of aerosol deposition and clearance. Selected references to available published works have been chosen to illustrate these factors rather than to serve as a complete bibliography. Much of the published information is based on studies of experimental animals, but there are usually significant differences in anatomical, morphological, and physiological characteristics between experimental animals and man. Although some supportive data from studies with experimental animals has been cited to illustrate basic phenomena, the emphasis is on deposition and clearance of potentially toxic particulate materials inhaled by people.

II. PROPERTIES OF AEROSOLS

A. General Description

An aerosol is a relatively stable suspension in a gas (usually air) of very small liquid or finely divided solid particles. This particulate dispersion is characterized by a high surface-to-mass ratio. Airborne particulate materials found in the environment, home, or workplace are examples of aerosols. Aerosols containing potentially toxic components may consist of particles with a variety of physical and chemical properties. In particular, a given aerosol may include particles with a spectrum of physical sizes, even if all the particles have similar chemical composition. Another important property, physical density of particles, may vary with size.[1] Also, the concentration or specific activity of toxic components in particles may be different for different sizes,[2] or morphologically identical particles may have totally different chemical compositions.[3] Commonly made assumptions that all particles in a given toxic aerosol have a relatively homogenous chemical composition, concentration, or specific activity, and physical density may adequately describe general aerosol behavior, but may be seriously misleading concerning specific aerosol toxicity.

If particles in an aerosol are smooth and spherical or nearly spherical, their physical sizes can be conveniently described in terms of their respective geometric diameters. Aerosols of solids rarely contain smooth, spherical particles, and various conventions for describing physical diameters have been based upon available methods of observing and measuring particle size. For example, the size of a particle may be described in terms of its projected area diameter (D_p), defined as the diameter of a circle with an area the same as the apparent cross-sectional area of the particle when lying on a collection surface and viewed with an optical or electron microscope. (Other conventions for describing physical size can be based on measurements of scattered light, surface area, electrical mobility, diffusional mobility, or other physical or chemical phenomena. Those methods have been discussed by Raabe[4] and by Mercer.[5])

Since aerosols rarely consist of particles of a single size, they must be described by size distribution. If either the diameter (D) of spherical particles or the projected area diameter is used to characterize particles, the distribution of particle sizes is most conveniently described as a probability density function f(D), with

$$\int_0^\infty f(D)dD = 1 \qquad (1)$$

One such generally useful function is the log-normal function described in detail by Raabe[6] and given in linear form as:

$$f_1(D) = \frac{1}{D\sqrt{(2\pi)}\ln \sigma_g} \, e^{-\left[\frac{(\ln D - \ln CMD)^2}{2(\ln \sigma_g)^2}\right]} \qquad (2)$$

with ln the natural logarithm, D the particle diameter, CMD the median (geometric mean) diameter, and σ_g the geometric SD of the distribution. The cumulative function describing the fraction of particles smaller than size D is given by:

$$F = \int_0^D f(D)dD \qquad (3)$$

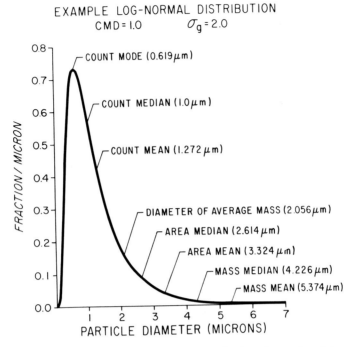

FIGURE 1.   Linear form of a log-normal distribution of aerosol particle sizes for count median (physical) diameter (CMD) equal to 1 μm (labeled micron) and geometric SD (σg) equal to 2. (From Raabe, O. G., *Aerosol Sci.*, 2, 289, 1971. With permission.)

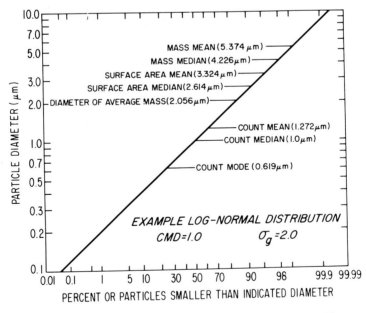

FIGURE 2.   Log-normal distribution of aerosol particle sizes from Figure 1 is plotted as the cumulative function on logarithmic probability coordinates.

The distribution of other physical characteristics of particles in an aerosol can be described similarly (see Figures 1 and 2). For example, particle surface area, which is important to such particle phenomena as surface adsorption and dissolution, might be

Table 1
AVERAGE DIFFUSIONAL
DISPLACEMENT IN ONE
DIRECTION AND
GRAVITATIONAL SETTLING
DISTANCE AT TERMINAL
SPEED IN 1 SEC FOR SPHERES
WITH DENSITY OF 1 G/CM³
AT 23°C IN AIR AT SEA
LEVEL[15]

Particle geometric diameter (μm)	Settling distance (cm)	Average diffusional displacement (cm)
0.002	1.31×10^{-6}	0.138
0.004	2.62×10^{-6}	6.40×10^{-2}
0.01	6.63×10^{-6}	2.58×10^{-2}
0.02	1.37×10^{-5}	1.31×10^{-2}
0.04	2.91×10^{-5}	6.75×10^{-3}
0.1	8.64×10^{-5}	2.95×10^{-3}
0.2	2.24×10^{-4}	1.68×10^{-3}
0.4	6.73×10^{-4}	1.03×10^{-3}
1.0	3.47×10^{-3}	5.90×10^{-4}
2.0	1.28×10^{-2}	4.02×10^{-4}
4.0	4.93×10^{-2}	2.78×10^{-4}
10.0	0.302	1.74×10^{-4}
20.0	1.21	1.23×10^{-4}

described with respect to diameter as log-normal with the surface area median diameter (SMD) and α_g. If the volume or mass distribution of the particles is being considered with respect to diameter, these can be described with the volume median diameter (VMD) or mass median diameter (MMD) and α_g. For aerosols consisting of potentially toxic components, the activity distribution of the toxic material may be described in terms of an appropriate activity median diameter (AMD).[5]

Use of the log-normal distribution function to describe aerosol property distributions with respect to size affords a number of useful mathematical transformations,[6-7] including $\ln \text{VMD} = \ln \text{CMD} + 3(\ln \sigma_g)^2$ and $\ln \text{SMD} = \ln \text{CMD} + 2(\ln \sigma_g)^2$ If the relationships between the volume and mass and/or specific toxic material activity of particles is known, similar equations can be developed to calculate the MMD and/or AMD from the CMD and σ_g.

B. Aerodynamic Properties

Aerodynamic properties of aerosol particles depend upon a variety of physical properties, including the size and shape of the particles and their physical densities. When particles are inhaled, their aerodynamic properties combined with various aspects of respiratory mechanics determine their fractional deposition and the deposition location in the respiratory tract.[8-14]

Two important aerodynamic properties of aerosol particles are the inertial properties, which are most important for particles larger than 0.5 μm in aerodynamic diameter (related to the settling speed in air under the influence of the gravity of the earth under normal conditions), and the diffusional properties, which are most important for particles smaller than 0.5 μm in physical diameter (related to the diffusion coefficient). Table 1 gives examples of the inertial and diffusional displacement for spherical particles (1 g/cm³ density) of various geometric diameters.

Bombardment of aerosol particles by gas molecules in air produces a random zig-zag (Brownian) motion, which tends to reduce particle concentration differences in an aerosol. The mean-square displacement $(\overline{X^2})$ of a large group of particles in a given time t is given by the Einstein equation:[15]

$$\overline{X^2} = 2\Delta t \tag{4}$$

where Δ is the particle diffusion coefficient, a function of the particle physical diameter, but independent of the particle physical density. Smaller particles have larger diffusion coefficients because they have less inertial and aerodynamic resistance to the impact of the gas molecules in air. This property of particles can be described in terms of a diffusive diameter. The diffusive diameter, D_{df}, is an artificial diameter dependent on surface characteristics representing the Brownian motion of an aerosol particle; D_{df} is equal to the geometric diameter of an ideal spherical particle with the same diffusivity as the actual particle under identical conditions. The D_{df} is primarily of value for particles smaller than 0.5 μm physical diameter.

An aerodynamic diameter customarily has been used to describe the inertial properties of an aerosol particle. The aerodynamic diameter is an artificial diameter dependent on particle shape, physical dimensions, and density representing the inertial behavior of an aerosol particle; either (1) aerodynamic equivalent diameter, D_{ae}, based upon equivalent unit density (1 g/cm³) sphere or (2) aerodynamic resistance diameter, D_{ar}, based upon aerosol mechanics under Stokes' law. Both of these definitions of aerodynamic diameter have been used and reported in inhalation toxicology research. The aerodynamic diameter most generally used is the D_{ae}, defined by Hatch and Gross[16] as "the diameter of a unit density sphere having the same settling speed (under gravity) as the particle in question of whatever shape and density". Raabe[17] has recommended the use of an D_{ar} defined with terms used in physics to describe inertial behavior and including all the factors, shape, size, and density that determine the inertial properties of a particle. Based on Stokes' law, the terminal settling speed of a spherical particle for viscous settling conditions is given by:

$$V_t = \frac{g\rho C(D)D^2}{18\eta} = \frac{g\rho^* D_{ar}^2}{18\eta} \tag{5}$$

where D is the physical (geometric) diameter of the sphere, g is the acceleration due to gravity (980 cm/s² at sea level), η is the viscosity of the gas (1.85 × 10⁻⁴ P for air at 25°C), ϱ is the particle physical density (more precisely, the difference in density of the particle and gas), D is the physical (geometric) diameter of the sphere, C(D) is its slip correction (a function of D), and D_{ar} is the aerodynamic (resistance) diameter defined by Raabe[17] as:

$$D_{ar} = \frac{D\sqrt{[\rho C(D)]}}{\sqrt{[\rho^*]}} = D_{ae}\sqrt{[C(D_{ae})]} \tag{6}$$

with D_{ae} the aerodynamic (equivalent unit density sphere) diameter and $C(D_{ae})$ the slip correction (a function of D_{ae}) associated with a unit density ($\varrho^* = 1$ g/cm³) sphere of diameter D_{ae}.

C(D) is a semiempirical factor that corrects the Stokes' law of viscous resistance for the effect of "slip" between the air molecules when the aerosol particles are almost as small as or smaller than the mean free path of air molecules. The C(D) is approximated for spheres by:

$$C(D) = 1 + 2A \left(\frac{\lambda}{D}\right) \tag{7}$$

with

$$A = \alpha + \beta e^{-(\gamma d/2\lambda)} \tag{8}$$

with λ the mean free path of the gas molecules, $\alpha = 1.26$, $\beta = 0.45$, and $\gamma = 1.08$. At sea level, the mean free path for air molecules is equal to about 0.0646 μm at 21°C and 0.0692 μm at 37°C.[17]

Particle characteristics described with respect to the physical diameter can also be described with respect to aerodynamic or diffusive diameters. The distribution functions can be described as $f(D_{ae})$, $f(D_{ar})$, or $f(D_{df})$. For example, count median diameter can be transformed to count median aerodynamic diameter (CMAD) or count median diffusive diameter (CMDD); mass median diameter, MMD, can be converted to mass median aerodynamic diameter (MMAD) or mass median diffusive diameter (MMDD); and toxicological activity median diameter, AMD, can be converted to activity median aerodynamic diameter (AMAD) and activity median diffusive diameter (AMDD). The AMAD and AMDD are the most generally useful size parameter for describing the distribution of a specific toxic component in an aerosol. For example, an environmental aerosol may consist primarily of $(NH_4)_2SO_4$ particles, but the presence of lead among these particles may be of primary concern. The aerosol size distribution of lead activity can be expressed as AMAD, where half of the lead is associated with particles bigger and half is associated with particles smaller than that AMAD (or AMDD for very small particles.)

C. Aerosol Dispersion Characteristics

Aerosols of potentially toxic materials that may be inhaled by man usually consist of particles of a wide variety of sizes. Such particle distributions are called polydisperse or heterodisperse to emphasize the various sizes or types of particles (see Figures 3A and B).[18] An aerosol of particles of but one size, shape, and type is referred to as monodisperse (see Figure 3C). In practice, monodisperse distributions are defined as those with a size coefficient of variation not exceeding 20%; for a log-normally distributed aerosol, this definition will include those distributions with σ_g less than 1.2. Monodisperse distributions are rarely found outside of controlled laboratory experiments.

In addition to particle characteristics, conditions of the medium gas influence the properties of aerosol dispersions. Such environmental conditions as relative humidity, temperature, barometric pressure, and fluid flow conditions (wind velocity, for example) affect the aerodynamics of aerosol particles. Another property of a given aerosol dispersion that can be of importance in affecting particle behavior is the state of electrostatic charge. In most cases, freshly generated aerosols have a large enough charge per particle to play a role in determining deposition, collection, or coagulation. In experimental studies, test aerosols are customarily mixed with bipolar ions or passed near a radioactive source to reduce the aerosol particle charge distribution to Boltzmann equilibrium.

The most basic dispersion properties of aerosols are those that relate to the particle concentration in air or other gaseous medium. The number of particles per unit volume of gas (number per cubic centimeter) provides information indicative of the coagulation rate for an aerosol. The mass concentration (mg/m³) and activity concentration (milligrams of constituent per cubic meter or μCi/m³ for radioactive constituents) provide the quantitative information needed for evaluating inhalation exposure levels.

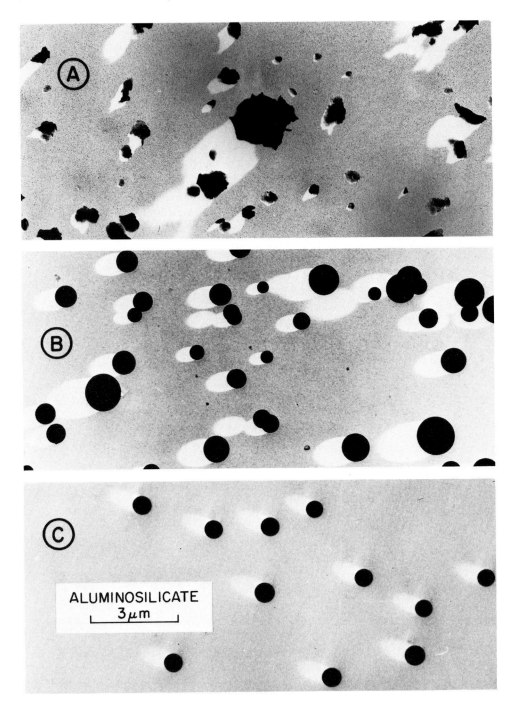

FIGURE 3.   Electron micrographs of aerosol samples shadowed with chromium vapor showing (A) poly-disperse, nonspherical, porous aluminosilicate particles of montmorillonite clay, (B) polydisperse, uniformly dense, fused aluminosilicate spheres, and (C) monodisperse particles of fused aluminosilicate spheres. (From Raabe, O. G., Yeh, H. C., Newton, G. J., Phalen, R. F., and Velasquez, D. J., *Inhaled Particles IV*, Walton, W. H., Ed., Pergamon Press, New York, 1977, 3. With permission.)

D. Chemical Properties

Information about the chemical characteristics of aerosol particles can be used in the evaluation of alterations in aerosol properties during inhalation, the clearance mechanism and rates from various regions of the respiratory tract, and the target organs and specific pathology associated with different particles. Particle chemistry would ideally include information on the exact chemical species, their proportions in various particles, the crystalline and amorphous states, and the uniformity. Realistically, heterodisperse aerosols may consist of complex mixtures of various inorganic and organic species that can affect their behavior and ultimate fate if inhaled. Such factors as the temperature history of aerosols also can markedly affect particle chemistry. Clearly, chemical identification, which may be difficult and complicated, remains an important aspect of aerosol characterization.

Physical properties that affect chemical properties include those that alter particle dissolution or degradation during reactions with body fluids after inhalation deposition. According to Mercer,[19] dissolution of sparingly soluble materials is not controlled by film diffusion kinetics, but instead depends on surface area, as in the following equation for a single particle or particle size:

$$\frac{dM}{dt} = -kS \tag{9}$$

where M is the particle mass, S is the particle surface area, t is the time, and k is the specific dissolution rate constant having units of mass dissolved per unit time and per unit surface area of the particle. From that relation, Raabe[20] calculated the fractional dissolution rate:

$$\frac{d\psi}{dt} = \frac{-k'}{D} \tag{10}$$

with ψ the mass fraction, D the particle physical diameter, and k' a constant equal to $k\alpha_s/\varrho\alpha_m$, with k the dissolution rate constant, α_s the particle surface shape factor, α_m the particle mass shape factor, and ϱ the physical density. Hence, the apparent dissolution rate, expressed as fraction of the mass, depends inversely on the particle size, with smaller particles dissolving faster.

Equilibrium solubility product and the dissolution rate constant describe different phenomena as illustrated in Figure 4. Although equilibrium solubility data would indicate that ZnO is less soluble in water than glass, the rate of dissolution of ZnO under nonequilibrium conditions (zero concentration environment) is very high, and the more "insoluble" ZnO dissolves more quickly than glass if placed in a large volume of solvent. Likewise, since the lung fluids are cleared of dissolved foreign materials by diffusion to the blood, ZnO would be expected to dissolve relatively rapidly in the lung.

Unfortunately, values of the dissolution rate constant cannot be calculated from equilibrium solubility data and have only been measured for a few chemical forms. Also, the dissolution rate constant for dissolution in the complex lung fluids may be different than for water. Hence, values of k frequently must be determined individually for each experimental study of inhalation hazards. Kanapilly et al.[21] and Kanapilly et al.[22] designed systems for measuring the in vitro dissolution rate constant in synthetic lung fluids.

III. RESPIRATORY AIRWAY GEOMETRY

A. Morphometric Measurements

In inhalation toxicology, measurements of the normal dimensions of each anatomi-

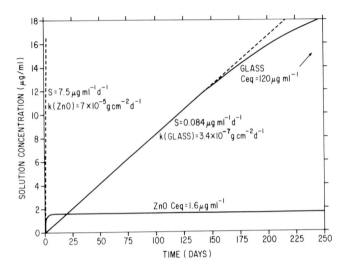

FIGURE 4.   Relationship of dissolution rate, $S(\mu g/m\ell^{-1}d^{-1})$, dissolution rate constant, $k(g/cm^{-2}/d^{-1})$, and equilibrium solubility concentration C_{eq} ($\mu g/m\ell^{-1}$), for 1 mg of 1 μm diameter ZnO and glass particles dissolving in 100 mℓ deionized and demineralized water.

cal section of human respiratory airways from nasal cavity to the parenchyma of the lung (see Figure 5) provide the foundation for predictive models of the deposition of inhaled particles. Clearly, differences among individuals and variability during the breathing cycle of one individual will exist.[23] However, nominal or representative descriptions of the variable anatomical features of the respiratory airways and airflow characteristics still can be beneficially used in general predictive models of deposition.

Morphometric measurements are usually made by

1.   Preparation of corrosion casts of the airspaces[24-27]
2.   Direct measurements in vivo, such as by endoscopy or radiography[28-30] or at autopsy[31]
3.   Two-dimensional measurements of cross-sectional cuts of tissue either by direct observation or with the aid of light and electron microscopy[32-36]

The respiratory airways include the passages of the nose, mouth, nasal pharynx, oral pharynx, epiglottis, larynx, trachea, bronchi, bronchioles, and small ducts and alveoli of the pulmonary acini. For consideration of the mechanisms associated with deposition and clearance of inhaled aerolsols, these airways can be divided into three functional regions:[37]

1.   Nasopharynx (NP), the airways extending from the nares down to the epiglottis and larynx at the entrance to the trachea (the mouth might be expected to the included in this region during mouth breathing)
2.   Tracheobronchial region (TB), the primary conducting airways of the lung from the trachea to the terminal bronchioles (i.e., that portion of the lung respiratory tract having a ciliated epithelium)
3.   Pulmonary region (P), the parenchymal airspaces of the lung, including the respiratory bronchioles, alveolar ducts, alveolar sacs, atria, and alveoli (i.e., the gas-exchange region)

In reality the anatomical and physiological divisions between these regions may be

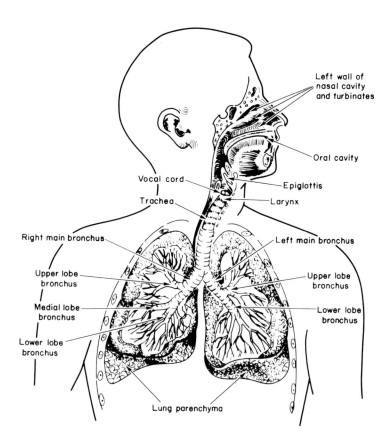

FIGURE 5. The respiratory airways of man.

gradual and difficult to distinguish. The formalized separation of the ciliated from the unciliated regions has a particularly useful application in studies of particle clearance.

The NP region consists primarily of hollow portions of the nose and throat. The nose is a complex structure of cartilage and muscle supported by bone and lined with mucosa.[38-40] The vestibule of the nares is unciliated, but contains a low-resistance filter consisting of small hairs. The nasal volume is separated into two cavities by a 2- to 7-mm-thick septum. The inner nasal fossae and turbinates are ciliated, with mucus flow in the direction of the pharynx. The turbinates are shelf-like projections of bone covered by ciliated mucous membranes with a high surface-to-volume ratio that facilitate humidifications of the incoming air.

The few measurements of the nasal region show that the total cross-sectional area of both nares in an adult is about 1.5 cm² of area.[41-42] The nasal cavity has a volume of about 8 cm³ and is about 7 cm long, with a maximum anteroposterior diameter of about 4 cm measured along the roof of the fossa.[43]

The larynx consists of two pairs of elevated mucosal folds that particularly obstruct the airway. The distance from the epiglottis to below the larynx is 5 to 7 cm with a vertical diameter of 3.6 to 4.4 cm;[43] females have smaller laryngeal regions than do males.

The trachea, an elastic tube supported by 16 to 20 cartilagenous rings that circle about three fourths of its circumference, is the first and largest of a series of conductive airway ducts into the lungs.[44] The trachea divides into two major bronchi. The caliber of the trachea and major bronchi is about 15% larger during inspiration than during expiration.[23,27,45]

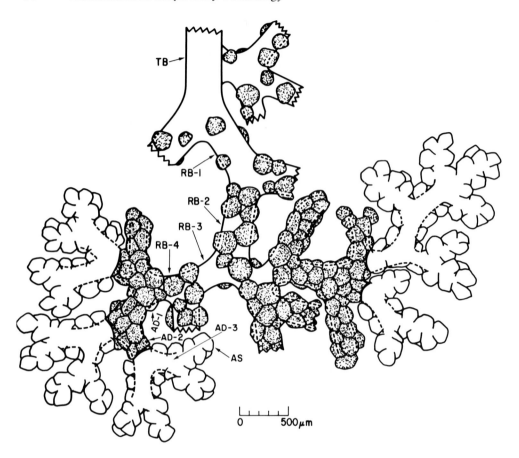

FIGURE 6.   Schematic representation of human respiratory acinus showing the terminal bronchiole (TB), four levels of respiratory bronchioles (RB-1 through RB-4), and four levels of alveolar ducts (AD-1 through AD-4) with bundles of adjoining alveoli. Unshaded acinar areas show alveoli in cross section. (From Schreider, J. P. and Raabe, O. G., *J. Anat.*, submitted. With permission.)

The lungs consist of two major parts, the left and right lungs, divided by the two major bronchi of the trachea. The left lung consists of two clearly separated lobes, the upper and lower lobes, and the right lung consists of three lobes, the upper, middle, and lower lobes. Each lobe is served by a bronchus from one of the two major bronchi.[46] Alavi et al.[47] have reported a mean branching angle of the trachea of 57°, with 95% limits from 45° to 69°. The conductive airways in each lobe of the lung consist of up to 18 to 20 dichotomous branches from the bronchi to the terminal bronchiole.[27,48] Bronchial caliber correlates to stature.[49] The caliber of the smaller conductive bronchioles may be up to 40% greater during inspiration than during expiration.[23,50]

The pulmonary, gas-exchange region of the lung begins with the partially alveolated respiratory bronchioles. Pulmonary branching proceeds through a few levels of respiratory bronchioles to completely alveolated ducts[51-53] and alveolar sacs.[45,54-56] The organization of a single human respiratory acinus from respiratory bronchiole to alveolar sacs is illustrated in Figure 6.[57] Alveoli are thin-walled polyhedron air pouches which cluster about the acinus through connections with respiratory bronchioles, alveolar ducts, or alveolar sacs. The tissue surfaces in the pulmonary region are coated with a complex aqueous liquid containing several biochemically specialized substances including pulmonary surfactants.[58]

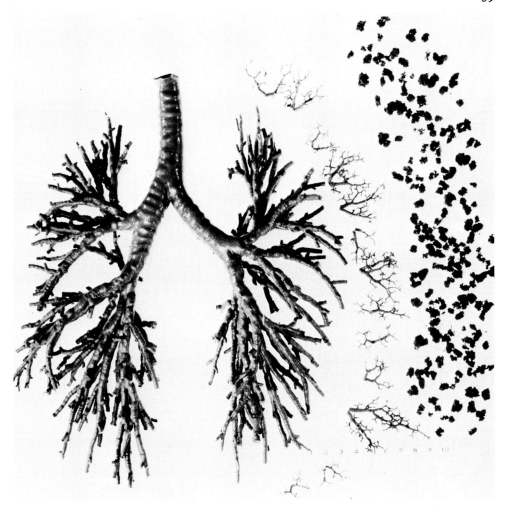

FIGURE 7. Silicon rubber cast of the human airways prepared by Raabe et al.[27] and divided into the conductive airway from trachea to bronchioles of 3 mm diameter, some separated segments from 3 mm diameter to terminal bronchioles, and some respiratory acinus bundles.

Several researchers have measured the conductive airways of the lung. Weibel[59] used a corrosion cast prepared by Liebow et al.[60] to make detailed measurements of unbroken segments to ten generations; he could not measure farther. Weibel[59] then combined those measurements with histological measurements[32] of the alveolar acinus to develop a consistent model of airway numbers and dimensions. Horsfield et al.[61-64] and Parker et al.[65] also measured casts of the human conductive airways. Raabe et al.,[27] using a method of Phalen et al.,[26] measured the conductive airways on casts of human lungs prepaired *in situ* at autopsy under conditions simulating end inspiration (see Figure 7), as well as of laboratory animals. These replicas purportedly were more faithful reproductions of the normal airway orientation than were those obtained with excised lungs. After determining the lengths, diameters, and branching angles for selected segments from trachea to terminal bronchioles (see Figure 8), Raabe et al.[27] demonstrated that the number of airway branches in the TB region from trachea to terminal bronchiole can range from 11 to 22. Also, different lobes had different average numbers of branches to terminal, with the apical or upper lobes having fewer than other lobes. These measurements reveal the diversity of branching angles, airway segment lengths, diameters, and branching patterns in mammalian species. Further, such factors as air-

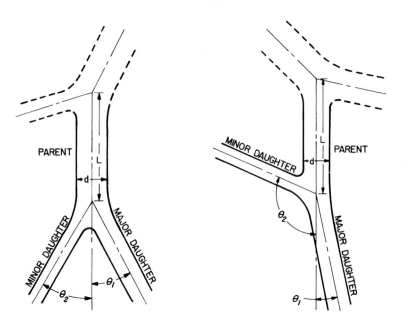

FIGURE 8.   Idealized model of isolated airway branches of lung showing segment diameter, d, segment length, L, and branching angles, θ_1 for major daughter and θ_2 for minor daughter. (From Raabe, O. G., Yeh, H. C., Schum, G. M., and Phalen, R. F., Tracheobronchial Geometry: Human, Dog, Rat, Hamster, LF-S3, Lovelace Foundation, Albuquerque, N. M., 1976. With permission.)

way closure, changes in caliber during breathing, bronchomotor tone, and constrictions can alter these dimensions.

The number of alveoli increases after birth until late childhood, reaching a maximum of about 300 million.[66-68] Other estimates of the total number of alveoli in man range from 100 million[69] to over 500 million.[70] Dimensions of the alveolar acinus are usually measured with light microscopy of histological preparations.[59] Schreider and Raabe[57] took acinus measurements from casts of the respiratory airways. Although the alveolus usually assumes an irregular shape because of the thin walls and close packing, alveolar size is usually described as the equivalent spherical diameter. Reported diameters range from 150 to 300 μm for man.[59,69,71-73] The alveolar dimensions vary under the influences of degree of inflation[74-75] and hydrostatic pressure that causes the alveoli of lower lobes in an upright person to be smaller at any given time than the alveoli of upper lobes.[76-77]

The total surface area of the alveoli in adult man was reported by Von Hayek[73] as 35 m² in expiration and 100 m² in deep inspiration. Weibel[59] estimated a surface area of 70 m² for a lung at three quarters capacity. This compares to 45.5 m² for 16-kg dogs[54] and 1.1 m² for guinea pigs.[78]

The deep lung parenchyma includes several types of tissue, circulating blood, lymphatic drainage pathways, and lymph nodes. In man the weight of the lung, including circulating blood, is about 1.4% of the total body; lung blood is equal to about 0.7% of total body weight (10% of total blood volume).[43] Because a portion of lung is occupied by air, the average physical density of the parenchyma is about 0.26 g/cm³ during normal breathing.[79]

B. Airway Models

Idealized or representative models of the airways, which simplify the complex array of branching and dimensions into workable mathematical functions, are useful in estimation of deposition. An early model of the airways of the human lung (see Table 2) for use in estimating the deposition of inhaled particles was described in a fundamental study reported in 1935 by Findeissen.[80] Findeissen's model assumed symmetry within the lung, with each generation consisting of airways of identical size. Other models based on a symmetry assumption have been proposed by Landahl[42] (see Table 3), Davies[71] (see Table 4), Weibel[59] (see Table 5). Horsfield and Cumming[62] developed a model to approximate the asymmetry of the airway branching scheme (see Table 6). A "nominal path" model which can be calculated from the measurements of Raabe et al.[27] integrates the important differences in lobar dimension (see Table 7). Taulbee and Yu[81] modeled the conductive airway as an imaginary continuously expanding tube to yield the appropriate correspondence of cross-sectional area with volume from trachea to alveoli. None of these models exactly describe the airways, but rather are more wieldy surrogates than the more complex reality.[82]

IV. RESPIRATORY AIRFLOW

A. Humidity and Temperature

Both the humidity and temperature of inhaled aerosol as well as the subsequent changes that occur as the aerosol passes through various parts of the airways have important influences on the inhalation deposition of airborne particles. Deposition of inhaled soluble, deliquescent, and hygroscopic aerosols will depend in part on the relative humidity in the airways, since the growth of such particles (with concomitant increase in aerodynamic size) will directly affect both the site and extent of inhalation deposition.

The relative humidity of inhaled air probably reaches near saturation in the nose.[83] Since the human nose is a relatively simple and short passageway, tranquil diffusion alone cannot account for rapid humidification. Rather, convective mixing must play a role. The lower temperature of inhaled air enhances the effectiveness of nasal humidification by convective mixing. Unlike humidity, the temperature of the inhaled air may not be equilibrated to the body temperature until relatively deep in the lung. Raabe et al.[27] found that the temperature of the air at the major bronchus in a nose-breathing dog averaged 35°C, 4°C less than the body temperature. The temperature of exhaled air at the nose of a dog averaged only 31°C.[84] Deal et al.[85-87] measured retrocardiac and retrotracheal temperatures in people and found airway cooling associated with the breathing of cool air.

B. Flow Dynamics

Inspiratory flow rate and depth of inhalation influences the deposition of inhaled particles. The average inspiratory flow rate, Q, and tidal volume, TV,[88-89] affect both inertial and diffusional deposition processes.[90] The total air remaining in the lungs at the end of normal expiration (functional residual capacity, FRC) affects the relative mixing of inhaled particles and, when compared with total lung capacity (TLC), is indicative of the extent of aerosol penetration into the lung. Weibel[91] developed relationships relating lung capacity to body weight, and Guyton[92-93] and Stahl[94] developed relationships describing respiratory volumes and patterns. An important difference between human beings and rodents is that small rodents breathe by inhaling shallowly and rapidly (for rats about 1.5 mℓ TV at 100 breaths per minute).

A graphical representation of respiration in man is illustrated in Figure 9 which incorporates definitions of various respiration terms.[95-96] The TV, the total volume of air inhaled per breath, times the respiratory rate, or breathing frequency (f_b) in breaths per minute (BPM) yields the minute volume (V_m). If half of the respiration time over the long-term is occupied by inspiration ($t_i = t_e$), the average flow rate (Q) is twice

Table 2
THE FINDEISEN MODEL[80] OF THE AIRWAYS OF THE HUMAN LUNG

	Part of the lung	Branching factor[a]	Number	Diameter (cm)	Length (cm)	Total cross-sectional area (cm²)	Flow velocity[b] (cm/s)	Residence time (s)
A	Trachea	1	1	1.3	11.0	1.3	150	0.07
B	Main bronchi	2	2	0.75	6.5	1.1	180	0.04
C	First-order bronchi	6	12	0.4	3.0	1.5	130	0.02
D	Second-order bronchi	8	100	0.2	1.5	3.1	65	0.02
E	Third-order bronchi	8	770	0.15	0.5	14	14	0.04
F	Terminal bronchi	70	5.4×10^4	0.06	0.3	150	1.3	0.22
G	Respiratory bronchioles	2	1.1×10^5	0.05	0.15	220	0.9	0.17
H	Alveolar ducts	240	2.6×10^7	0.02	0.02	8,200	0.025	0.82
I	Alveolar sacs	2	5.2×10^7	0.03	0.03	(147,000)[c]	ca. 0	1.2

b   For inspiratory flow rate (Q) = 12 ℓ/min.

c   Total surface of the spherical alveolar sacs.

Table 3
THE LANDAHL MODEL[42] OF THE HUMAN RESPIRATORY AIRWAYS

Region	Number	Diameter (cm)	Cross length (cm)	Total section area (cm²)	Flow volume[a] (cm³)	Residence velocity (cm/s)	Time (sec)
(1) Mouth	1	2	7	3	20	100	0.07
(2) Pharynx	1	3	3	7	20	45	0.07
(3) Trachea	1	1.6	12	2	25	150	0.08
(4) Primary bronchi	2	1.0	6	0.8	10	190	0.032
(5) Secondary bronchi	12	0.4	3	0.12	4	210	0.014
(6) Tertiary bronchi	100	0.2	1.5	0.12	5	100	0.015
(7) Quarternary bronchi	770	0.15	0.5	0.018	7	22	0.023
(8) Terminal bronchioles	6×10^4	0.06	0.3	2.8×10^{-3}	50	1.8	0.17
(9) Respiratory bronchioles	1.5×10^5	0.04	0.15	1.2×10^{-3}	30	1.7	0.09
(10) Alveolar ducts I	3×10^6	0.03	0.05	7×10^{-4}	100	0.14	0.36
(11) Alveolar ducts II	4×10^7	0.025	0.03	4.9×10^{-4}	600	0.015	2.0
(12) Alveolar sacs	10^8	0.033	0.033	—	(2000)	—	—

[a] For inspiratory flow rate (Q) = 18 ℓ/min; TV = 450 cm³.

Table 4
THE DAVIES MODEL[71] OF THE HUMAN RESPIRATORY AIRWAYS

Region		Number	Diameter of lumen (cm)	Length (cm)	Cross-sectional area (cm²)	Total cross-sectional area (cm²)	Total volume (cm³)
Mouth		1	2	7	3.1	3	22
Pharynx		1	3	3	7	7	21
Trachea		1	1.7	12	2.3	2.3	27
Main bronchi	R	1	1.4	2.5	1.54	2.67	9.5
	L	1	1.2	5	1.13		
Lobar bronchi	RU	1	0.8	2	0.5		
	RM	1	0.8	3	0.5		
	RL	1	0.8	4	0.5	2.5	7.0
	LU	1	0.8	2	0.5		
	LL	1	0.8	3	0.5		
Segmental bronchi		18	0.5	6	0.2	3.6	21.6
Intrasegmental bronchi		252	0.3	2.5	0.071	17.9	45.4
Bronchioles		504	0.2	2.0	0.032	16.1	31.7
Secondary bronchioles		3,024	0.1	1.5	0.0079	24	36.3
Terminal bronchioles		12,096	0.07	0.5	0.0039	47	23
Respiratory bronchioles		169,400	0.05	0.2	0.002	339	68
Alveolar ducts		847,000	0.08	0.125	0.005	4,240	534
Atria		4,240,000	(sphere 0.06 cm diam)		0.0028	11,900	479
Alveolar sacs		21,200,000	0.03	0.05	0.0007	14,800	741
Alveoli		530,000,000	(sphere 0.015 cm diam)		0.00018	95,400	939

Table 5

THE WEIBEL MODEL[59] OF THE AIRWAYS OF THE HUMAN LUNG (WITH REGULAR DICHOTOMY)[a]

Region	Generation	Number per generation	Diameter (cm)	Length (cm)	Total cross-sectional area (cm²)	Total volume (cm³)
Trachea	0	1	1.8	12.0	2.54	30.5
Main bronchi	1	2	1.22	4.76	2.33	11.3
Lobar bronchi	2	4	0.83	1.90	2.13	4.0
	3	8	0.56	0.76	2.00	1.5
Segmental bronchi	4	16	0.45	1.27	2.48	3.5
	5	32	0.35	1.07	3.11	3.3
	6	64	0.28	0.90	3.96	3.5
Bronchi with cartilage in wall	7	128	0.23	0.76	5.10	3.9
	8	256	0.186	0.64	6.95	4.5
	9	512	0.154	0.54	9.56	5.2
	10	1,024	0.130	0.46	13.4	6.2
Terminal bronchi	11	2,048	0.109	0.39	19.6	7.6
	12	4,096	0.095	0.33	28.8	9.8
Bronchioles with muscle in wall	13	8,192	0.082	0.27	44.5	12.5
	14	16,384	0.074	0.23	69.4	16.4
	15	32,768	0.066	0.20	113.0	21.7
Terminal bronchioles	16	65,536	0.060	0.165	180.0	29.7
Respiratory bronchioles	17	131,072	0.054	0.141	300.0	41.8
	18	262,144	0.050	0.117	534.0	61.1
	19	524,288	0.047	0.099	944.0	93.2
Alveolar ducts	20	1,048,576	0.045	0.083	1,600.0	139.5
	21	2,097,152	0.043	0.070	3,220.0	224.3
	22	4,194,304	0.041	0.059	5,880.0	350.0
Alveolar sac	23	8,388,608	0.041	0.050	11,800.0	591.0
Alveoli		300,000,000	0.028	0.023	—	—

[a] Average adult lung with volume 4800 mℓ at about three fourths maximal inflation.

V_m. During individual breaths, the inspiratory flow rate, V_I, is the time derivative of the lung volume (dv/dt).[89] Pauses may occur, but they are of little significance under conditions of moderate activity in describing inhaled particle deposition. The inspiratory reserve volume (IRV) is the maximum volume of air that can be inhaled after a given normal inspiration. Likewise, the expiratory reserve volume (ERV) is the maximum volume of air that can be exhaled after a given normal expiration. The inspiratory capacity (IC), the maximum volume of air that can be inhaled after a given normal expiration, is contrasted to the vital capacity (VC) which is the maximum volume of air that can be expelled from the lungs with effort after maximum forced inspiration. Air that remains in the conductive airways (from nose to terminal bronchioles) at end expiration is considered to occupy the respiratory dead space (V_D), since the conductive airways are not involved in gas exchange.[97-99]

Gas flow dynamics within the upper airways may be expected to be turbulent in humans and dogs, but laminar everywhere in the airways of small rodents.[100-105] For a 2-cm diameter human trachea at Q of 43.5 ℓ/min, the Reynolds' number is about 3000, higher than the critical Reynolds' number of 2300 for initiation of turbulence in a straight cylinder. The larynx introduces an air flow disturbance.[106-107] Turbulent conditions are also produced by constrictions to flow in sections of the nasopharyngeal region, around the larynx, and at the tracheal carina. For these reasons, those regions can be foci for the deposition of labeled particles and critical regions with respect to ultimate pathological responses. In the major bronchi, the Reynolds' number is below

Table 6

THE HORSFIELD AND CUMMING ASYMMETRICAL
MODEL[62] OF THE AIRWAYS OF THE HUMAN LUNG

Structure	Generation[a]	Number	Diameter (cm)	Length (cm)
Trachea	25	1	1.6	10.0
Bronchus	24	1	1.2	4.0
Bronchi	23	2	1.03	2.6
	22	2	0.89	1.8
	21	2	0.77	1.4
	20	3	0.66	1.1
	19	6	0.57	1.0
	18	8	0.49	1.0
	17	12	0.42	1.0
	16	14	0.35	1.0
	15	20	0.33	0.96
	14	30	0.31	0.91
	13	37	0.29	0.86
	12	46	0.28	0.82
	11	64	0.26	0.78
	10	85	0.24	0.74
	9	114	0.23	0.70
	8	158	0.22	0.67
	7	221	0.20	0.63
	6	341	0.178	0.57
	5	499	0.151	0.50
	4	760	0.129	0.44
	3	1,104	0.110	0.39
	2	1,675	0.093	0.35
	1	2,843	0.079	0.31
Terminal bronchioles	(−2)	27,992	0.060	—
Distal respiratory bronchioles	(−5)	223,941	0.040	—

[a] Based on last bronchi before terminal bronchiole as 1.

2300 at Q of 43.5 ℓ/min, but some turbulence may be transmitted from the trachea. West[105] observed that the gas flow was probably turbulent in a hollow cast of the bronchial tree. Schroter and Sudlow[102] and Olson et al.[103] observed secondary flow patterns and highly asymmetric velocity profiles in trachea and major bronchi. Martin and Jacobi[104] characterized air flow in the trachea or major bronchi as nonlaminar. In the smaller bronchi and bronchioles, where Reynolds' numbers are quite small, laminar flow does prevail, but branching patterns, filling patterns,[108] and flow reversals with varying velocity profiles complicate a description of flow in the small airways.[109-110]

Because actual flow in the respiratory airways currently cannot be described, simplified assumptions, such as laminar or bulk flow and uniform velocity profiles, are usually incorporated into analytic descriptions. Clearly, such assumptions are a major shortcoming in such analyses and limit accurate description of the physics of aerosol behavior in the respiratory airways. Still, such analyses may be sufficiently accurate descriptions of the dynamic conditions to yield applicable estimates of regional aerosol deposition.

Even though there is great variability in anatomical and physiological factors between individuals of different ages and sexes and of different physical proportions and states of health, it is desirable to be able to utilize reasonably representative values of respiratory characteristics for general estimation purposes. Reference values for

Table 7

"NOMINAL PATH" MODEL BASED ON MEASUREMENTS OF CAST OF THE AIRWAYS AT END INSPIRATION OF A MAN BASED ON RAABE ET AL.[27] GIVING SEGMENT LENGTH (L), DIAMETER (d), AND BRANCH ANGLE (θ) FOR THE LOBULAR PATHS HAVING THE MEDIAN NUMBER OF GENERATIONS TO TERMINAL BRONCHIOLES

Generation number	Right lung — Upper lobe			Middle lobe			Lower lobe			Left lung — Upper lobe			Lower lobe		
	L (mm)	d (mm)	θ (°)	L (mm)	d (mm)	θ (°)	L (mm)	d (mm)	θ (°)	L (mm)	d (mm)	θ (°)	L (mm)	d (mm)	θ (°)
Trachea							120.0	20.1							
2	12.2	10.2	60	30.9	17.5	25	8.8	10.1	5	56.3	13.8	40	14.2	11.5	25
3	8.7	7.15	39	(30.2)	13.3	15	11.40	9.0	5	14.5	10.3	35	15.3	9.9	10
4	13.2	6.18	32	22.7	7.2	25	11.04	7.84	3	11.1	8.46	26	9.8	8.9	5
5	10.7	5.08	13	13.24	6.16	17	8.16	8.54	3	10.1	6.70	16	10.49	9.23	30
6	8.59	4.12	18	13.07	5.85	10	12.18	8.04	8	14.0	5.76	13	17.44	6.57	19
7	12.74	3.68	17	10.24	4.24	45	13.02	5.96	17	10.9	4.52	19	10.28	4.67	21
8	8.09	2.91	31	8.53	3.51	30	15.29	5.31	19	11.0	3.91	16	8.49	4.50	9
9	5.92	2.29	31	11.23	3.25	47	9.29	4.25	17	12.9	3.41	22	13.76	4.00	17
10	4.56	1.80	41	6.06	2.47	64	7.76	3.42	18	6.76	2.65	20	8.03	3.22	26
11	3.60	1.24	50	5.10	1.80	52	8.13	2.79	35	6.60	2.13	26	7.19	2.91	25
12	2.64	0.96	51	3.24	1.19	40	5.41	1.91	45	5.10	1.64	34	6.60	2.21	31
13	2.02	0.79	49	2.55	1.03	44	3.59	1.39	55	3.80	1.14	40	4.60	1.61	44
14	1.56[a]	0.59	52	2.04	0.79	45	2.76	1.09	56	2.83	0.88	49	3.36	1.06	46
15	—	—	—	1.53	0.64	45	2.35	0.87	62	2.16[a]	0.62	54	2.05	0.88	43
16	—	—	—	1.20[a]	0.50	—	1.64[a]	0.67	57	—	—	—	1.98[a]	0.61	57
17	—	—	—	—	—	—	—	—	—	—	—	—	—	—	—
18	—	—	—	—	—	—	—	—	—	—	—	—	—	—	—

[a] Terminal bronchiole segment for the lobe.

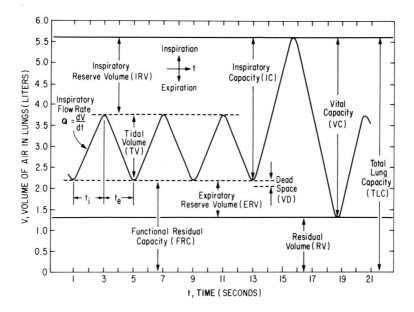

FIGURE 9. Parameters used in respiratory physiology are illustrated on a hypothetical spirometric record of breathing patterns.

normal human respiratory parameters[37,43] have been developed for a young adult weighing 70 kg with a height of 175 cm and a body surface area of 1.8 m². His lungs, including circulating blood, weigh 1000 g. At rest, his breathing rate (f_b) is 12 BPM with minute volume (V_m) of 7.5 ℓ/min. During light activity, f_b is 16 to 17 BPM with V_m of 20 ℓ/min. Reference values of respiratory parameters under an average condition of moderate activity are summarized in Table 8. It is understood that these values do not describe any particular person, and considerable variability in respiratory parameters may occur among individuals. However, these reference values provide a valuable tool for general deposition and dosimetric predictions.

V. DEPOSITION

A. Physical Factors Affecting Deposition

The behavior of inhaled airborne particles in the respiratory airways and their alternative fates of either deposition or exhalation depend upon aerosol mechanics under the given physiological and anatomical condition.[111-112] Figure 10 illustrates the five primary physical processes that lead to particle contact with the wall of the airways. Contact of a particle with those typically moist surfaces results in irreversible removal of the particle from the airstream. The contact process can occur during inspiration or expiration of a single breath or subsequently if a particle has been transferred to unexhaled lung air.[113-115] Deposition increases with duration of breath holding and depth of breathing.[115-117]

Electrostatic forces on particles in the airway may cause particles to be attracted to and contact airway surfaces. Electrostatic attraction is probably a minor mechanism of deposition in most circumstances. Pavlik[118] predicted that light air ions would be deposited by electrostatic attraction in the mouth and throat and suggested that the tonsils were naturally charged for this purpose. Fraser[119] found that an average of 1000 electronic units of charge per aerosol particle resulted in double the inhalation deposition in experimental animals. Melandri et al.[120] reported enhanced deposition of inhaled monodisperse aerosols by people when the particles were charged. Longley[121] and Londley and Berry[122] found the charge of the individual to have an influence on

Table 8

REFERENCE VALUES FOR RESPIRATORY
PHYSIOLOGY IN AN AVERAGE MAN
UNDER CONDITIONS OF MODERATE
ACTIVITY OR WORK[37,43]

Parameter	Symbol	Value
Weight	W	70 kg
Height	h	175cm
Age		20—30 years
Body surface area	SA	1.8 m²
Lung weight	W_L	1000 g
Lung surface area		80 m²
Trachea weight	W_T	10 g
Trachea length	L_T	12 cm
Total lung capacity	TLC	5.6 ℓ
Functional residual capacity	FRC	2.2 ℓ
Vital capacity	VC	4.3 ℓ
Residual volume	RV	1.3 ℓ
Respiratory dead space	V_D	160 mℓ
Breathing rate	f_b	15 BPM
Tidal volume	TV	1450 mℓ
Average inspiratory flow rate	Q	43.5 ℓ/min
Minute volume	V_m	21.75 ℓ/min
Inspiratory period	t_i	2 sec
Expiratory period	t_e	2 sec

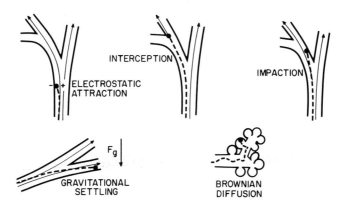

FIGURE 10.   Representation of five major mechanisms of deposition of inhaled airborne particles in the respiratory tract.

deposition. However, the airways are covered by a relatively conductive electrolytic liquid that probably precludes the buildup of forceful electric fields. Charged particles are therefore collected primarily by image charging as they near the wall of an airway or by mutual repulsion for a unipolarly charged cloud with a high concentration of particles.[123] The charge-to-mass ratio (and associated electrical mobility) of an aerosol particle determines the extent to which the mechanisms may play a role in deposition.

Interception consists of noninertial incidental meeting of a particle and the lining of the airway and thus depends on the physical size of the particle. This process would have a zero probability if the particles were only points rather than extended bodies. This mechanism of deposition is important primarily for particles with large aspect ratios, such as long fibrous particles of asbestos.[124]

Impaction dominates deposition of particles larger than 3 μm D_{ar} in the nasopharyngeal and tracheobronchial regions.[125] In this process, changes in direction or magnitude of air velocity streamline or eddy components are not duplicated by airborne particles because of their inertia. For example, if air is directed towards an airway surface (such as a branch carina), but the velocity is suddenly reduced because of change in flow direction, inertial momentum may carry larger particles across the air streamlines and into the surface of the airway. Aerodynamic separation of this type is generally characterized by the distance a particle travels after cessation of forward air flow. This stopping distance (L_s) is given by:

$$L_s = \frac{\rho^* V_o \, D_{ar}^2{}^2}{18\eta} \qquad (11)$$

with ϱ^* the standardizing density equal to 1 g/cm³, V_o the initial velocity of the particle with respect to the airstream, D_{ar} the aerodynamic (resistance) diameter, and η the viscosity of air.[17] The importance of a given stopping distance in a cylindrical tube depends on the tube diameter. This relationship is represented by the dimensionless Stokes' number given by Stk $= 2L_s/d$, where d is the tube diameter.

Impaction at an airway branch also has been likened to impaction at the bend of a bent tube;[126] Yeh[127] calculated the probability of deposition by impaction alone as:

$$P_I = 1 - \frac{2}{\pi} \arccos(\theta \, \text{Stk}/2) + \frac{1}{\pi} \sin[2\arccos(\theta \, \text{Stk}/2)] \text{ for } [\theta \, \text{Stk}/2 < 1] \qquad (12)$$

with θ the bend angle for the bent tube. Though not as rigorous as similar expressions derived by Cheng and Wang,[128] Yeh's equation is much easier to apply. Also Cheng and Wang[128] consider only a right angle bend. If impaction in the respiratory airways is likened to collection of aerosols in a round-jet impactor, the 50% collection efficiency would occur at Stk equal to 0.2. This yields a value of 18 μm D_{ar} for the tracheal bifurcation for Q of 45 ℓ/min and indicates little impaction effect on particles smaller than 6 μm D_{ar}. However, the airflow in the trachea and major bronchi in human beings is turbulent and disturbed by the larynx so that turbulent impaction involving particles smaller than 6 μm D_{ar} plays an important role in the deposition in these larger airways.[107] Breathing patterns involving higher volumetric flow rates would tend to impact smaller particles. Also, the passages of the nose contain smaller airways, and the convective mixing spaces of the nasal turbinates would be expected to collect some particles as small as 1 or 2 μm D_{ar} by impaction.

Gravitational settling occurs because of the influence of the earth gravity on small particles. Deposition by gravitational settling of particles can occur in all airways except those very few that are exactly vertical. The probability of this deposition (P_s) is usually estimated with equations describing gravitational settling of particles in an inclined cylindrical tube of diameter, d, under laminar flow conditions:[129-130]

$$P_s = \frac{2}{\pi} [2\kappa(1-\kappa^{2/3})^{1/2} - \kappa^{1/3}(1-\kappa^{2/3})^{1/2} + \arcsin \kappa^{1/3}] \qquad (13)$$

where κ is the characteristic parameter given by:

$$\kappa = \frac{3t V_s \cos \beta}{4d} = \frac{t\rho^* g \, D_{ar}^2 \cos \beta}{24\eta d} \qquad (14)$$

with β the incline angle, and t the time in the tube. Hence, the deposition probability for sedimentation is also dependent on the aerodynamic resistance diameter, D_{ar}.

Deposition by diffusion results from the random (Brownian) motion of very small particles caused by bombardment of the gas molecules in air. The magnitude of this property can be described by the diffusion coefficient for a given physical particle diameter. Since larger particles have relatively greater inertia, diffusion primarily effects deposition of particles with physical diameters smaller than 0.5 μm. For a 0.5-μm diameter spherical particle with a physical density of about 1 g/cm³, the influences of inertial properties and diffusional properties on lung deposition are about equal.

Accurate calculation of the diffusional deposition of aerosols in the airways requires information concerning the three-dimensional velocity profile of air flow in each airway segment. If the flow of a given segment is laminar and approximately Poiseuille, the probability of desposition by diffusion (P_D) in a tube of length L is given by the Thomas modification[131] of the Gormley-Kennedy[132] equation:

$$P_D = 1 - 0.819e^{-1.828u} + 0.097e^{-11.15u} + 0.032e^{-28.5u} + 0.027e^{-61.5u} + 0.025e^{-375u} \quad (15)$$

where u is a function of volumetric flow rate Q, tube length L, and particle diffusion coefficient Δ: $u = 2\pi\Delta L/Q$. Equation 15, which assumes the aerosol is mixed at the entrance of the cylinder, might overestimate deposition in lung segments where there is minimal mixing between branches and laminar flow between segments.

It is important to note that the diffusivity (and D_{df}), electrical mobility, and interception potential of a particle depend on its physical size, while the inertial properties of settling and impaction depend on its aerodynamic diameter. These two measures of size may be quite different, depending on particle shape and physical density. Because the main mechanism of deposition is diffusion for small particles, less than 0.5 μm D_{df} and impaction and settling above 0.5 μm D_{ar}, it is convenient to use 0.5 μm as the boundary between two regions. Although this convention may lead to confusion in the case of very dense particles, most potentially toxic aerosols have densities below 3 g/m³, and the deposition probability tends to plateau between 0.5 μm and 1 μm D_{ar} (the equivalent D_{ar} for a spherical particle with physical diameter 0.5 μm and with density 3 g/m³). Of course, a comparison of deposition probabilities is desirable between the aerodynamic diameter and diffusive diameter of submicrometer particles.

Deposition calculations usually group lung regions without regard to nonuniformity of the pattern of deposited particles within the regions. Schlesinger and Lippmann[133] found nonuniform deposition in the trachea could be caused by the air flow disturbance of the larynx. Bell and Friedlander[134,135] studied the nonuniform deposit that actually is found at a single airway bifurcation. Raabe et al.[18] observed that the relative lobar pulmonary deposition of monodisperse aerosols was up to 60% higher in the right apical lobes of small rodents (corresponding to the human right upper lobe) and that the difference was most pronounced for 3.15- and 2.19-μm D_{ar} particles than for smaller particles. In addition, they showed that these differences in relative lobar deposition were related to the geometric mean number of airway bifurcations between trachea and terminal bronchioles in each lobe. Since similar morphometric differences occur in human lungs (see Table 7), nonuniform lobar deposition should also occur in human lungs. Schlesinger et al.[136] found nonuniform deposition in the lobular branches of a hollow model of the tracheobronchial airways and were able to demonstrate a correlation of higher lobular deposition and the reported incidence of bronchogenic carcinoma in different human lung lobes.

Most deposition studies and models tend to focus on insoluble and stable test aerosols whose properties do not change during the course of inhalation and deposition. However, many toxic aerosols consist of deliquescent or hygroscopic particles that may grow in size in the humid airways. That growth will affect deposition properties. The International Commission on Radiological Protection (ICRP) Task Group on Lung

Dynamics[37] addressed this problem by considering the equilibrium diameter for deliquescent materials at relative humidities near, but less than, 100%. However, residence times in the respiratory tract may be too short for large particles to reach their equilibrium size, and humidities at complete saturation may be encountered.

Ferron[137] has described the factors affecting soluble particle growth in the airways during breathing. Basically, his results suggest that particles 1 μm in aerodynamic diameter will increase by a factor of three to four in aerodynamic diameter during passage through the airways. NP, TB, and pulmonary deposition of those enlarged particles would be greater than the deposition expected for the original particle size. Submicronic particles, including those as small as 0.05 μm, will grow by a factor of two in physical diameter with relatively little effect on deposition; the particles smaller than 0.3 μm D may even have some reduced pulmonary deposition with growth because of reduced diffusivity.

B. Theoretical Models of Regional Deposition

Deposition of inhaled aerosols in a given region of the respiratory tract or in the entire tract is expressed as deposition fraction of inhaled particles. Deposition fraction is the ratio of the number or mass of particles deposited in the respiratory tract to the number or mass of particles inhaled. The undeposited fraction represents those particles that are exhaled after inhalation. Pulmonary deposition (sometimes called alveolar deposition) is the ratio of the number or mass of particles deposited in the unciliated small airways and gas-exchange spaces of the parenchyma of the lung to the number or mass of particles entering the nose or mouth. The fraction not deposited in the pulmonary region is either deposited in some other region or exhaled. Similarly, deposition fractions can be defined for the NP and TB regions of the respiratory airways.

The probability of deposition is calculated as the difference between unity and the product of the probabilities of transmission through a given duct or series of ducts. Hence, the probability of deposition for the combination of impaction, settling, and diffusion (see Equations 12, 13, and 15) for a single segment is given by $P = 1 - (1 - P_I)(1 - P_S)(1 - P_D)$. Likewise, the probability of deposition in the total respiratory tract can be computed from the deposition probabilities in each segment.

Using available models of the morphometric anatomy of the airways and various plausible assumptions concerning airflow and particle dynamics, various investigators have developed theoretical models of the deposition of inhaled particles in the respiratory tract of man.[42,80,138-141] In such calculations, deposition is a function of physical size for particles primarily affected by diffusion and aerodynamic size for particles primarily affected by inertial properties. For simplicity, most models are based on the assumption that the particles do not change in size during breathing; appropriate modifications are needed for deliquescent or hygroscopic particles.

Apparently, the earliest theoretical model and calculations of deposition by impaction, gravitational settling, and diffusion were developed by Findeissen.[80] Other pioneering work was done by Landahl,[42] and later he developed improved equations.[141] Beekmans[138] performed similar computations with a computer to evaluate the effects of changes in particle density and breathing parameters.

The most widely used models of regional deposition vs. particle size were developed by the ICRP Task Group on Lung Dynamics under the chairmanship of Morrow.[37] Although the purpose of those models was the determination of radiation exposure from inhaled radioactive aerosols, the aerosol deposition and clearance models are generally applicable to all aerosols. The ICRP Task Group[37] used the anatomical model and general methods of Findeissen,[80] and Landahl[42,138-141] for calculating deposition in the TB and pulmonary regions and the Gormley-Kennedy[132] equation for cylindrical tubes was used for calculating diffusional deposition. Particles were assumed to be insoluble, stable, and spherical with physical densities of 1 g/cm^3. Regional dep-

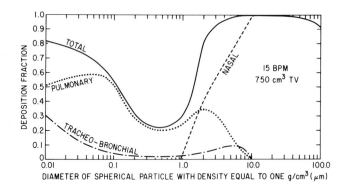

FIGURE 11.   Total and regional deposition fractions for various sizes of inhaled airborne spherical particles with physical density of 1 g/cm³ in the human respiratory tract as calculated by the ICRP Task Group on Lung Dynamics[37] for a breathing rate of 15 BPM and a tidal volume of 750 cm³.

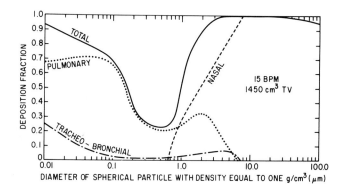

FIGURE 12.   Total and regional deposition fractions for various sizes of inhaled airborne spherical particles with physical density of 1 g/cm³ in the human respiratory tract as calculated by the ICRP Task Group on Lung Dynamics[37] for a breathing rate of 15 BPM and a tidal volume of 1450 cm³.

osition for reference man[43] was calculated for a breathing rate of 15 BPM for three representative TVs:

1.   TV 750 cm³, at rest (see Figure 11)
2.   TV 1450 cm³, moderate activity (see Figure 12)
3.   TV 2150 cm³, fairly strenuous activity[37]

The ICRP Task Group[37] used the calculated deposition fractions for individual particle sizes to predict deposition of log-normally distributed aerosols consisting of unit density spherical particles with geometric standard deviations (σ_g) as high as 4.5. When the results were expressed in terms of the MMD for these various size distributions of unit density aerosols (equivalent to the MMAD), the loci of the expected deposition values spanned relatively narrow limits (see Figure 13).

Most model calculations treat the various mechanisms of deposition as independently occurring phenomena. However, such processes as Brownian diffusion and gravitational settling will interfere with each other when their effects are of comparable

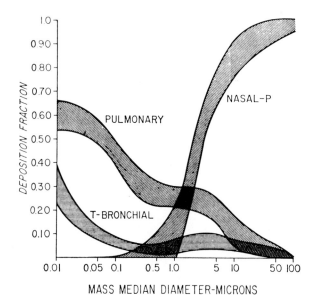

FIGURE 13.   The range of regional deposition fractions (shaded areas) for log-normally distributed spherical aerosols in human nose breathing at 15 BPM and 1450 cm³ TV. Geometric SDs range between 1.2 and 4.5; particle physical density is 1 g/cm³. (From Morrow, D. E. (Chairman), *Health Phys.*, 12, 173, 1966. With permission.)

magnitude, and that interference can reduce the combined deposition to less than the sum of the separate depositions.[142] Taulbee and Yu[143] have developed a theoretical deposition model which allows for the combined effects of the primary deposition mechanisms and features an imaginary expanding tube model of the airway system based on cross-sectional areas and airway lengths taken from Weibel.[59]

C. Experimental Measurements of Deposition

The ICRP Task Group on Lung Dynamics[37] compared the calculated regional and total deposition fractions for inhaled particles with the available human data. Those data were primarily total deposition values for polydisperse and sometimes unstable aerosols.[12,41,139,144-149] Since then, the deposition in people of monodisperse stable aerosols of different sizes has been measured under different breathing conditions. The most extensive of these studies are those of Lippmann and Albert,[150] Heyder et al.,[151] and Giacomelli-Maltoni et al.[152] Additional useful data are reported by Palmes and Wang,[153] Shanty,[154] George and Breslin,[155] Altshuler et al.,[90] Hounam et al.,[156-157] and Foord et al.,[158] among others.[159-169]

These human deposition data have been collected from volunteers inhaling test aerosols through either mouthpieces or nose tubes. Differences between those artificially controlled inhalations and normal spontaneous mouth or nose breathing are possible. Also, the f_b, FRC, and TV used in those experiments affected deposition data.

If the quantity of aerosol exhaled is compared with that inhaled, the data can be expressed as total deposition, but regional involvement cannot be distinguished.[151] If the test aerosols are radiolabeled, deposition can be separated by region, beginning with nasal-pharyngeal deposition for nose breathing or pharyngeal deposition for mouth breathing.[170] Further, the measurement of clearance of the radiolabel from the thorax can be used to separate early clearance, indicative of TB deposition, from more slowly cleared pulmonary (P) deposition.[150]

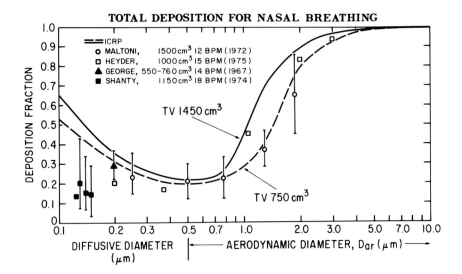

FIGURE 14.   Selected data[151,152,154,155] reported for the deposition in the entire respiratory tract of monodisperse aerosols inhaled through the nose by people are compared with predicted values calculated by the ICRP Task Group on Lung Dynamics.[37] (RPM refers to respirations or breaths per minute, BPM.)

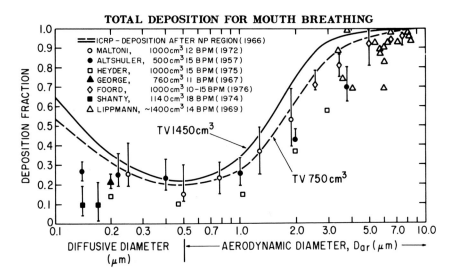

FIGURE 15.   Selected data[150-152,154,155,158,167] reported for the deposition in the respiratory tract of monodisperse aerosols inhaled through the mouth by people are compared with predicted values calculated by the ICRP Task Group on Lung Dynamics.[37]

Selected portions of the available data on total and regional aerosol deposition have been compared with the calculated deposition values of the ICRP Task Group on Lung Dynamics[37] (see Figures 14 to 18).* In these comparisons, their values either agree well with or represent the upper limit of the observed deposition values. The greatest overall

---

*In these figures, D_{ar}, is used to describe particles bigger than 0.5 μm and D_{df} for the smaller particles. The D_{ar} primarily determines deposition for particles bigger than 0.5 μm, whereas the D_{df} primarily controls deposition for smaller particles. Little discontinuity occurs at the junction, since the deposition values for spheres whose physical density is not far from 1 g/cm^3 tend to plateau at or near 0.5 μm.

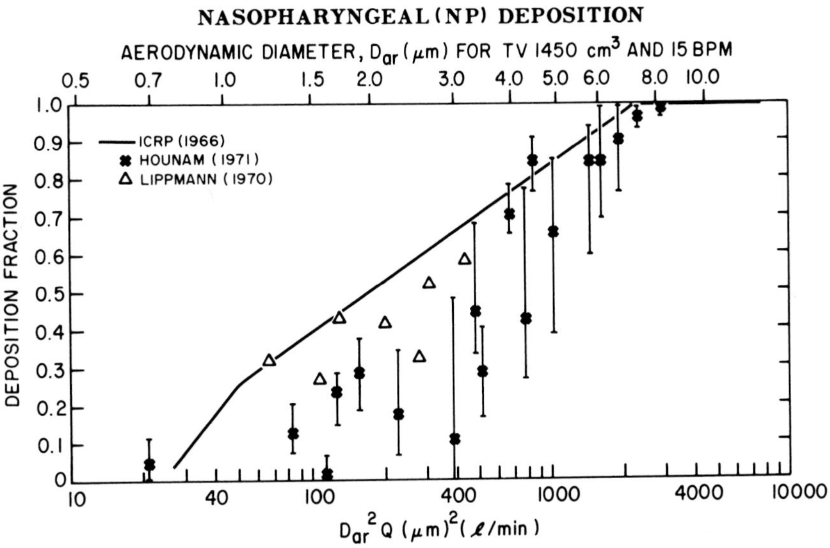

NASOPHARYNGEAL (NP) DEPOSITION

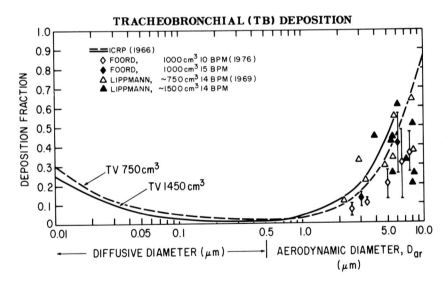

FIGURE 16.   Selected data[156-157,168] reported for the deposition fraction of monodisperse aerosols in the human region of the respiratory tract are plotted against the characteristic term (D_{ar}^2F) that controls inertial impaction; for reference, the calculated value[37] is shown for 15 BPM at 1450 cm³ TV.

TRACHEOBRONCHIAL (TB) DEPOSITION

FIGURE 17.   Selected data[150,158] reported for TB deposition of monodisperse aerosols inhaled through the mouth by people are compared with predicted values calculated by the ICRP Task Group on Lung Dynamics.[37]

discrepancy between actual and calculated values occurs for particles smaller than 0.2 μm; fractional pulmonary deposition measured for those particles during mouth breathing is about 0.1 to 0.2, compared with the 0.3 to 0.6 predicted by the Task Group.[37] However, actual data for these smaller particles are based on only a few experiments, and future studies may modify this discrepancy.

Davies[171] suggests that, in general, experimental errors tend to lead to overestimates of deposition. However careful, laboratory experiments under controlled and sometimes somewhat nonphysiological conditions might yield artificially low deposition val-

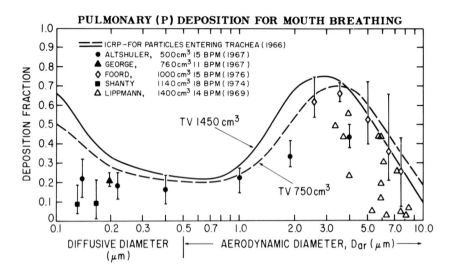

FIGURE 18.   Selected data[90,150,154,155,158] reported for pulmonary (P) deposition of monodisperse aerosols inhaled through the mouth by people are compared with predicted values calculated by the ICRP Task Group on Lung Dynamics.[37]

ues. As a particular example, the lower deposition fractions measured by Heyder et al.[151] for mouth breathing (see Figure 15) are probably a reflection of the fact that the test aerosol was humidified and heated to near body temperature prior to inhalation. Consequently, convective mixing in the airways would have been less than normal. Normal convective mixing leads to transfer of inhaled airborne particles to unexhaled air.[115,172] Subsequently particles can be directly deposited on airway surfaces by one of the normal physical mechanisms.

Considering the limitations of the models used by the ICRP Task Group on Lung Dynamics,[37] their results are generally useful for health protection purposes, especially since they do not underestimate deposition fraction for the chosen respiratory parameters. Those models may be quite satisfactory representations of other breathing conditions as well, considering that individuals can exhibit differences in deposition depending on the physiological parameters.

Since many data concerning inhalation toxicology are collected with beagle dogs or small rodents, it is important to consider the comparative regional deposition in these experimental animals. Cuddihy et al.[173] measured the regional deposition of polydisperse aerosols in beagles with TV about 170 mℓ at about 15 BPM and expressed the results as mass deposition percentage vs. mass median aerodynamic resistance diameter (MMAD$_{ar}$) that ranged from 0.42 to 6.6 μm, with geometric SD $\sigma_g = 1.8$. Their results showed beagle deposition to be comparable to the Task Group value for man with TV 1450 cm³.

Raabe et al.[18] have measured the regional deposition of 0.1 to 3.15 μm D$_{ar}$ monodisperse aerosols in rats (TV about 2 mℓ, 70 BPM) and Syrian hamsters (TV about 0.8 mℓ at about 40 BPM). Their results are summarized in Figure 19. The deposition in small rodents is about one half the Task Group[37] estimates for people at TV 1450 cm³. Some values are comparable to deposition vs. particle size in man measured by Heyder et al.[151] The distributions among the respiratory regions during nose breathing follow a pattern very similar to human regional deposition during nose breathing. The use of rodents or dogs in inhalation toxicology research for extrapolation to nose-breathing people does not seem to entail significant problems associated with differences in regional deposition of inhaled aerosols based on particle size for inert insoluble particles during nose breathing.

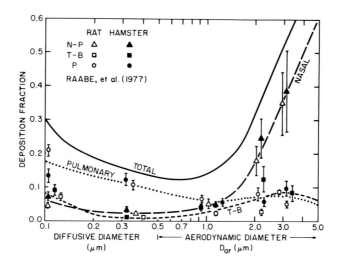

FIGURE 19. Deposition of inhaled monodisperse aerosols of fused aluminosilicate spheres in small rodents showing the deposition in the NP (nasal) region, the (TB) region, the pulmonary region, and in the total respiratory tract.[18]

When aerosols are inhaled via the nose, the relatively efficient filtration action of the nasopharyngeal region prevents the passage of particles larger than 10 μm D_{ar} to the lung and markedly reduces the pulmonary deposition of particles between 1 and 10 μm D_{ar} (see Figures 11 to 13). On the other hand, during mouth breathing the filtration action of the NP region is circumvented, and the deposition in the TB and pulmonary region is increased for particles larger than 1 μm D_{ar} (see Figures 17 and 18). Total deposition is not significantly altered, with the mouth and oral pharynx becoming the site of deposition of larger particles (see Figures 14 and 15). Lippmann[174] has calculated with his earlier data[150] that some particles as large as 15 μm D_{ar} may deposit (10%) in the upper TB region during slow mouth breathing (Q = 30 ℓ/min) in contrast to 0% during nose breathing.

An active person breathing with 15 BPM and TV = 1450 cm³ would be expected to deposit in the deep lung about 35, 25, 10, and close to 0% of inhaled aerosols of unit density (1 g/cm³) spherical particles of 0.2, 1, 5, and 10 μm, respectively, during nose breathing. On the other hand, the deposition in the deep lung would be expected to be about 35, 30, 55, and 10%, respectively, for the same particles during mouth breathing.

VI. CLEARANCE

A. Factors Affecting Clearance

Particulate material deposited in the respiratory tract may eventually be cleared via the TB ciliary mucus flow or nasal mucus flow (to the GI tract or expectorated), the lymphatic system, or by transfer to the blood. The importance of clearance as a protective mechanism for the respiratory tract critically depends on the physicochemical characteristics of the particles, site of deposition, and respiratory physiology. If the particles are soluble in body fluids, their deposition in the nasal turbinates with subsequent absorption into the blood may be more important than pulmonary deposition, and total deposition of soluble particles may be more important than regional deposition. For relatively insoluble particles, deposition in the pulmonary region, where they may be tenaciously retained, would be the most potentially hazardous. If the particles can chemically react with body fluids, possible transformations of the material can introduce intermediate control over further clearance. Consequently, there must be careful consideration given to the relative importance of physiological and biochemical processes and the inherent properties of the deposited particles. In all respiratory regions, the dissolution (or equivalent fragmentation to diffusible ultrafine pieces) of particles competes with other clearance processes for temporal advantage.

For clearance of particulate material from the nonciliated respiratory tract, the natural respiratory defense mechanisms appear to be primarily poised for immunological responses. Hence, microbiologically inert particles may be treated as if they were living bacterial invaders rather than misplaced mineralogical refuse. Since many inhaled particles are comparable in size to microbiological intruders, the common response of the human system may be congruous.

Because clearance from the three airway regions (NP, TB, and P) is physiologically and temporally different, the ICRP Task Group on Lung Dynamics[37] systematized clearance from the respiratory tract by region of deposition as well as characteristic chemical classes of particles (i.e., by solubility in body fluids). An understanding of regional deposition is requisite to an evaluation of respiratory clearance and the description of the retention of deposited particulate materials. In addition, there may be significant differences in the relative importance of clearance mechanisms in different mammalian species.

B. Nasal Clearance

Particle deposition in the NP region is primarily limited to the larger particles deposited by intertial impaction (see Figure 16). Deposition of various aerosols in this region may lead to inflammation, congestion, ulceration, and even cancer in the case of long-term repeated exposures to carcinogenic materials. For particles that do not quickly dissolve or react with body fluids, clearance from this region is mechanical. The anterior one third of the nose (where most particles bigger than 5 μm may deposit) does not clear except by blowing, wiping, sneezing, or other extrinsic means, and particles may not be removed for 1 or more days after deposition.[38,39,175-177]

The posterior portions of the nose, including the nasal turbinates, have mucociliary clearance averaging 6 mm/min.[175-177] Particles are moved with this natural mucus drainage to the throat and swallowed or expectorated. Various reactions can occur in the GI tract, and some assimilation into the blood is possible, even for particles that were relatively insoluble in the nose. The ICRP Task Group[37] adopted a 4-min half-time for physical clearance from the NP region by mucociliary transport to the throat and subsequent swallowing.

Soluble particles or droplets are readily assimilated via the mucous membranes of the NP region directly into the blood. Solubility is graded from extremely insoluble through to instantly soluble, and the dissolution rate constant for the particles must be considered for each aerosol. Partial dissolution with important ramifications may occur in the nasal turbinate section of the NP region even for some only moderately soluble particles.

C. Tracheobronchial Clearance

Since the TB region includes both very large and very small conductive airways, particles of all sizes can be deposited in this region. If deposited in sufficient quantity and over a sufficiently long period, some of these particles can lead to bronchospasms, allergic reactions (pollen aerosols), obstructive disorders, bronchial congestion, bronchitis, and cancer in the case of inhaled carcinogenic particulate materials.[28,178] The temporal retention of deposited materials in this region can differ markedly between individuals and can be affected by such factors as cigarette smoking, pathological abnormalities, or responses to inhaled air pollutants. Clearly, the more rapid the clearance, the less time available for untoward responses or latent injury. In mouth breathing of aerosols, such as during smoking or under physical exertion, the beneficial filtering of large particles in the NP region is lost, and a greater fraction of these large particles can be deposited in the TB region (as noted earlier).

An important characteristic of the TB region is that it is both ciliated and equipped with mucus-secreting cells. The detailed nature of the mucociliary clearance mechanism has been reviewed by Schlesinger.[179] For relatively insoluble and inert particles, the primary clearance mechanism for the TB region is mucociliary transport to the glottis, with subsequent expectoration or swallowing and passage through the GI tract. Mucus flow consists of adhesive globules carried along by the cilia.[180-185] The rate of mucus movement is slowest in the finer, more distal airways and greatest in the major bronchi and trachea. Linear speed of mucus movement in the human trachea averaged 2.15 cm/min (Santa Cruz et al.)[186] On the other hand, Yeates et al.[187] observed mean tracheal mucus rates of only 4.7 and 5.9 mm/min. Particles depositing in the TB tree are distributed differently with respect to size, with smaller particles generally depositing deeper in the lung. Hence, the clearance of small particles from the TB tree is slower than for larger particles that deposit primarily in the larger airways.[188-191]

Hence, the clearance of material in the TB compartment cannot be described by a single rate. Data from experimental studies imply that the larger airways clear with a half-time of about 0.5 hr, intermediate airways with a half-time of 2.5 hr, and finer airways with a half-time of 5 hr.[10,182] There is also considerable variability among individuals.[188,193-194] Material with slow dissolution rates in the TB compartment will usually not persist for longer than about 24 hr in healthy humans. Cigarette smoking may increase, decrease, or have little effect on the efficiency and speed of TB clearance.[125,193,195-197]

D. Pulmonary (Alveolar) Clearance

All particles smaller than about 10 μm in aerodynamic diameter are deposited to some extent in the pulmonary region of the lung upon inhalation, although the deposition of particles much smaller than 0.01 μm may be quite small because of diffusional deposition in the NP and TB regions. Particles that deposit in the pulmonary region land on surfaces kept moist by a complex liquid containing pulmonary surfactants.[55,198-201] There are no ciliated cells in the epithelium of this region, and flow of liquid from pulmonary airspaces into the TB region is minimal in humans (unlike murine species).[202] Hence, insoluble materials that deposit in the pulmonary region are usually retained for extended periods in that region. Particles deposited in the pulmonary region may be responsible for fibrogenic diseases, emphysema, functional disorders, and cancer.[203]

A description of the clearance of particles from the pulmonary region includes a characterization of their distribution and redistribution. Relatively insoluble particles commonly are rapidly engulfed and phagocytized by pulmonary macrophages,[204-213] but smaller particles may not be as efficiently collected.[214] Some particles may enter the alveolar interstitium by pinocytosis.[215] Pulmonary macrophages are primarily responsible for engulfment, killing, and digestion of bacterial aerosols. Inert particles in the size range of bacteria, usually larger than 1 μm in physical diameter, are reasonable surrogates,[216] but are not digested; instead they accumulate in macrophages and may be cytotoxic to that cell.[217] Macrophages show chemotactic response to particles.[216] Migration and grouping of macrophages laden with particles can lead to redistribution of evenly dispersed particles into clumps and focal aggregations of particles in the deep lung. Some macrophages containing particles may enter the boundary region between the ciliated bronchioles and the respiratory ducts and then can be carried with the mucociliary flow of the TB region and cleared via the GI tract. However, that process is inefficient in man (or dogs or primates in contrast to murine species), with a probable clearance half-time of 1 to 2 years. Small rodents demonstrate pulmonary clearance half-times from only 50 to 100 days.

Some insoluble particles deposited in the lungs are eventually trapped in the pulmonary interstitium,[215] impeding the possibility of mechanical redistribution or removal.[218] Only the very smallest particles (smaller than 10 nm in physical diameter) can readily move by diffusion through available pores directly into the blood, passing intact through the air-to-blood cellular barrier of the gas-exchange regions of the lung.[219-221]

Another possible route of clearance of migrating particles and particle-laden macrophages is via the pulmonary lymph drainage system with translocation to the TB lymph nodes.[222-224] Little information is available about the clearance rates for transfer from lung to lymph nodes in man, but half-times of 1 to 2 years seem to fit the available data for dogs and monkeys.[225-226] Like transfer to the TB region with clearance via the mucociliary escalator, transfer to lymph nodes may affect only a portion of the material deposited in the lung.

Waligora[227] studied the pulmonary clearance of extremely insoluble and inert particles of zirconium oxide radiolabeled with ^{95}Nb. Although his results were not precise, the biological clearance half-life in man was about 1 year, about the same as for beagles. Leach et al.[225-226] exposed experimental animals to insoluble UO_2 ($MMAD_{ar}$ of about 3.5 μm) and observed lung retention half-times of 19.9 months for dogs and 15.5 months for monkeys. Ramsden et al.[228] measured the retention of accidentally inhaled, relatively insoluble[239] PuO_2 in a man's lungs and found the clearance half-time to be about 240 to 290 days; some of that material was dissolved into blood and excreted in the urine. Pulmonary clearance half-times as long as 1000 days have been reported for extremely insoluble particles of plutonium dioxide in dogs.[229] Because of the slow clearance via the various mechanical pathways, dissolution and associated physical and biochemical transformations are often the dominant mechanisms of clearance from the pulmonary region.[230] The term "dissolution" is taken in its broadest context to include whatever processes cause material in a discrete particle to be dispersed into the lung fluids and the blood. Many chemical compounds deposited in the lung in particulate form are mobilized faster than can be explained by known chemical properties at the normal lung fluid pH of about 7.4.[231] Raabe et al.[220] suggested that the apparent dissolution of highly insoluble PuO_2 actually may be fragmentation to particles small enough to move readily into the blood, rather than true dissolution.

Mercer[19] developed an analysis of pulmonary clearance based on particle dissolution under nonequilibrium conditions (see Equation 9). If the dissolution rate constant, k, is known for the particular material, the time required to dissolve half the mass of (monodisperse) particles of initial physical diameter, D_o, is given by:

$$T_{1/2} = 0.618\, \alpha_v\, \rho D_o / \alpha_s k \qquad (16)$$

with ϱ the physical density of the particles and α_v and α_s the volume and surface shape factors, respectively (for spherical particles $\alpha_s/\alpha_v = 6$). The particles would be expected to be completely dissolved at a time, t_f, given by:

$$t_f = 3\alpha_v\, \rho\, D_o / \alpha_s k \qquad (17)$$

Mercer[19] also calculated the expected dissolution half-time for polydisperse particles when their (physical) MMD in the lung is known:

$$T_{1/2} = 0.6\, \alpha_v\, \rho (MMD) / \alpha_s k \qquad (18)$$

Table 9
HYPOTHETICAL PULMONARY
CLEARANCE BY DISSOLUTION OF
DEPOSITED AEROSOLS OF GLASS
SPHERES OF DIFFERENT MONODISPERSE
SIZES (ϱ = 2.47 g/cm^3; k = 3.44 × 10^{-7} g cm^{-2}/
d^{-1} at 37°C

Geometric diameter, D (μm)	Aerodynamic diameter, D_{ar} (μm)	Half-time (days)	Total dissolution time (days)
0.001	—	0.07	0.4
0.01	—	0.7	3.6
0.05	—	3.7	18
0.1	0.27	7.4	36
0.2	0.44	15	72
0.5	0.91	37	180
1.0	1.7	74	360
2.0	3.3	150	720

Further, he showed that the resulting apparent lung retention function R(t) could be described as the sum of two exponentials of the form:

$$R(t) = M/M_O = f_1 e^{-\lambda_1 \beta} + f_2 e^{-\lambda_2 \beta} \qquad (19)$$

where $f_1 = (1 - f_2)$, $\beta = \alpha_s Kt/\alpha_v \varrho (MMD)$ and f_1, f_2, λ_1, and λ_2 are functions of the geometric SD. Therefore, for dissolution-controlled pulmonary clearance, smaller particles will exhibit proportionately shorter clearance half-times. When the dissolution half-times are much shorter than the half-times associated with the translocations of particles to the TB region or to lymph nodes (i.e., much less than 1 year), dissolution will dominate retention characteristics. Materials usually thought to be relatively insoluble may have high dissolution rate constants and short dissolution half-times for the small particles found in the lung (see Table 9). Also, changes in structure or chemical properties, such as by heat treatment of aerosols,[232] can lead to important changes in dissolution rates and observed pulmonary retention.

E. Retention Models and Translocation

Although many investigators have used radiographic techniques to directly measure the retention with respect to time of the burden of material in the respiratory tract,[190,191,233-240] calculation of estimated retention involves the combination of deposition and clearance functions. Since respiratory tract clearance may begin immediately after the initial deposition, the dynamics of retention can become quite complicated when additional deposition is superimposed on clearance phenomena. Extended or chronic exposures can lead to accumulation of particulate material in the lungs.[145,241-243]

The lung burden or respiratory tract burden can be represented by an appropriate retention function with time as the independent variable.[11,12] For models based on simple first-order kinetics, the lung burden, y, at a given time during exposure is controlled by the instantaneous equation:[244]

$$\frac{dy}{dt} = E - \lambda_1 y \qquad (20)$$

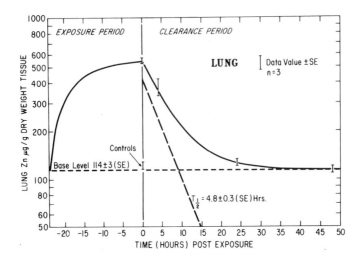

FIGURE 20.   Single exponential model, fit by weighted least squares, of the build-up (based on text Equation 19) and retention (based on text Equation 21) of zinc in rat lungs. From Hollinger, M. A., Raabe, O. G., Giri, S. N., Freywald, M., Teague, S. V., and Tarkington, B., *J. Toxicol. Appl. Pharmacol.*, 49, 53, 1979. With permission.)

where E is the instantaneous deposition rate of particulate material deposited in the lung per unit time during an inhalation exposure and λ_1 is the fraction of material in the lung cleared from the lung per unit time. For an exposure that lasts a time t_e, the lung burden during the exposure is given by:

$$y_e = (E - Ee^{-\lambda_1 t_e})/\lambda_1 \tag{21}$$

where E is the average exposure rate.

After the exposure ends, the clearance is governed by:

$$\frac{dy}{dt} = -\lambda_1 y \tag{22}$$

and the lung burden is given by:

$$y = y_e e^{-\lambda_1 t} \tag{23}$$

where y_e is the lung burden at the end of exposure period, t_e. Hollinger et al.[245] used this simple model to describe the deposition and clearance of inhaled submicronic ZnO in rats (see Figure 20), where the concentration of zinc (as Zn) in the lungs (as described by Equations 19 and 21) is superimposed on the natural background concentration of zinc in lung tissue. The normally insoluble zinc (compare Figure 4) had only a 4.8-hr dissolution half-time $\lambda_1 = 0.21\ h^{-1}$) for this aerosol.

If several deposition and clearance regions, subregions, or special pools are involved, a more complicated multicompartmental model may be required to describe lung or respiratory tract buildup and retention of inhaled aerosols. If each compartment can be described by first order kinetics as given in Equations 19 and 21, the lung burden during exposure is given by:

$$y_e = \sum_{i=1}^{n} y_i = \sum_{i=1}^{n} (E_i - E_i e^{-\lambda_i t_e})/\lambda_i \tag{24}$$

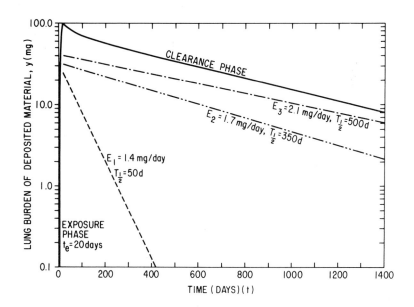

FIGURE 21. Example of the use of the sum of exponential models for describing lung uptake during inhalation exposure (See Equation 28) and retention (clearance phase) after exposure ends (see Equation 23) for three lung compartments with half-lives of 50 day, 350 day, and 500 day and 20-day exposure rates of 1.4 mg/day (E_1), 1.7 mg/day (E_2), and 2.1 mg/day (E_3), respectively.

where the subscript i is the index associated with each of the n different clearance compartments. Likewise the retention when exposure ends is given by:[244]

$$y = \sum_{i=1}^{n} (y_i e^{-\lambda_i t})$$ (25)

where each of the λ_i values translates to a clearance rate for each of the compartments given by half-time $T_{1/2} = \ln 2/\lambda_i$ (see Figure 21).

For chronic exposures where the several pools are in complex arrays of change, a simple power function may serve as a satisfactory model of pulmonary retention.[246] In such a model, the pulmonary region is treated as one complex, well-mixed pool into which material is added and removed during exposure as given by the instantaneous equation:

$$\frac{dy}{dt} = E - \lambda_p y/t \; [y = 0 \text{ at } t = 0]$$ (26)

where y is the total lung burden at a given time, t, E is the average deposition rate of inhaled particulate material in the lung, and λ_p is the fraction of available lung burden being cleared. Unlike the λ_i of the exponential retention models, λ_p is dimensionless. Also the time coordinate is not arbitrary; time is taken as zero only at the beginning of the inhalation exposure when the lung burden is nil. Thus, during an exposure lasting until time, t_e, the pulmonary burden, y_e, is given by:[244]

$$y_e = Et_e/(\lambda_p + 1)$$ (27)

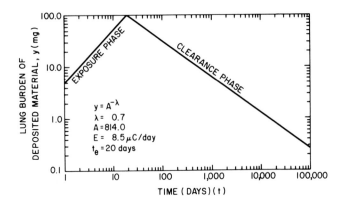

FIGURE 22. Example of the use of the power function model for describing lung uptake during inhalation exposure (text Equation 27) and retention (clearance phase) after exposure ends (text Equation 28) for a 20-day exposure at 8.5 mg/day (E).[244]

and the lung burden, y, after the exposure ends is given by:[244]

$$y = y_e t_e^{\lambda_p} t^{-\lambda_p} = At^{-\lambda_p} \quad [t = t_e + t_p] \tag{28}$$

where time, t, is reckoned from the beginning of exposure and is equal to the sum of the t_e, and the time after exposure, t_p. This model is illustrated in Figure 22.

Deposited particulate material cleared from the lung is usually transformed chemically and transferred to other tissues of the body. The injurious properties of a toxic material translocated from the lung may therefore be expressed in other organs. Identification of the potential hazards associated with inhalation exposures to toxicants is compounded when the respiratory tract is not the only target for injury, but still serves as the portal of entry into the body. The metabolic behavior and excretion of inhaled toxicants after deposition in the lung could define the probable target organs and indicate potential pathogenesis of resulting disease.

Multicompartmental models that describe the biological behavior can become quite complex. Each toxicant or component of aerosol particles deposited in the respiratory tract may need to be described by a separate rate constant and pool or compartment. A general model of the metabolic behavior of inhaled particles (see Figure 23) shows 39 different places where rate constants may need to be determined.[247] In this general model, the pulmonary region of the lung is visualized as consisting of three independent clearance compartments, and the particles are presumed to be converted from their original particulate state to some other physicochemical form or transformed state prior to clearance from the respiratory tract. Such a transformed state can be used to describe, for example, the behavior of hydrolytic aerosols in the respiratory tract.

A more specific model of the systemic metabolism of inhaled aerosols is shown (see Figure 24) for $^{144}CeCl_3$ contained in particles of CsCl with a $MMAD_{ar}$ of about 2 μm.[248] The resultant pattern of combined uptake and retention in various organs after inhalation exposure is shown in Figure 25. In this case, the potentially toxic ^{144}Ce is more likely to injure bone or liver rather than the lung.

VII. DISCUSSION AND SUMMARY

When aerosols are inhaled by man, different fractions of the inhaled materials are deposited by a variety of mechanisms in various locations in the respiratory tract.

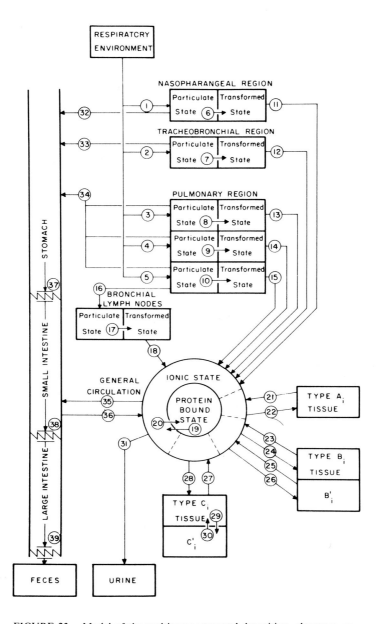

FIGURE 23. Model of the multicompartmental deposition, clearance, retention, translocation, and excretion of inhaled particulate material in the respiratory tract and tissues of the body; the numbered circles represent the transfer rate constants. (From Cuddihy, R. G., Fission Product Inhalation Program Annual Report 1968-1969, LF-41, Lovelace Foundation, Albuquerque, N.M., 1969, 136. With permission.)

Particle size distribution, particle chemical properties, respiratory tract anatomy, and airflow patterns in the lung airways all influence the deposition. Subsequent to deposition, the inhaled material will be translocated by processes that depend on its character and site of deposition. If the material is quite soluble in body fluids, it will readily enter the blood stream. Relatively insoluble material that lands on ciliated epithelium, either in the NP region or TB airways, will be translocated with mucus flow to the throat and be swallowed. Depending on particle size, inhaled relatively insoluble material that deposits on nonciliated surfaces in the pulmonary (P) region may be phag-

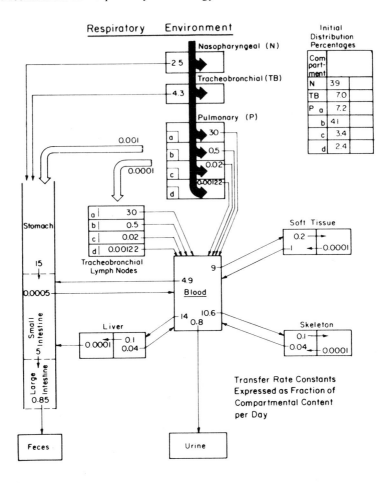

FIGURE 24.   Multicomponental model of the deposition clearance, retention, translocation, and excretion of [144]C inhaled as [144]CeCl$_3$ in a soluble carrier aerosol of CsCl; the rate constants are based on first order kinetics (as in text Equation 20). (From Boecker, B. B. and Cuddihy, R. G., *Radiat. Res.*, 60, 133, 1974. With permission.)

ocytized or may enter the interstitium and remain in the lung for an extended period or be translocated via lymphatic drainage. Some material from the pulmonary region may enter the TB region and be cleared via the mucociliary conveyor.

Both deposition and retention play roles in determining the effects of inhaled particulate toxicants.[249] In our modern society, virtually everyone is exposed occupationally, avocationally, or environmentally to a variety of dusts, fumes, sprays, mists, smoke, photochemical particles, and combustion aerosols. Particulate toxic aerosols, which may have detrimental effects on the lung, include asbestos, silica, metal fumes, infectious agents, pollen, acid mists, fibrous glass, tobacco smoke, insecticides, herbicides, organic carcinogens, and from the nuclear industry, radioactive aerosols. The particle size distribution and chemical and physical composition of airborne particulate material require special attention in evaluation of respiratory toxicology, since a wide variability of physicochemical properties may be encountered in both experimental and actual inhalation exposures.

The three functional regions (NP, TB, and P) of the respiratory airways each can be characterized by major mechanisms of deposition, clearance, and potential harmful effects to the respiratory tract (see Table 10). In addition, the respiratory tract is not

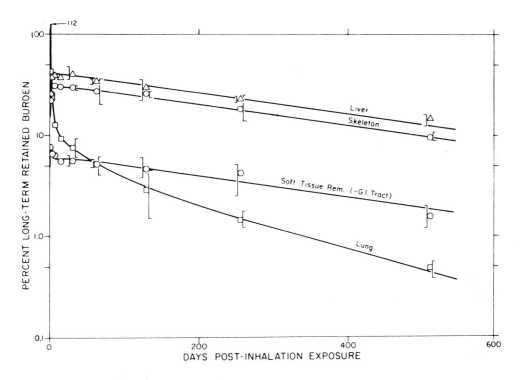

FIGURE 25. Retention of ^{144}C in major organs based on the multicomponent model in Figure 24. (From Boecker, B. B. and Cuddihy, R. G., *Radiat. Res.*, 60, 133, 1974. With permission.)

Table 10
SUMMARY OF THE DEPOSITION, CLEARANCE, AND POSSIBLE RESPIRATORY EFFECTS OF INHALED TOXIC AEROSOLS[8]

Region	Deposition	Clearance	Pathology
NP, nasopharyngeal	Impaction diffusion, interception, attraction	Mucociliary sneezing, blowing, dissolution	Inflammation, congestion, ulceration, cancer
TB, tracheobronchial	Impaction, diffusion, settling, interception, attraction	Mucociliary, coughing, dissolution	Bronchospasm, obstruction, congestion, bronchitis, cancer
P, pulmonary	Diffusion, settling, attraction, interception	Dissolution, phagocytosis, lymph flow	Inflammation, edema, fibrosis, emphysema, cancer

only one target of inhaled toxicants, but also the portal of entry by which other organs may be affected. An appreciation of the mechanisms and patterns of translocation to other organ systems is required for evaluation of the potential for injury or response in those organs.

ACKNOWLEDGMENT

The author is indebted to Evelyn E. Raabe for encouragement and support, Dr. Jay

P. Schreider for beneficial advice and assistance in assembly of deposition data, Jerry Azevedo for editorial assistance, and to Dr. Marvin Goldman for generous leadership as the Director of the Laboratory for Energy-Related Health Research. Ken Shiomoto and Shirley Coffelt drew and photographed most of the illustrations. Nancy Hardaker and Charles Baty prepared the typescript. Marion Lundquist supervised the clerical activities. This report was made possible by the support of the Office of Health and Environmental Research (OHER) of the U.S. DOE under Contract EY-76-C-03-0472 with the University of California, Davis and has been assigned document number UCD-472-503.[250]

REFERENCES

1. **Raabe, O. G., Boyd, H. A., Kanapilly, G. M., Wilkinson, C. J., and Newton, G. J.,** Development and use of a system for the routine production of monodisperse particles of $^{238}PuO_2$ and evaluation of gamma emitting labels, *Health Phys.,* 28, 655, 1975.

2. **Natusch, D. F. S., Wallace, J. R., and Evans, C. A., Jr.,** Toxic trace elements: preferential concentration in respirable particles, *Science,* 183, 202, 1974.

3. **Pawley, J. B. and Fisher, G. L.,** Using simultaneous three colour X-ray mapping and digital-scan-stop for rapid elemental characterization of coal combustion by-products, *J. Microsc.,* 110, 87, 1977.

4. **Raabe, O. G.,** Generation and characterization of aerosols, Inhalation Carcinogenesis, CONF-691001, Hanna, M. G., Jr., Nettesheim, P., and Gilbert, J. R., Eds., U.S. Atomic Energy Commission, Division of Technical Information, Washington, D.C., 1970, 123.

5. **Mercer, T. T.,** *Aerosol Technology in Hazard Evaluation,* Academic Press, New York, 1973, 66.

6. **Raabe, O. G.,** Particle size analysis utilizing grouped data and the log-normal distribution, *Aerosol Sci.,* 2, 289, 1971.

7. **Hatch, T. and Choate, S. P.,** Statistical description of the size properties of non-uniform particulate substances, *J. Franklin Inst.,* 207, 369, 1929.

8. **Phalen, R. F. and Raabe, O. G.,** Aerosol particle size as a factor in pulmonary toxicity, Proc. 5th Conf. on Environ. Toxicol., AMRL-TR-74-125, Aerospace Medical Research Laboratory, Wright-Patterson Air Force Base, Dayton, Ohio, 1974.

9. **Morrow, P. E., Gibb, F. R., and Johnson, L.,** Clearance of insoluble dust from the lower respiratory tract, *Health Phys.,* 10, 543, 1964.

10. **Morrow, P. E.,** Theoretical and experimental models for dust deposition and retention in man, *Rev. Environ. Health,* 1, 186, 1974.

11. **Morrow, P. E.,** Experimental studies of inhaled materials, *Arch. Intern. Med.,* 126, 466, 1970.

12. **Morrow, P. E.,** Models for the study of particle retention and elimination in the lung, in *Inhalation Carcinogenesis,* Hanna, M. G., Nettesheim, P., Gilbert, J. R., Eds., U.S. Atomic Energy Commission, Oak Ridge, Tenn., 1970, 103.

13. **Lippmann, M., Albert, R. E., and Peterson, H. T., Jr.,** The regional deposition of inhaled aerosols in man, in *Inhaled Particles III,* Walton, W. H., Ed., Unwin Brothers, Surrey, England, 1971, 105.

14. **Hamilton, R. J. and Walton, W. H.,** The selective sampling of respirable dust, in *Inhaled Particles and Vapours,* Davies, C. N., Ed., Pergamon Press, Oxford, 1961, 465.

15. **Fuchs, N. A.,** *The Mechanics of Aerosols,* MacMillan, New York, 1964.

16. **Hatch, T. E. and Gross, P.,** *Pulmonary Deposition and Retention of Inhaled Aerosols,* Academic Press, New York, 1964.

17. **Raabe, O. G.,** Aerosol aerodynamic size conventions for inertial sampler calibration, *J. Air Pollut. Control Assoc.,* 26, 856, 1976.

18. **Raabe, O. G., Yeh, H. C., Newton, G. J., Phalen, R. F., and Velasquez, D. J.,** Deposition of inhaled monodisperse aerosols in small rodents, in *Inhaled Particles IV,* Walton, W. H., Ed., Pergamon Press, New York, 1977, 3.

19. **Mercer, T. T.,** On the role of particle size in the dissolution of lung burdens, *Health Phys.,* 13, 1211, 1967.

20. **Raabe, O. G.,** Instruments and methods for characterizing radioactive aerosols, *IEEE Nucl. Sci.,* NS-19, 64, 1972.

21. Kanapilly, G. M., Raabe, O. G., Goh, C. H. T., and Chimenti, R. A., Measurement of in vitro dissolution of aerosol particles for comparison to in vivo dissolution in the lower respiratory tract after inhalation, *Health Phys.*, 24, 497, 1973.

22. Kanapilly, G. M., Raabe, O. G., and Boyd, H. A., A method for determining the dissolution characteristics of accidentally released radioactive aerosols, in Proc. 3rd Int. Congr. International Radiation Protection Association, U.S. Atomic Energy Commission, Oak Ridge, Tenn., 1974, 1237.

23. Marshall, R. and Holden, W., Changes in calibre of the smaller airways in man, *Thorax*, 18, 54, 1963.

24. Tompsett, D. H., *Anatomical Techniques*, Livingstone, Edinburgh, 1970.

25. Frank, N. R. and Yoder, R. E., A method of making a flexible cast of the lung, *J. Appl. Physiol.*, 21, 1925, 1966.

26. Phalen, R. F., Yeh, H. C., Raabe, O. G., and Velasquez, D. J., Casting the lungs *in situ, Anat. Rec.*, 177, 255, 1973.

27. Raabe, O. G., Yeh, H. C., Schum, G. M., and Phalen, R. F., *Tracheobronchial Geometry: Human, Dog, Rat, Hamster*, LF-53, Lovelace Foundation, Albuquerque, N.M., 1976.

28. Nadel, J. A., Corn, M., Zwi, S., and Flesch, G. P., Location and mechanism of airway constriction after inhalation of histamine aerosol and inorganic sulfate aerosol, in *Inhaled Particles and Vapours II*, Davies, C. N., Ed., Pergamon Press, Oxford, 1967, 55.

29. Adams, R., and Davenport, L., The technique of bronchography and a system of bronchial nomenclature, *JAMA*, 188, 111, 1942.

30. Yeh, H. C., Hulbert, A. J., Phalen, R. F., Velasquez, D. J., and Harris T. D., A steroradiographic technique and its application to the evaluation of lung casts, *Invest. Radiol.*, 10, 351, 1975.

31. Berg, A. M., Boyden, E. A., and Smith, F. R., An analysis of the segmental bronchi of the left lower lobe of fifty dissected and ten injected lungs, *J. Thorac. Surg.*, 18, 216, 1949.

32. Weibel, E. R. and Elias, H., Introduction to stereologic principles, in *Quantitative Methods in Morphology*, Weibel, E. R. and Elias, H., Eds., Springer-Verlag, Berlin, 1967, 89.

33. Nagashi, C., *Functional Anatomy and Histology of the Lung*, University Park Press, Baltimore, 1972.

34. Hansen, J. E. and Ampaya, E. P., Lung morphometry: a fallacy in the use of the counting principle, *J. Appl. Physiol.*, 37, 951, 1974.

35. Hansen, J. E. and Ampaya, E. P., Human air space, shapes, sizes, areas, and volumes, *J. Appl. Physiol.*, 38, 990, 1975.

36. Hansen, J. E., Ampaya, E. P., Bryant, G. H., and Navin, J. J., Branching pattern of airways and air spaces of a single human terminal bronchiole, *J. Appl. Physiol.*, 38, 983, 1975.

37. Morrow, P. E., (Chairman), International Commission on Radiological Protection (ICRP) Task Group on Lung Dynamics, Deposition and retention models for internal dosimetry of the human respiratory tract, *Health Phys.*, 12, 173, 1966.

38. Proctor, D. F., Swift, D. L., Quinlan, M., Salman, S., Takagi, Y., and Evering, S., The nose and man's atmospheric environment, *Arch. Environ. Health*, 18, 671, 1969.

39. Proctor, D. F. and Swift, D., The nose — a defence against the atmospheric environment, *Inhaled Particles III*, Vol. 1, Walton, W. H., Ed., Unwin Brothers, Surrey, England, 1971, 59.

40. Holmes, T. H., Goodell, H., Wolf, S., and Wolff, H. G., *The Nose*, Charles C. Thomas, Springfield, Ill., 1950.

41. Landahl, H. and Black, S., Penetration of air-borne particulates through the human nose, *J. Ind. Hyg. Toxicol.*, 29, 269, 1947.

42. Landahl, H. D., On the removal of airborne droplets by the human respiratory tract. I. The lung, *Bull. Math. Biophys.*, 12, 43, 1950.

43. Snyder, W. S., (Chairman), International Commission on Radiological Protection (ICRP) Task Group on Reference Man, *Report of the Task Group on Reference Man*, Pergamon Press, Oxford, 1975.

44. Tenney, S. M. and Bartlett, D., Comparative quantitative morphology of the mammalian lung: trachea, *Respir. Physiol.*, 3, 130, 1967.

45. Frasier, R. G. and Paré, J. A. P., *Structure and Function of the Lung*, W. B. Saunders, Philadelphia, 1971.

46. Ryan, S. F., The structure of the primary lobe lobule, *Ann. Clin. Lab Sci.*, 3, 147, 1973.

47. Alavi, S. M., Keats, T. E., and O'Brien, W. M., The angle of tracheal bifurcation: its normal mensuration, *An. J. Roentgenol.*, 108, 547, 1970.

48. Pump, K. K., The morphology of the finer branches of the bronchial tree of the human lung, *Dis. Chest*, 46, 379, 1964.

49. Thurlbeck, W. M. and Haines, J. B., Bronchial dimensions and stature, *Am. Rev. Respir. Dis.*, 112, 142, 1975.

50. Hughes, J. M., Hoppin, F. G., and Mead, J., Effect of lung inflation on bronchial length and diameter in excised lungs, *J. Appl. Physiol.*, 32, 25, 1972.

51. **Smith, F. A. and Boyden, E. A.,** An analysis of the segmental bronchi of the right lower lobe of fifty injected lungs, *J. Thorac. Surg.,* 18, 195, 1949.

52. **Whimster, W. F.,** The microanatomy of the alveolar duct system, *Thorax,* 25, 141, 1970.

53. **Krahl, V.,** Microstructure of the lung, *Arch. Environ. Health,* 6, 37, 1963.

54. **Tenney, S. M. and Remmers, J. E.,** Comparative quantitative morphology of the mammalian lung: diffusing area, *Nature (London),* 197, 54, 1963.

55. **Pattle, R. E.,** The lining complex of the lung alveoli, in *Inhaled Particles and Vapours,* Davies, C. N., Ed., Pergamon Press, Oxford, 1961, 70.

56. **Machlin, C. C.,** The alveoli of the mammalian lung: an anatomical study with clinical correlations, *Proc. Inst. Med.,* 18, 78, 1950.

57. **Schreider, J. P. and Raabe, O. G.,** Structure of the human respiratory acinus, *J. Anat.,* submitted.

58. **Green. G. M.,** In defense of the lung, *Am. Lung Assoc. Bull.,* 60, 4, 1974.

59. **Weibel, E. R.,** *Morphometry of the Human Lung,* Academic Press, New York, 1963.

60. **Liebow, A. A., Hales, M. R., Gustaf, E. L., and Bloomer, W. E.,** Plastic demonstrations of pulmonary pathology, *Bull. Int. Assoc. Med. Mus.,* 27, 116, 1947.

61. **Horsfield, K. and Cumming, G.,** Angles of branching and diameters of branches in the human bronchial tree, *Bull. Math. Biophys.,* 29, 245, 1967.

62. **Horsfield, K. and Cumming, G.,** Morphology of the bronchial tree in man, *J. Appl. Physiol.,* 24, 373, 1968.

63. **Horsfield, K., Dart, G., Olson, D., Filley, G., and Cumming, G.,** Models of the human bronchial tree, *J. Appl. Physiol.,* 31, 207, 1971.

64. **Horsfield, K.,** Analysis and Modeling of Branching Systems, Dissertation, University of Birmingham, Department of Medicine, England, 1972.

65. **Parker, M., Horsefield, K., and Cumming, G.,** Morphology of distal airways in the human lung, *J. Appl. Physiol.,* 31, 386, 1971.

66. **Charnock, E. L. and Doershuk, C. F.,** Developmental aspects of the human lung, *Pediatr. Clin. North Am.,* 20, 275, 1973.

67. **Davies, G. and Reid, L.,** Growth of the alveoli and pulmonary arteries in childhood, *Thorax,* 23, 669, 1970.

68. **Dunnill, M. S.,** Postnatal growth of the lung, *Thorax,* 17, 329, 1962.

69. **Kliment, V.,** Similarity and dimensional analysis, evaluation of aerosol deposition in the lungs of laboratory animals and man, *Folia Morphol.,* 21, 59, 1973.

70. **Angus, G. E. and Thurlbeck, W. M.,** Number of alveoli in the human lung, *J. Appl. Physiol.,* 32, 483, 1972.

71. **Davies, C. N.,** A formalized anatomy of the human respiratory tract, in *Inhaled Particles and Vapours,* Davies, C. N., Ed., Pergamon Press, Oxford, 1961, 82.

72. **Crosfill, M. L. and Widdicombe, J. G.,** Physical characteristics of the chest and lungs and the work of breathing in different mammalian species, *J. Physiol.,* 158, 1, 1961.

73. **Von Hayek, H.,** *The Human Lung,* Hafner, New York, 1960.

74. **D'Angelo, E.,** Local alveolar size and transpulmonary pressure *in situ* and in isolated lungs, *Respir. Physiol.,* 14, 251, 1972.

75. **Forrest, J. B.,** The effect of changes in lung volume on the size and shape of alveoli, *J. Physiol.,* 210, 533, 1970.

76. **Glazier, J. B., Hughes, J. M. B., Maloney, J. E., and West, J. B.,** Vertical gradient of alveolar size in lungs of dogs frozen intact, *J. Appl. Physiol.,* 21, 416, 1966.

77. **Glazier, J. B., Hughes, J. M., Maloney, J. E., and West, J. B.,** Vertical gradient of alveolar size in lungs of dogs frozen intact, *J. Appl. Physiol.,* 23, 694, 1967.

78. **Schreider, J. P.,** Lung Anatomy and Characteristics of Aerosol Retention of the Guinea Pig, Ph.D . thesis, University of Chicago, 1977.

79. **Fowler, J. F. and Young, A. E.,** The average density of healthy lung, *Am. J. Roentgenol. Radium Ther.,* 81, 312, 1959.

80. **Findeissen, W.,** Uber das Absetzen kleiner, in der Luf t suspendieter Teilchen in der menschlichen lunje bei der atmung, *Pflugers Arc h. Physiol.,* 236, 367, 1935.

81. **Taulbee, D. B. and Yu, C. P.,** A theory of aerosol deposition in the human respiratory tract, *J. Appl. Physiol.,* 38, 77, 1975.

82. **Yeates, D. B. and Aspin, N.,** A mathematical description of the human lungs, *Respir. Physiol.,* 32, 91, 1978.

83. **Verzar, F., Keith, J., and Parchet, V.,** Temperatur und Feuchtigkeit der Luft in den Atemwegen, *Pflugers Arch.,* 257, 400, 1953.

84. **Raabe, O. G. and Yeh, H. C.,** Principles for inhalation exposure systems using concurrent flow spirometry, *J. Aerosol Sci.,* 7, 233, 1976.

85. Deal, E. C., McFadden, E. R., Ingram, R. H., and Jaeger, J. J., Hyperpnea and heat flux: initial reaction sequence in exercise-induced asthma, *J. Appl. Physiol. Respir. Environ. Exercise Physiol.*, 46, 476, 1979.

86. Deal, E. C., McFadden, E. R., Ingram, R. H., and Jaeger, J. J., Esophageal temperature during exercise in asthmatic and nonasthmatic subjects, *J. Appl. Physiol. Respir. Environ. Exercise Physiol.*, 46, 484, 1979.

87. Deal, E. Chandler, McFadden, E. R., Ingram, R. H., Strauss, R. H., and Jaeger, J. J., Role of respiratory heat exchange in production of exercise-induced asthma, *J. Appl. Physiol. Respir. Environ. Exercise Physiol.*, 46, 467, 1979.

88. Bake, B., Wood, L., Murphy, B., Macklem, P., and Milic-Emili, J., Effect of inspiratory flow rate on regional distribution of inspired gas, *J. Appl. Physiol.*, 37, 8, 1974.

89. Clement, J., Afschrift, M., Pardens, J., and Van de Woestline, K., Peak expiratory flow rate and rate of change of pleural pressure, *Respir. Physiol.*, 18, 222, 1973.

90. Altshuler, B., Palmes, E. D., and Nelson, N., Regional aerosol deposition in the human respiratory tract, in *Inhaled Particles and Vapours II,* Davies, C. N., Ed., Pergamon Press, 1967, 323.

91. Weibel, E. R., Morphometric estimation of pulmonary diffusion capacity, *Respir. Physiol.*, 14, 26, 1972.

92. Guyton, A. C., Measurement of the respiratory volumes of laboratory animals, *Am. J. Physiol.*, 150, 20, 1947.

93. Guyton, A. C., Analysis of respiratory patterns in laboratory animals, *Am. J. Physiol.*, 150, 78, 1947.

94. Stahl, W. R., Scaling of respiratory variables in mammals, *J. Appl. Physiol.*, 22, 453, 1967.

95. West, J. B., *Respiratory Physiology: the Essentials,* Williams & Wilkins, Philadelphia, 1974.

96. Luft, U. C., Spirometric methods, in *Aviation Medicine — Selected Reviews,* White, C. S., Lovelace, W. R., and Hirsch, F. G., Eds., Pergamon Press, New York, 1958, 168.

97. Paiva, M. and Paiva-Veretennicoff, I., Stochastic simulation of the gas diffusion in the air phase of the human lung, *Bull. Math. Biophys.*, 34, 457, 1972.

98. Paiva, M., Gas transport in the human lung, *J. Appl. Physiol.*, 35, 401, 1973.

99. Palmes, E. D., Measurement of pulmonary air spaces using aerosols, *Arch. Intern. Med.*, 131, 76, 1973.

100. Dekker, E., Transition between laminar and turbulent flow in human trachea, *J. Appl. Physiol.*, 16, 1060, 1961.

101. Fry, D., A preliminary model for simulating the aerodynamics of the bronchial tree, *Comp. Biomed. Res.*, 2, 111, 1968.

102. Schroter, R. C. and Sudlow, M. F., Flow patterns in models of the human bronchial airways, *Respir. Physiol.*, 7, 341, 1969.

103. Olson, D. E., Sudlow, M. F., Horsefield, K., and Filley, G. F., Convective patterns of flow during inspiration, *Arch. Intern. Med.*, 131, 51, 1973.

104. Martin, D. and Jacobi, W., Diffusion deposition of small-sized particles in the bronchial tree, *Health Phys.*, 23, 23, 1972.

105. West, J. B., Observations on gas flow in the human bronchial tree, in *Inhaled Particles and Vapours,* Davies, C. N., Ed., Pergamon Press, Oxford, 1961, 3.

106. Bartlett, D., Remmers, J. E., and Gautier, H., Laryngeal regulation of respiratory airflow, *Respir. Physiol.*, 18, 194, 1973.

107. Schlesinger, R. and Lippmann, M., Particle deposition in the trachea: in vivo and in hollow casts, *Thorax*, 31, 678, 1976.

108. Grant, B. J., Jones, H. J., and Hughes, J. M., Sequence of regional filling during a tidal breath in man, *J. Appl. Physiol.*, 158, 108, 1974.

109. Silverman, L. and Billings, C. E., Pattern of airflow in the respiratory tract, in *Inhaled Particles and Vapours,* Davies, C. N., Ed., Pergamon Press, Oxford, 1961, 9.

110. Cinkotai, F. F., Fluid flow in a model alveolar sac, *J. Appl. Physiol.*, 37, 249, 1974.

111. Yeh, H. C., Phalen, R. F., and Raabe, O. G., Factors influencing the deposition of inhaled particles, *Environ. Health Perspect.*, 15, 147, 1976.

112. DuBois, A. B. and Rogers, R. M., Respiratory factors determining the tissue concentrations of inhaled toxic substances, *Respir. Physiol.*, 5, 34, 1968.

113. Engel, L. A., Wood, L. D., Utz, G., and Macklem, P. T., Gas mixing during inspiration, *J. Appl. Physiol.*, 35, 18, 1973.

114. Davies, C. N., An algebraical model for the deposition of aerosols in the human respiratory tract during steady breathing, *J. Aerosol Sci.*, 3, 297, 1972.

115. Altshuler, B., The role of the mixing of intrapulmonary gas flow in the deposition of aerosols, in *Inhaled Particles and Vapours,* Davies, C. N., Ed., Pergamon Press, Oxford, 1961, 47.

116. Palmes, E. D., Altshuler, B., and Nelson, N., Deposition of aerosols in the human respiratory tract during breath holding, in *Inhaled Particles and Vapours II*, Davies, C. N., Ed., Pergamon Press, Oxford, 1967, 339.

117. Palmes, E., Wang, C., Goldring, R., and Altshuler, B., Effect of depth of inhalation on aerosol persistence during breath holding, *J. Appl. Physiol.*, 34, 356, 1973.

118. Pavlik, I., The fate of light air ions in the respiratory pathways, *Int. J. Biometeorol.*, 11, 175, 1967.

119. Fraser, D. A., The deposition of unipolar charged particles in the lungs of animals, *Arch. Environ. Health*, 13, 152, 1966.

120. Melandri, C., Prodi, V., Tarroni, G., Formigani, M., DeZaiacomo, T., Bompane, G. R., Maestri, G., and Giaconelli-Malton, G. G., On the deposition of unipolarly charged particles in the human respiratory tract, in *Inhaled Particles IV*, Walton, W. H., Ed., Pergamon Press, New York, 1977, 193.

121. Longley, M. Y., Pulmonary deposition of dust as affected by electric charges on the body, *Am. Ind. Hyg. Assoc. J.*, 21, 187, 1960.

122. Longley, M. Y. and Berry, C. M., Pulmonary deposition of aerosols: effect of electrostatic charging of the animal body and the aerosol, *Arch. Environ. Health*, 2, 533, 1961.

123. Yu, C. P., Precipitation of unipolarly charged particles in cylindrical and spherical vessels, *J. Aerosol Sci.*, 8, 237, 1977.

124. Harris, R. L. and Fraser, D. A., A model for deposition of fibers in the human respiratory system, *Am. Ind. Hyg. Assoc. J.*, 37, 73, 1976.

125. Bohning, D. E., Albert, R. E., Lippman, M., and Foster, W. M., Tracheobronchial particle deposition and clearance, *Arch. Environ. Health*, 30, 457, 1975.

126. Johnston, J. and Muir, D., Inertial deposition of particles in the lung, *J. Aerosol Sci.*, 4, 269, 1973.

127. Yeh, H. C., Use of a heat transfer analogy for a mathematical model of respiratory tract deposition, *Bull. Math. Biol.*, 36, 105, 1974.

128. Cheng, Y. S. and Wang, C. S., Inertial deposition of particles in a bend, *J. Aerosol Sci.*, 6, 139, 1975.

129. Wang, C. S., Gravitational deposition from laminar flows in inclined channels, *J. Aerosol Sci.*, 6, 19, 1975.

130. Heyder, J. and Gebhart, J., Gravitational deposition of particles from laminar aerosol flow through inclined circular tubes, *J. Aerosol Sci.*, 8, 289, 1977.

131. Thomas, J. W., Particle loss in sampling conduits, in *Assessment of Airborne Radioactivity*, International Atomic Energy Agency, Vienna, 1967, 701.

132. Gormley, P. G. and Kennedy, M., Diffusion from a stream flowing through a cylindrical tube, *Proc. R. Ir. Acad.*, A52, 163, 1949.

133. Schlesinger, R. B. and Lippmann, M., Selective particle deposition and bronchogenic carcinoma, *Environ. Res.*, 15, 424, 1978.

134. Bell, K. and Friedlander, S., Aerosol deposition in models of a human lung bifurcation, *Staub Reinhalt. Luft*, 33, 183, 1973.

135. Bell, K. A., Local particle deposition in respiratory airways models, in *Recent development in Aerosol Science*, Shaw, D. T., Ed., John Wiley & Sons, New York, 1978, Chap. 6.

136. Schlesinger, R. B., Bohning, D. E., Chan, T. L., and Lippmann, M., Particle deposition in a hollow cast of the human tracheobronchial tree, *J. Aerosol Sci.*, 8, 429, 1977.

137. Ferron, G. A., The size of soluble aerosol particles as a function of the humidity of the air; application to the human respiratory tract, *J. Aerosol Sci.*, 8, 251, 1977.

138. Beekmans, J. B., The deposition of aerosols in the respiratory tract, *Can. J. Physiol. Pharmacol.*, 43, 157, 1965.

139. Landahl, H. and Herrmann, R., On the retention of air-borne particulates in the human lung, *J. Ind. Hyg. Toxicol.*, 30, 181, 1948.

140. Landahl, H., Tracewell, T., and Lassen, W., On the retention of airborne particulates in the human lung. II, *AMA Arch Ind. Health Occupat. Med.*, 3, 359, 1951.

141. Landahl, H., Particle removal by the respiratory system, *Bull. Math. Biophys.*, 25, 29, 1963.

142. Goldberg, I. S., Lam, K. Y., Bernstein, B., and Hutchens, H. O., Solution to the Fokker-Planck equations governing simultaneous diffusion and gravitational settling of aerosol particles from stationary gas in a horizontal tube, *J. Aerosol Sci.*, 9, 209, 1978.

143. Taulbee, D. B. and Yu, C. P., Simultaneous diffusion and sedimentation of aerosols in channel flows, *J. Aerosol Sci.*, 6, 433, 1975.

144. Davies, C. N., Deposition and retention of dust in the human respiratory tract, *Ann. Occup. Hyg.*, 7, 169, 1964.

145. Davies, C. N., A comparison between inhaled dust and the dust recovered from human lungs, *Health Phys.*, 10, 1029, 1964.

146. Van Wijk, A. M. and Patterson, H. S., The percentage of particles of different sizes removed from dust-laden air by breathing, *J. Ind. Hyg. Toxicol.*, 22, 31, 1940.

147. Brown, J. H., Cook, K. M., Nex, F. G., and Hatch, T., Influence of particle size upon the retention of particulate matter in the human lung, *Am. J. Public Health,* 40, 450, 1950.
148. Dautrebande, L. and Walkenhurst, W., New studies on aerosols. XXIV, *Arch. Int. Pharmacodyn.,* 162, 194, 1966.
149. Morrow, P., Mehrhof, E., Casarett, L., and Morken, D., An experimental study of aerosol deposition in human subjects, *AMA Arch. Ind. Health,* 18, 292, 1958.
150. Lippmann, M. and Albert, R., The effect of particle size on the regional deposition of inhaled aerosols in the human respiratory tract, *Am. Ind. Hyg. Assoc. J.,* 30, 257, 1969.
151. Heyder, J., Arbruster, L., Gebhart, J., Grein, E., and Stahlhofen, W., Total deposition of aerosol particles in the human respiratory tract for nose and mouth breathing, *J. Aerosol Sci.,* 6, 311, 1975.
152. Giacomelli-Maltoni, G., Melandri, C., Prodi, V., and Tarroni, G., Deposition efficiency of monodisperse particles in human respiratory tract, *Am. Ind. Hy. Assoc. J.,* 33, 603, 1972.
153. Palmes, E. D. and Wang, C. S., An aerosol inhalation apparatus for human single breath deposition studies, *AM. Ind. Hyg. Assoc. J.,* 32, 43, 1971.
154. Shanty, F., Deposition of Ultrafine Aerosols in the Respiratory Tract of Human Volunteers, Doctoral dissertation, School of Hygiene and Public Health of the Johns Hopkins University, Baltimore, 1974.
155. George, A. C. and Breslin, A. J., Deposition of natural radon daughters in human subjects, *Health Phys.,* 13, 375, 1967.
156. Hounam, R. F., Black, A., and Walsh, M., The deposition of aerosol particles in the nasopharyngeal region of the human respiratory tract, *J. Aerosol Sci.,* 2, 47, 1971.
157. Hounam, R. F., Black, A., and Walsh, M., The deposition of aerosol particles in the nasopharyngeal region of the human respiratory tract, in *Inhaled Particles III,* Walton, W. H., Ed., Unwin Brothers, Surrey, England, 1971, 71.
158. Foord, N., Black, A., and Walsh, M., Regional deposition of $2.5 - 7.5 \mu m$ diameter inhaled particles in healthy male non-smokers, AERE Harwell, ML. 76/2892, 1976.
159. Pavia, D., Thomson, M., and Shannon, H. S., Aerosol inhalation and depth of deposition in the human lung, *Arch. Environ. Health,* 32, 131, 1977.
160. Muir, D. C. and Davies, C. N., The deposition of 0.5μ diameter aerosols in the lungs of man, *Ann. Occup. Hyg.,* 10, 161, 1967.
161. Taulbee, D., Yu, C., and Heyder, J., Aerosol transport in the human lung from analysis of single breaths, *J. Appl. Physiol.,* 44, 803, 1978.
162. Lourenco, R. V., Klimek, M. F., and Borowski, C. J., Deposition and clearance of 2μ particles in the tracheobronchial tree of normal subjects — smokers and nonsmokers, *J. Clin. Invest.,* 50, 1411, 1971.
163. Hounam, R. F., The deposition of atmospheric condensation nuclei in the nasopharyngeal region of the human respiratory tract, *Health Phys.,* 20, 219, 1971.
164. Heyder, J. and Davies, C. N., The breathing of half micron aerosols. III. Dispersion of particles in the respiratory tract, *J. Aerosol Sci.,* 2, 437, 1971.
165. Heyder, J., Conditions for the determination of aerosol particle deposition in the human respiratory tract, *Staub Reinhalt. Luft,* 31, 11, 1971.
166. Fry, F. A. and Black, A., Regional deposition and clearance of particles in the human nose, *J. Aerosol Sci.,* 4, 113, 1973.
167. Altshuler, B., Yarmus, L., Palmes, E., and Nelson, N., Aerosol deposition in the human respiratory tract, *AMA Arch. Ind. Health,* 15, 293, 1957.
168. Lippmann, M., Deposition and clearance of inhaled particles in the human nose, *Ann. Otol.,* 79, 519, 1970.
169. Altshuler, B., Calculation of regional deposition in the respiratory tract, *Bull. Math. Biophys.,* 21, 257, 1959.
170. Albert, R., Lippmann, M., Spiegelman, J., Liuzzi, A., and Nelson, N., The deposition and clearance of radioactive particles in the human lung, *Arch. Environ. Health.,* 14, 10, 1967.
171. Davies, C. N., Deposition of inhaled particles in man, *Chem. Ind.,* 441, 1974.
172. Altshuler, B., Palmes, E. D., Yarmus, L., and Nelson, N., Intrapulmonary mixing of gases studied with aerosols., *J. Appl. Physiol.,* 14, 321, 1959.
173. Cuddihy, R. G., Brownstein, D. G., Raabe, O. G., and Kanapilly, G. M., Respiratory tract deposition of inhaled polydisperse aerosols in beagle dogs, *Aerosol Sci.,* 4, 35, 1973.
174. Lippmann, M., Regional deposition of particles in the human respiratory tract, in *Handbook of Physiology,* Agents, Lee, D. H. K., Falk, H. L., and Murphy, S. D., Eds., The American Physiology Society, Bethesda, 1977, 213.
175. Proctor, D. F. and Wagner, H. N., Clearance of particles from the human nose, *Arch. Environ. Health,* 11, 366, 1965.
176. Proctor, D. F. and Wagner, H. N., Mucociliary clearance in the human nose, in *Inhaled Particles and Vapours II,* Davies, C. N., Ed., Pergamon Press, Oxford, 1967, 25.

177. Proctor, D. F., Andersen, I., and Lundquist, G., Clearance of inhaled particles from the human nose, *Arch. Intern. Med.,* 131, 132, 1973.

178. Ulmer, W. T., Reaction of the lungs to various broncho-irritating substances, in *Inhaled Particles and Vapours II,* Davies, C. N., Ed., Pergamon Press, 1967, 87.

179. Schlesinger, R. B., Mucociliary interaction in the tracheobronchial tree and environmental pollution, *Biol. Sci.,* 23, 567, 1973.

180. Van As, A. and Webster, I., The organization of ciliary activity and mucus transport in pulmonary airways, *S. A. Med. J.,* 46, 347, 1972.

181. Van As, A. and Webster, I., The morphology of mucus in mammalian pulmonary airways, *Environ. Res.,* 7, 1, 1974.

182. Besarab, A. and Litt, M., Model studies on the adhesive properties of mucus and similar polymer solutions, *Arch. Intern. Med.,* 126, 504, 1970.

183. Dadaian, J. H., Yin, S., and Laurenzi, G. A., Studies of mucus flow in the mammalian respiratory tract, *Am. Rev. Respir. Dis.,* 103, 808, 1971.

184. Camner, P., Strandberg, K., and Philipson, K., Increased mucociliary transport by adrenergic stimulation, *Arch. Environ. Health,* 79, 1976.

185. Barton, A. D. and Lourenco, R.V., Bronchial secretions and mucociliary clearance, *Arch. Intern. Med.,* 131, 146, 1973.

186. Santa Cruz, R., Landa, J., Hirsch, J., and Sackner, M., Tracheal mucus velocity in normal man and patients with obstructive lung disease; effects of terbutaline, *Am. Rev. Respir. Dis.,* 109, 458, 1974.

187. Yeates, D. B., Aspin, N., Levison, H., Jones, M. T., and Bryan, A. C., Mucociliary tracheal transport rates in man, *J. Appl. Physiol.,* 39, 487, 1975.

188. Albert, R. E., Lippmann, M., Spiegelman, J., Strehlow, C., Briscoe, W., Wolfson, P., and Nelson, N., The clearance of radioactive particles from the human lungs, in *Inhaled Particles and Vapours II,* Davies, C. N., Ed., Pergamon Press, Oxford, 1967, 361.

189. Albert, R. E., Lippmann, M., Peterson, H. T., Berger, J., Sanborn, K., and Bohning, D., Bronchial deposition and clearance of aerosols, *Arch. Intern. Med.,* 131, 115, 1973.

190. Camner, P., Philipson, K., Friberg, L., and Holma, B., Human tracheobronchial clearance studies, *Arch. Environ. Health,* 22, 444, 1971.

191. Luchsinger, P. G., LaGarde, B., and Kilfeather, J. E., Particle clearance from the human tracheobronchial tree, *Am. Rev. Respir. Dis.,* 97, 1046, 1968.

192. Morrow, P. E., Gibb, F. R., and Gazioglu, K. M., A study of particulate clearance from the human lungs, *Am. Rev. Respir. Dis.,* 96, 1209, 1967.

193. Camner, P. and Philipson, K., Tracheobronchial clearance in smoking-discordant twins, *Environ. Health,* 474, 1972.

194. Camner, P., Philipson, K., and Friberg, L., Tracheobronchial clearance in twins, *Arch. Environ. Health,* 24, 82, 1972.

195. LaBelle, C. W., Bevilacqua, M. A., and Brieger, H., The influence of cigarette smoke on lung clearance, *Arch. Environ. Health,* 12, 588, 1966.

196. Albert, R. E., Berger, J., Sanborn, K., and Lippmann, M., Effects of cigarette smoke components on bronchial clearance in the donkey, *Arch. Environ. Health,* 29, 96, 1974.

197. Thomson, M. L. and Davia, D., Long-term tobacco smoking and mucociliary clearance, *Arch. Environ. Health,* 26, 86, 1973.

198. Blank, M., Goldstein, A. B., and Lee, B. B., The surface properties of lung extract, *J. Colloid Interface Sci.,* 29, 148, 1969.

199. Balis, J. V., Shelley, S. A., McCue, M. J., and Rappaport, E. S., Mechanisms of damage to the lung surfactant system, *Exp. Mol. Pathol.,* 14, 243, 1971.

200. Kott, A. T., Gardner, J. W., Schecter, R. S., and DeGroot, W., The elasticity of pulmonary lung surfactants, *J. Colloid. Interface Sci.,* 47, 265, 1974.

201. Henderson, R. F., Waide, J. J., and Pfleger, R. C., Replacement time for alveolar lipid removed by pulmonary lavage: effects of multiple lavage on lung lipids, *Arch. Intern. Physiol. Biochem.,* 83, 261, 1975.

202. Gross, P., Pfitzer, E. A., and Hatch, T. F., Alveolar clearance: its relation to lesions of the respiratory bronchiole, *Am. Rev. Respir. Dis.,* 94, 10, 1966.

203. Dunworth, D. L., Schwartz, L. W., Tyler, W. S., and Phalen, R. F., Morphological methods for evaluation of pulmonary toxicity in animals, in *Annual Review of Pharmacology and Toxicology,* Elliott, H. W., Ed., Annual Reviews, Palo Alto, 1976, 381.

204. LaBelle, C. W. and Brieger, H., Patterns and mechanisms in the elimination of dust from the lung, in *Inhaled Particles and Vapours,* Davies, C. N., Ed., Pergamon Press, Oxford, 1961, 356.

205. Sanders, C. L. and Adee, R. R., Phagocytosis of inhaled plutonium oxide ^{239}Pu particles by pulmonary macrophages, *Science,* 162, 918, 1968.

206. Green, G. M., Alveolobronchiolar transport observations and hypothesis of a pathway, *Chest*, 59, 15, 1971.
207. Green, G. M., Alveolobronchiolar transport mechanisms, *Arch. Intern. Med.*, 131, 109, 1973.
208. Green, J. F., The pulmonary circulation, in *The Peripheral Circulations*, Zelis, R., Ed., Grune & Stratton, New York, 1975, 9.
209. Ferin. J., Urbankova, G., and Vlckova, A., Pulmonary clearance and the clearance of macrophages, *Arch. Environ. Health*, 10, 790, 1965.
210. Camner, P., Hellstrom, P., and Lundborg, M., Coating 5 μ particles with carbon and metals for lung clearance studies, *Arch. Environ. Health*, 27, 331, 1973.
211. Camner, P., Hellstrom, P., and Philipson, K., Carbon dust and mucociliary clearance, *Arch. Environ. Health*, 26, 294, 1973.
212. Camner, P., Lundborg, M., and Hellstrom, P., Alveolar macrophages and 5 μm particles coated with different metals, *Arch. Environ. Health*, 29, 211, 1974.
213. Chapman, M. A. and Hibbs, J. B., Macrophage tumor killing: influence of the local environment, *Science*, 197, 279, 1977.
214. Hahn, F. F., Newton, G. J., and Bryant, P. L., In vitro phagocytosis of respirable-sized monodisperse particles by alveolar macrophages, in *Pulmonary Macrophage and Epithelial Cells*, CONF-760927, U.S. Department of Commerce, Springfield, Va., 1977, 424.
215. Strecker, F. J., Tissue reactions in rat lungs after dust inhalation with special regard to bronchial dust elimination and to the penetration of dust into the lung interstices and lymphatic nodes, in *Inhaled Particles and Vapours II*, Davies, C. N., Ed., Pergamon Press, Oxford, 1967, 141.
216. Metzger, G., Some Environmental Factors Influencing the In Vitro Phagocytosis of Inert Test Particles, Doctoral dissertation, University of Rochester, N.Y., 1968.
217. Allison, A. C., Harington, J. S., Birbeck, M., and Nash, T., Observations on the cytotoxic action of silica on macrophages, in *Inhaled Particles and Vapours II*, Davies, C. N., Ed., Pergamon Press, Oxford, 1967, 121.
218. Muggenburg, B. A., Felicetti, S. A., and Silbaugh, S. A., Removal of inhaled radioactive particles by lung lavage — a review, *Health Phys.*, 33, 213, 1977.
219. Gross, P. and Westrick, M., The permeability of lung parenchyma to particulate matter, *Am. J. Pathol.*, 30, 195, 1954.
220. Raabe, O. G., Teague, S. V., Richardson, N. L., and Nelson, L. S., Aerodynamic and dissolution behavior of fume aerosols produced during the combustion of laser-ignited plutonium droplets in air, *Health Phys.*, 35, 663, 1978.
221. Raabe, O. G., Newton, G. J., Wilkinson, C. J., and Teague, S. V., Plutonium aerosol characterization inside safety enclosures at a demonstration mixed-oxide fuel fabrication facility, *Health Phys.*, 35, 649, 1978.
222. Thomas, R. G., Transport of relatively insoluble materials from lung to lymph nodes, *Health Phys.*, 14, 111, 1968.
223. Lauweryns, J. M. and Baert, J. H., Alveolar clearance and the role of the pulmonary lymphatics, *Am. Rev. Respir. Dis.*, 115, 625, 1977.
224. Leeds, S. E., Reich, S., Uhley, H. N., Sampson, J. J., and Friedman, M., The pulmonary lymph flow after irradiation of the lungs of dogs, *Chest*, 59, 203, 1971.
225. Leach, L. J., Maynard, E. A., Hodge, H. C., Scott, J. K., Yuile, C. L., Sylvester, G. E., and Wilson, H. G., A five year inhalation study with natural uranium-dioxide (UO_2) dust. I. Retention and biological effect in the monkey dog and rat, *Health Phys.*, 18, 599, 1970.
226. Leach, L. J., Yuile, C. L., Hodge, H. C., Sylvester, G. E., and Wilson, H. B., A five-year inhalation study with natural uranium dioxide (UO_2) dust. II. Postexposure retention and biological effects in the monkey, dog, and rat, *Health Phys.*, 25, 239, 1973.
227. Waligora, S. J., Jr., Pulmonary retention of zirconium oxide (^{95}Nb) in man and beagle dogs, *Health Phys.*, 20, 89, 1971.
228. Ramsden, D., Bains, M. E. D., and Fraser, D. C., In vivo and bioassay results from two contrasting cases of plutonium-239 inhalation, *Health Phys.*, 19, 9, 1970.
229. Raabe, O. G. and Goldman, M., A predictive model of early mortality following acute inhalation of PuO_2 aerosols, *Radiat. Res.*, 78, 264, 1979.
230. Morrow, P. E., Alveolar clearance of aerosols, *Arch. Intern. Med.*, 131, 101, 1973.
231. Kanapilly, G. M., Alveolar microenvironment and its relationship to the retention and transport into blood of aerosols deposited in the alveoli, *Health Phys.*, 32, 89, 1977.
232. Raabe, O. G., Kanapilly, G. M., and Newton, G. J., New methods for the generation of aerosols of insoluble particles for use in inhalation studies, in *Inhaled Particles III*, Walton, W. H., Ed., Unwin Brothers, Surrey, England, 1971, 3.
233. Sanchis, J., Dolovich, M., Chalmers, R., and Newhouse, M., Quantitation of regional aerosol clearance in the normal human lung, *J. Appl. Physiol.*, 33, 757, 1972.

234. Barclay, A. E., Franklin, K. J., and Macbeth, R. G., Roentgenographic studies of the excretion of dusts from the lungs, *Am. J. Roentgenol. Radiat. Ther.*, 39, 673, 1938.

235. Aldas, J. S., Dolovich, M., Chalmers, R., and Newhouse, M. T., Regional aerosol clearance in smokers and nonsmokers, *Chest*, 59, 25, 1971.

236. Edmunds, L. H., Graf, P. D., Sagel. S. S., and Greenspan, R. H., Radiographic observations of clearance of tantalum and barium sulfate particles from airways, *Invest. Radiol.*, 5, 131, 1970.

237. Ferin, J., The mechanism of elimination of deposited particles from the lungs, *Ann. Occupat. Hyg.*, 10, 207, 1967.

238. Friberg, L. and Holma, B., External measurement of lung clearance, *Arch. Environ. Health*, 3, 56, 1961.

239. Holma, B., Lung clearance of mono- and di-disperse aerosols determined by profile scanning and whole-body counting, *Acta Med. Scand.*, (Suppl. 473), 1967.

240. Morrow, P. E., Gibb, F. R., and Gazioglu, K., The clearance of dust from the lower respiratory tract of man: An experimental study, in *Inhaled Particles and Vapours*, Davies, C. N., Ed., Oxford, Pergamon Press, 1967, 351.

241. Davies, C. N., The handling of particles by the human lungs, *Br. Med. Bull.*, 19, 49, 1963.

242. Walkenhorst, W., Untersuchungen an einem nach Teilchengrossen geordneten Michstaub im Atembarden korngrossenboreich, in *Inhaled Particles and Vapours II*, Davies, C. N., Ed., Pergamon Press, Oxford, 1967, 563.

243. Einbrodt, H. J., Experiments on the elimination of dust from human lungs, *Ann. Occupat. Hyg.*, 10, 47, 1967.

244. Raabe, O. G., Some important consideration in use of power function to describe clearance data, *Health Phys.*, 13, 293, 1967.

245. Hollinger, M. A., Raabe, O. G., Giri, S. N., Freywald, M., Teague, S. V., and Tarkington, B., Effect of the inhalation of zinc and dietary zinc on paraquat toxicity in the rat, *J. Toxicol. Appl. Pharmacol.*, 49, 53, 1979.

246. Downs, W. L., Wilson, H. B., Sylvester, G. Z., Leach, L. J., and Maynard, E. A., Excretion of uranium by rats following inhalation of uranium dioxide, *Health Phys.*, 13, 445, 1967.

247. Cuddihy, R. G., Analog simulation of the biological behavior of inhaled radionucludes, in *Fission Product Inhalation Program Annual Report 1968-1969*, LF-41, Lovelace Foundation, Albuquerque, N.M., 1969, 136.

248. Boecker, B. B. and Cuddihy, R. G., Toxicity of ^{144}Ce inhaled as ^{144}CeCl$_3$ by the beagle: metabolism and dosimetry, *Radiat. Res.*, 60, 133, 1974.

249. Muir, D. C., *Clinical Aspects of Inhaled Particles*, William Heinemann, London, 1972.

250. Raabe, O. G., Deposition and Clearance of Inhaled Aerosols, UCD-472-503, U.S. Department of Energy, National Technical Information Service, Springfield, Va., 1979.

Chapter 3

STRUCTURE OF THE BLOOD AND LYMPHATIC VASCULAR SYSTEMS IN THE LUNG

Lee V. Leak

TABLE OF CONTENTS

I. INTRODUCTION

In vertebrates, components of the circulatory system consist of the heart and blood vessels. In addition, the lymphatic vessels provide a drainage system which returns extravascular fluids and proteins to the blood circulatory system. The heart is responsible for continuously supplying oxygenated blood to the systemic circulation to reach the various tissue components throughout the body. This muscular pump also provides the power for propelling deoxygenated blood to the lungs for oxygenation (pulmonary circulation) and subsequently returning it to the heart for redistribution to the systemic circulation.[76,96]

The blood vascular supply to the lung is divided into pulmonary and bronchial systems. The pulmonary system functions mainly to regulate gas exchange, while the bronchial system serves as nutrient vessels.[19,139] The distribution of blood from the heart to the systemic circulation occurs at a high pressure and velocity, while the flow to the pulmonary circulation is approximately one sixth of that in the systemic circulation.[11] The bronchial arteries carrying blood from the systemic circulation also reflect the higher pressure of this system by having a thicker muscular wall than pulmonary vessels of a comparable size.[5,78] In common with the systemic circulation, the distribution of blood from the heart to the lungs takes place through a series of arteries in which a transition from elastic to muscular components takes place in the arterial wall. The smaller pulmonary arteries have a thin media which is composed of smooth muscles bounded internally and externally by thin elastic laminae. Blood continues through the arterial tree to arteries of about 70 μm in diameter from which the blood enters the capillary bed. Branching from the arterioles, the capillaries are reported to be wide in comparison to those of the systemic circulation. This segment is composed of an extensive network of microscopic vessels with extremely attenuated walls.

Like the microvascular bed in the systemic circulation, pulmonary capillaries serve as the site of action for the transfer of gases, nutrients, metabolites, and hormones. Gases move to and from the alveoli when blood flows through the alveolar capillaries, providing a uniform pool model for respiratory gas transfer.[218]

Leaving pulmonary capillaries, blood flows into vessels with a diameter of less than 100 μm which pass into the connective tissue septa between secondary lobules to enter pulmonary veins. Unlike the arterial vessels, pulmonary veins are located away from the bronchial tree and drain into the larger veins within the interlobular septa.[139] From pulmonary veins within the interlobular septa, blood flows into larger trunks that are formed near the hilus and lie in close association with bronchi and pulmonary arteries. From the larger veins within the interlobular septa, the venous outflow is in general carried by the superior and inferior pulmonary veins of each lung. These in turn connect directly with the left atrium for returning oxygenated blood back to the heart and subsequent distribution to the systemic circulation.

The bronchial vascular supply to the lung consists of arterial branches from the descending thoracic aorta or vessels arise from the upper posterior aortic intercostal arteries.[19,120,121,139] Entering the lung at the hilus, the bronchial arteries follow each bronchus as it enters the lobe and interconnect to form a plexus of vessels around each bronchus. Accompanying the bronchial tree to the level of the respiratory bronchiole, they ramify to supply smooth muscle of the airway, bronchial glands, mucous coats, the surface of the lung, and lymph nodes.[52,206,207] The bronchial capillary plexus communicates with a network of venules which flow into veins that drain into the azygos and hemiazygos veins near the hilar region of the lung.[194]

Like the interstitial areas in other regions of the body, there is also a continuous fluid flow from blood capillaries toward the interstitium in the lung.[187,188] If left undisturbed, fluid and protein accumulations would be considerable in the interstitial spaces leading to edema and subsequently altering the hemodynamics of interstitial fluid pressure within the lung tissue. To prevent the accumulation of excess fluid within the pulmonary interstitial areas and the alveoli for maintenance of an efficient gas exchange across the air-blood barrier, the interstitium is efficiently drained via lymphatic vessels located within the pulmonary fluid-flow pathway.

The past decade has seen the introduction of new techniques and methods for observing lymphatic vessels. Likewise, the use of radiopaque injections[28,200] has provided a method for delineating boundaries of large lymphatic vessels for topographic studies of pulmonary lymphatics within individual lobes as well as providing information on the direction of lymph flow. In addition, the techniques of electron microscopy have been brought to bear on delineating the ultrastructure of pulmonary blood and lymphatic vessels. Since the early 1960s, electron microscopic studies have revealed much information concerning the structure and arrangement of both blood and lymphatic vessels in various regions throughout the body. Likewise, concepts have been advanced to explain how fluids and materials pass across the blood vascular endothelium into the interstitium with subsequent drainage by the lymphatic vascular system. Concepts have also been advanced to explain how materials are retained within the lymphatic lumen for subsequent drainage to larger collecting vessels. Such information provides a framework for analyzing the structural features which underlie the process of gaseous exchange within and across the air-blood barrier and the removal of fluids and proteins from the interstitial areas of the lungs under normal and edematous conditions. This report will review briefly the organization and morphology of the pulmonary blood and lymphatic vasculatures. The ultrastructural aspects of the various segments of the blood and lymphatic vessels of the lungs will also be presented. In addition, the recent findings presented by a number of investigators that relate to the structural basis of exchange across the pulmonary vascular wall and the role of the lymphatic in the removal of fluids, large molecules, and particulate materials from the lung will also be given.

II. GENERAL ORGANIZATION OF BLOOD VESSELS IN THE LUNG

The use of angiocardiographic methods in the visualization of the cardiovascular system has greatly improved with the development of electronic devices and improved roentgenographic techniques.[168,190] Its use has given rise to detailed and useful information on the normal pulmonary circulation and is now routinely employed for diagnosis of acquired and congenital diseases of the pulmonary vasculature.[169,171]

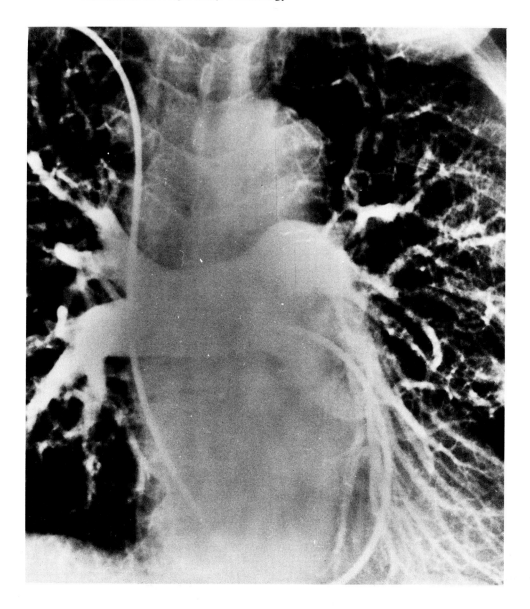

FIGURE 1.   A normal angiocardiogram (anterior/posterior view) which shows the pulmonary trunk and its bifrication into right and left main pulmonary arteries. The larger and lower branch of the right main artery is seen passing into the right middle and lower lobes while the smaller upper branch supplies the right upper lobe of the right lung. The branches of the left main pulmonary artery are also demonstrated. The lobar and segmental branches from both right and left pulmonary arteries are demonstrated. (Courtesy of Dr. E. C. Chapman, Howard University Hospital).

A. Pulmonary Blood Vessels

In pulmonary angiograms, the anatomic features of the pulmonary arteries are clearly delineated (see Figure 1). Leaving the right ventricle as a short tube, the pulmonary trunk extends for a short distance and bifurcates into right and left main pulmonary arteries which supply the right and left lungs. Branches from the right and left main pulmonary arteries divide into lobar branches to supply the right upper, middle, and lower lobes and upper and lower lobes of the left lung. The branches supplying each lobe show a great deal of variability; they accompany the bronchi, with subsequent branches of the pulmonary arteries coursing along its dorsal surface to supply bronchial pulmonary segments.[9]

By using angiographic methods to study the pulmonary and bronchial circulation in dogs, Lauweryns[104] showed that the pulmonary arteries follow a course in close proximity to the bronchial tree and appear as large, broad vessels (see Figure 2). Lying within the peribronchial and peribronchiolar connective tissue, the pulmonary arteries ramify to follow the branching pattern of the bronchi and bronchioles (see Figure 2). Ramifications from the segmental branches arise at various angles to accompany the successive branching of the bronchioles, and radiologic images of vessels with diminishing calibers can be followed to the level of small arterioles.[104]

In latex cast of the pulmonary circulation, branches of the pulmonary artery can be traced to the smaller arterioles as well as into capillaries in the peripheral region of the lung. Resin cast observed in the scanning electron microscope discloses the finer ramifications of the smaller arterioles into a rich capillary network (see Figure 3). The capillary network consists of numerous vessels of uniform size. Draining the rich capillary network are numerous fine vessels which empty into lobar veins that become large in caliber as they extend to the peripheral portion of the pulmonary lobule to form the larger interlobular pulmonary veins (see Figures 3 and 4). The extensive ramifications of the pulmonary veins also provide for drainage of the alveolar capillary network as well as the pleural capillaries and to some extent the bronchial venous network. Each lobule of the lung is drained by a pulmonary vein. Angiographic images of the pulmonary vein confirm that location within the intersegmental or interlobular spaces (See Figures 4 and 5). The venous outflow from each lung is in general provided by a superior and inferior pulmonary vein which empties into the left atrium (see Figure 6).

B. Bronchial Blood Vessels

By using angiographic methods, it is evident that the bronchial arteries follow very closely the ramification of the air conducting passages (see Figure 7). They run a parallel course with each bronchus (see Figure 8) and continue beyond the level of the segmental bronchi extending to the terminal airways as indicated by their termination at the respiratory bronchiole (see Figure 9).[104,194] Injection studies have also indicated a direct connection between bronchial arteries and pulmonary veins (see Figure 9) (i.e., bronchial pulmonary veins of Lefort) and provide evidence in support of the concept that a large part of the intrapulmonary venous blood is drained into the pulmonary veins.[109,118,119,198]

In addition to the larger-caliber bronchial arteries which run in the adventitia of bronchi and bronchioles, there are ramifications into the muscular layer, the secretory glands, mucous membrane, and branches which preforate the bronchial wall to form a fine network of vessels beneath the ciliated epithelium. The bronchial arteries also supply the pulmonary pleura and the walls of the pulmonary artery and vein as the *vasa vasorum*.[42,73,206]

III. THE WALL OF BLOOD VESSELS IN THE LUNG

As in the systemic circulation, the organization of the vascular wall in the lung follows a common plan. In general, the wall of the larger vessels is composed of three distinct layers. These include an inner layer, which is termed the tunica intima; a middle layer, the tunica media; and an outer layer, the tunica adventitia. In some segments of the vascular tree, various aspects of the common plan are prominent, while in others they are greatly reduced or absent from the vascular wall.

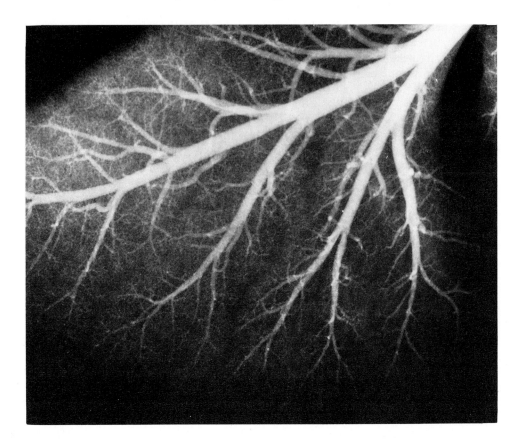

FIGURE 2.   Radiograph of pulmonary arteries of right lung of a beagle injected with a barium sulfate suspension (at 10 cm H_2O pressure) (magnification × 2.1.) (From Lauweryns, J. M., *Pathol. Annu.*, 4, 125, 1971. With permission.)

A. Tunica Intima

This layer is found in all vessels (arteries, the microcirculation, and veins). It consists of a specialized simple squamous epithelial tissue and is termed the endothelium. It forms a continuous lining for blood vessels as well as for the various chambers of the heart. Although forming a continuous layer in all vessels, there is structural variability which reflects the functional activities along various segments of blood vessels throughout the lung. The endothelial cells rest on a basal lamina that overlie a subendothelial layer which is composed of fibrous elastic tissue. For the pulmonary arteries, this layer is in the form of an internal elastic lamina consisting of narrow bands of elastic fibers intermixed with collagen fibers (see Figure 24). In veins the elastic fibers are greatly reduced in the internal elastic lamina and are replaced by numerous collagen fibers within this subendothelial area (see Figures 18 and 37).

B. Tunica Media

The tunica media lies between the intima and adventitia and consists of circularly or spirally organized components. In the pulmonary trunk, there are large amounts of elastic fibers arranged in sheet-like plates which alternate with smooth muscle cells and collagen fibers (see Figure 10). In the larger muscular pulmonary arteries, the media is composed of circularly oriented smooth muscle cells which is bounded by internal and external elastic laminae (see Figures 11B and 13A). In veins the media is slightly irregular in thickness, with smooth muscle cells obliquely and circularly arranged (see

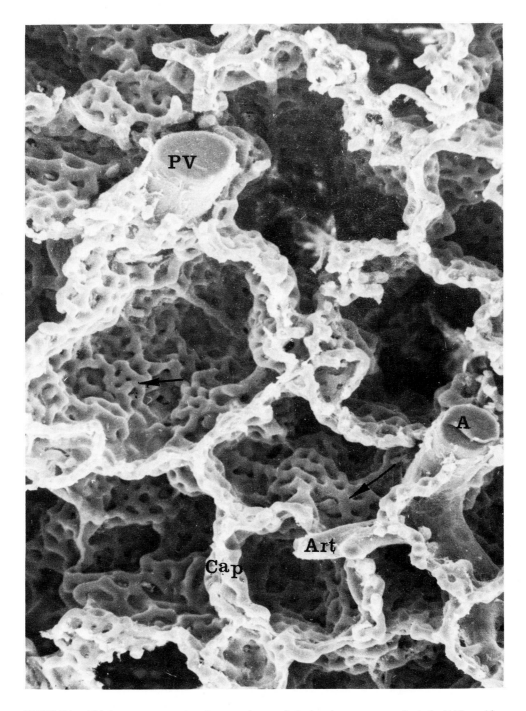

FIGURE 3.   This low power scanning electron micrograph depicts the appearance of arteries (A) branching into arterioles (Art) which supply alveolar capillaries (Cap) which form a rich network within the alveolar wall. These in turn are drained by venules which drain into larger pulmonary veins (Pv). The alveolar capillaries consist of an anastomosing network of short capillaries that are interconnected within the alveolar wall (arrows). (Magnification × 240.)

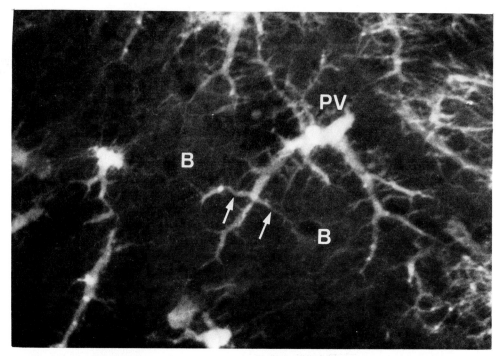

FIGURE 4.   Micrograph of bronchial pulmonary veins (arrows) of a beagle filled after injection of the pulmonary veins (Pv) which courses throughout the lung parenchyma toward the radioluscent bronchiolar ramifications (B). The bronchial pulmonary veins are side branches of the pulmonary veins which probably drain the major part of the blood of the intrapulmonary peribronchial and peribronchiolar venus plexus. Injection of a barium sulfate suspension left upper lung lobe. (Magnification × 11.9.) (From Lauweryns, J. M., *Lymphology,* 4, 125, 1971. With permission.)

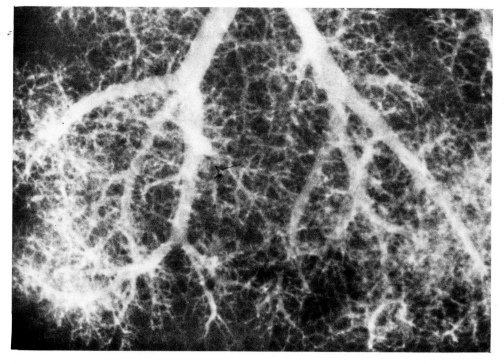

FIGURE 5.   This radiograph illustrates the terminal meshwork formed by the fine terminal ramifications of the pulmonary veins of a beagle. Injected with a barium sulfate suspension (left upper lung lobe). (Magnification × 7.) (From Lauweryns, J. M., *Lymphology,* 4, 125, 1971. With permission.)

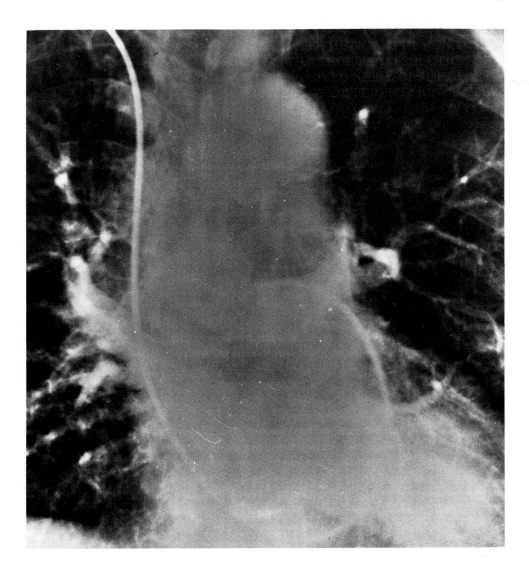

FIGURE 6. A normal angiocardiogram (anterior/posterior view) showing contrast medium in the pulmonary veins which run into the left atrium. (Courtesy of Dr. E. C. Chapman, Howard University Hospital).

Figure 18), and consists of both smooth and cardiac muscle in the main pulmonary vein in some species (see Figures 35 and 36).

C. Tunica Adventitia

Like blood vessels of the systemic circulation, the tunica adventitia is longitudinally arranged. It lies immediately adjacent to the tunica media. In muscular arteries and veins, it is bounded by an external elastic lamina (see Figures 11A and 36). It is larger in arteries than in veins and is composed of fibroelastic tissue which blends into the adjoining loose connective tissue which surrounds the blood vessels. For the larger-sized vessels, it is very prominent and contains fibroblasts, collagen, and elastic fibers. In addition, it contains small blood vessels (*vasa vasorum*), lymphatics, and nerves which blend with the adjacent loose connective tissue surrounding the blood vessels (see Figures 12A and B).

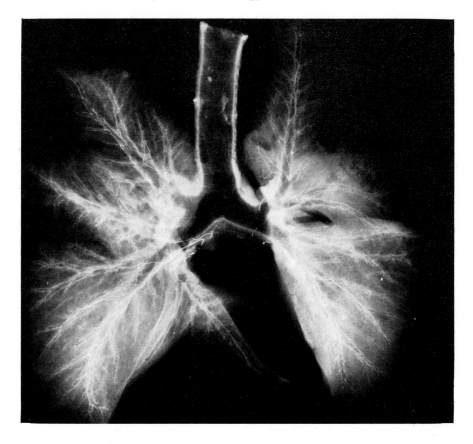

FIGURE 7.   Radiograph of bronchial arteries in both lungs of a beagle injected with a barium sulfate suspension. The bronchial arteries follow closely the ramifications of the bronchi to form a parallel type of bronchial vascular supply. (From Lauweryns, J. M., *Pathol. Annu.,* 1971. With permission.)

IV. CLASSIFICATION OF BLOOD VESSELS IN THE LUNG

In addition to size and functional differences between the pulmonary and bronchial circulatory systems, the blood vessels of the lung also show size and morphological differences that are related to segmental specializations along the vascular tree of each system.

The arterial system of the pulmonary circulation not only serves as a conducting system, but it also provides an elastic buffering system for a rapid and continuous flow of blood to the lungs. Using size, structural features and functional activities, Brenner[11] outlined a means for classifying pulmonary blood vessels into elastic pulmonary arteries, muscular pulmonary arteries, pulmonary arterioles, pulmonary venules, and veins.

Using precise measuring techniques, the recent studies of Elliott,[39] Elliott and Reid,[40] and Reid[163] outlined the structure and branching pattern of pulmonary arteries of normal rats. Using both light optical and electron microscopy, Meyrick et al.[136] further classified the arterial pathway into five structural categories: elastic, transitional, muscular, partially muscular, and nonmuscular. The repeated branching pattern along the arterial tree gives rise to arterioles and vessels of progressively smaller diameter and wall structure. At this level of dichotomous branching, the vessels join the pulmonary capillary network which is drained by venules which in turn lead into veins.

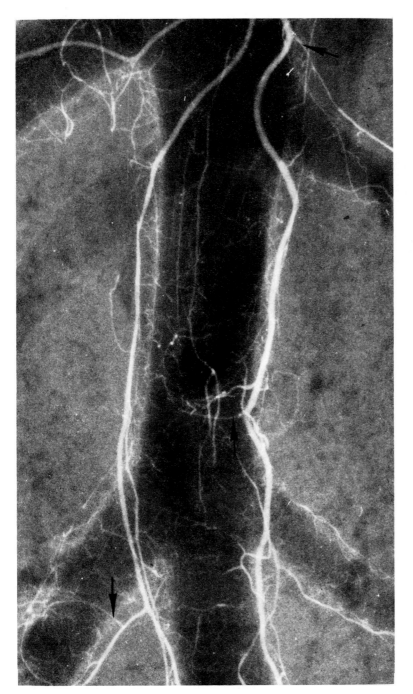

FIGURE 8. Microradiograph of bronchial arteries demonstrating the parallel course followed by the bronchus and its ramifications. The smaller branching vessels of the bronchial arteries are also demonstrated (arrows). (From Lauweryns, J. M., *Pathol. Annu.,* 4, 125, 1971. With permission.)

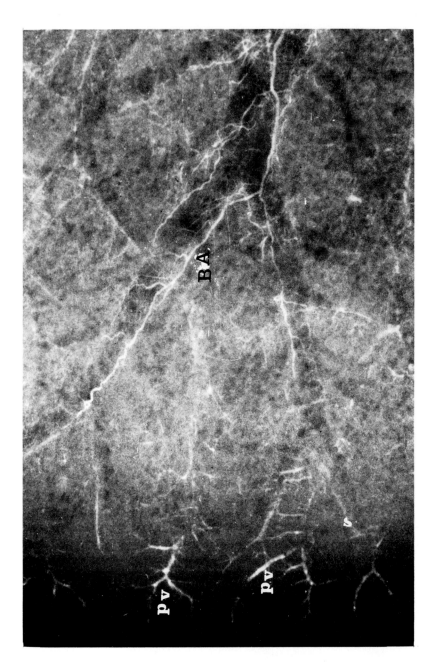

FIGURE 9.   Microradiograph illustrating the filling of some radicals of the pulmonary veins (Pv) after injection of bronchial arteries (BA) with a barium sulfate suspension. The drainage of the injected solutions into veins indicate that the major part of the blood of the intrapulmonary peribronchial venus plexus is drained off by bronchial pulmonary veins toward the pulmonary veins. (Magnification × 7.2.) (From Lauweryns, J. M., *Pathol. Annu.*, 4, 125, 1971. With permission.)

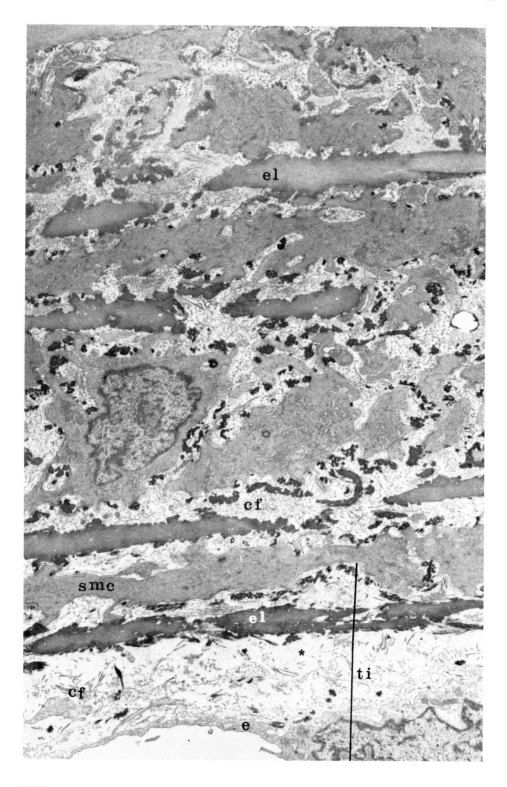

FIGURE 10. An electron micrograph of a main pulmonary artery from the rat. The tunica intima (ti) consist of an endothelial lining (e) and a subendothelial connective tissue of collagen fibers (cf), elastic fibers (el) and ground substance. The tunica media contains wide plaques of elastic fibers surrounded by collagen fibers (cf) which alternate with layers of smooth muscle cells (smc). (Magnification × 9500.)

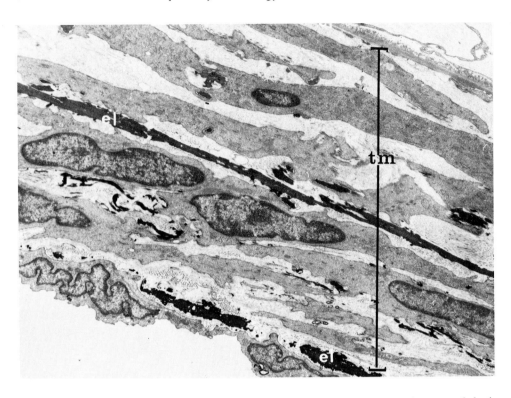

FIGURE 11A.   Electron micrograph of an intrapulmonary artery showing the reduced amount of elastic fibers (el) within the tunica media (tm). (Magnification × 6300.)

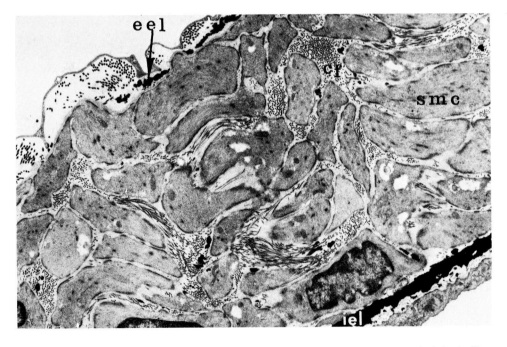

FIGURE 11B.   Electron micrograph of a muscular pulmonary artery with a dense band of elastic fibers forming the internal elastic lamina (iel) and a thin band of elastic fibers forming the external elastic lamina (eel). The media contains several layers of smooth muscle cells (smc) many of which are surrounded by collagen fibers (cf) and a few strands of elastic fibers. (Magnification × 9300.)

A. Pulmonary Elastic Arteries

The pulmonary trunk and arteries with an external diameter exceeding 1 mm are of the elastic or conducting type with a structure very similar to that of arteries in the systemic circulation (i.e., the aorta) (see Figure 10). Considered as shock absorbers, elastic arteries are able to withstand rapid and large changes in the pulse pressure by rapidly dilating with each systole.[10,74,87] The media of elastic vessels consists predominantly of elastic fibers which alternate with smooth muscle cells and collagen fibers (see Figures 10 and 11A).

In the pulmonary trunk segment, elastic laminae are irregularly arranged (see Figure 10), while the intrapulmonary segment of the elastic fibers shows a more regular pattern with circularly arranged elastic laminae and smooth muscles (see Figure 11A). A thick internal elastic lamina lies within the subendothelial layer (see Figure 10), and the outermost layer of elastic fibers comprises the external elastic lamina (see Figure 11A). This outermost layer is most prominent in the smaller-sized elastic arteries as they approach the muscular pulmonary arteries (see Figure 11A), i.e., the transitional area between elastic and muscular-type arteries.[78]

The number of elastic laminae within the media ranges from 3 to 4 in arteries of 1000-μm external diameter to 16 to 20 in arteries of 5000 μm in diameter.[11] The recoil of large amounts of elastic laminae within the vessel wall causes a contraction of the vessel which narrows its lumen and thus propels blood onward during diastole of the heart. The recoil of pulmonary elastic vessels would be similar to that in the aorta which is greatly facilitated by the contraction of smooth muscle cells intermixed between collagen fibers and elastic fibers within the tunica media.[2]

B. Muscular Arteries

Beyond the transitional regions of elastic arteries, the tunica media merges into a typical muscular artery in which the media is composed of circularly oriented smooth muscle fibers bounded by internal and external elastic laminae (see Figure 11B). This transition usually occurs in arteries of sizes of 100 to 1000 μm in diameter.[11]

Muscular pulmonary arteries differ from those in the systemic circulation of a comparable caliber in that the pulmonary arteries have a wide lumen and thinner media which is bounded by two distinct elastic laminae. In contrast, the external elastic membrane is usually very thin, incomplete, or absent in most systemic muscular arteries (compare Figures 13 and 39).

Percentage medial wall thickness is used to compare the thickness of the media in arteries of various sizes[11,79,134,135,208] and indicates the thickness of the media in terms of the diameter of the external elastic lamina. Muscular pulmonary arteries follow closely bronchioles, respiratory bronchioles, and alveolar ducts. The thin media and wide lumen of muscular arteries suggest a low resistance to flow.[44,51]

Pulmonary muscular arteries are characterized by the presence of a prominent internal elastic membrane beneath the endothial lining cells (see Figure 11B). For the large- and medium-sized muscular arteries, the tunica media contains circularly to obliquely oriented smooth muscle cells that alternate with collagenous fibers and elastic fibers. The media is bounded by an external elastic lamina which marks the inner margin of the tunica adventitia and forms a distinct border in the large- and medium-sized muscular arteries (see Figures 11B and 13A).

The adventitia in pulmonary muscular arteries consists of a dense fibrous connective tissue in which collagen and elastic fibers are longitudinally or spirally arranged. The extracellular fibers of this layer blend with the connective tissue components of the peribronchial sleeve (see Figure 13A). For the larger vessels, a network of smaller blood vessels (*vasa vasorum*) as well as nerves and lymphatic vessels lie within and in close apposition to the tunica adventitia of the larger arteries (see Figures 12A and B).

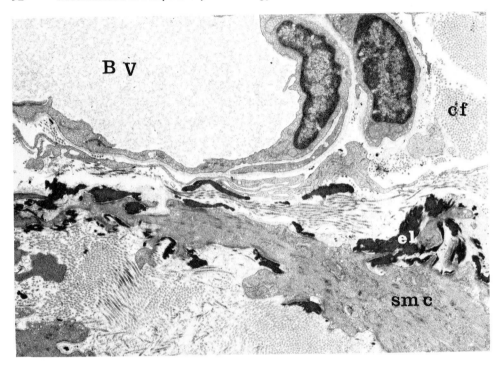

FIGURE 12A.   Electron micrograph showing portion of the pulmonary arterial wall which illustrates blood
vessels (Bv) within the tunica adventitia which is surrounded by collagen fibers (cf). The outer boundary of
the tunica media is indicated by smooth muscle cells (smc) and elastic fibers (el). (Magnification × 7300.)

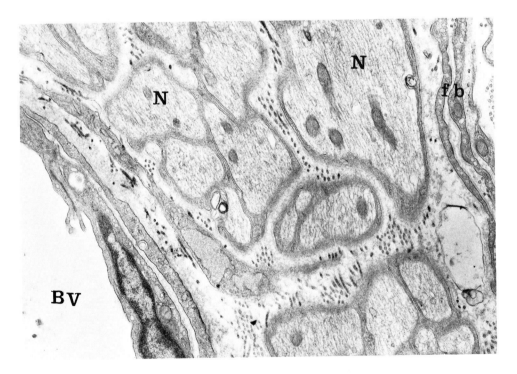

FIGURE 12B.   This electron micrograph shows a portion of the tunica adventitia from the pulmonary
artery illustrating a part of a blood vessel (Bv) and nerve axon (N). Thin cytoplasmic processes from fiberblasts (fb) are indicated at the right portion of the micrograph. (Magnification × 20,520.)

C. Pulmonary Arterioles

In arterial vessels below 100 μm in diameter, the transition from muscular to arterioles is apparent when the medial layer gradually changes from a single continuous layer of muscle cells to an incomplete layer which spirals about the vessel (see Figure 13A). At the points of origin of the pulmonary arterioles, two elastic laminae are present on the inner and outer aspects of the smooth muscle layer.[11] As the vessels decrease in caliber (16 to 18 μm in external diameter), a single elastic lamina is found under the endothelium.[36,79,122] With the gradual transition from muscular to nonmuscular arterioles (see Figures 14A and B), the adventitia is also decreased in content and thickness.[134]

D. Pulmonary Capillaries

The tapering of pulmonary arterioles into an elaborate capillary network is unlike the capillary bed in other organ systems. Those in the lung are not supported or surrounded by large masses of solid tissues, but are intimately exposed to air over extensive areas which consist only of a very thin tissue membrane serving as a barrier.[216] The alveolar network of blood vessels is interlaced with connective tissue fibers and cells to provide an extensive surface area which facilitates the rapid exchange of gases across an exceedingly thin tissue membrane (see Figures 15, 28, and 29). Like the capillaries in other organs, this network of microscopic vessels (microvascular bed) is situated between arterioles and venules. They provide for a rapid transfer of gases, nutrients, metabolites, and waste products. The pulmonary capillaries are arranged into communicating networks with segments of 10 to 14 μm in length and 7 to 9 μm in diameter.[216,217] The alveolar capillaries join with each other to drain into vessels of increasingly larger diameters (see Figures 27 and 28).

E. Postcapillary Venules

Postcapillary venules[60,230] measure less than 100 μm and are similar to pulmonary arterioles (see Figure 16). They originate near branches of bronchioles and pass into the connective tissue septa between secondary lobules to drain into pulmonary veins (see Figures 16 and 17).

F. Pulmonary Veins

The pulmonary veins are located at some distance from the bronchial tree, with the larger veins lying in the interlobular septa (see Figure 16). While it is difficult to distinguish the smaller veins from smaller arteries, the larger veins are more easily identified by the absence of a definitive internal elastic lamina between the endothelium and smooth muscles (see Figures 17 and 18). The media is irregular in thickness and consists of obliquely and circularly arranged smooth muscle cells that are separated by collagen fibers and small strands of elastic fibers.

The adventitia contains collagen bundles and elastic fibers and small vessels (vasa vasorum) and nerves. Like the larger veins in other organ systems, pulmonary veins are also thin walled and collapsable and offer very little resistance to flow.

V. STRUCTURE OF THE PULMONARY VASCULAR WALL

Although routine histological and histochemical studies demonstrated that the vascular wall is organized into a repeating pattern of concentric lamellae, there was no sharp line of demarcation between the cell types or the connective tissue components within the wall of large blood vessels.[5,11] Likewise, it was difficult to distinguish segmental variations within the microcirculatory vessels of the lung in routine paraffin sections.[11]

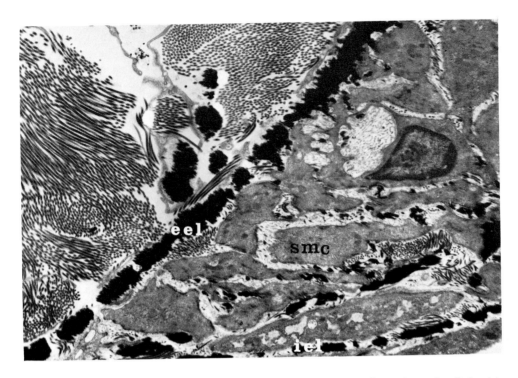

FIGURE 13A.   The transition from a pulmonary artery with several layers of smooth muscle cells (smc) to a single layer is illustrated in this electron micrograph. Both internal (iel) and external elastic laminae (eel) are indicated. (Magnification × 6700.)

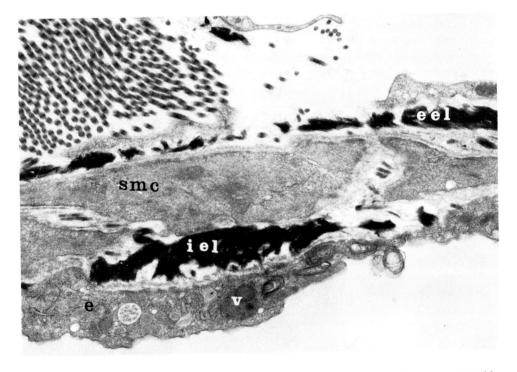

FIGURE 13B.   A single layer of smooth muscle cells (smc) comprise the tunica media and is separated by an internal elastic lamina (iel) and an external elastic lamina (eel). The endothelialPcell (e) contains electron dense vesicles (v) of various sizes. (Magnification × 23,600.)

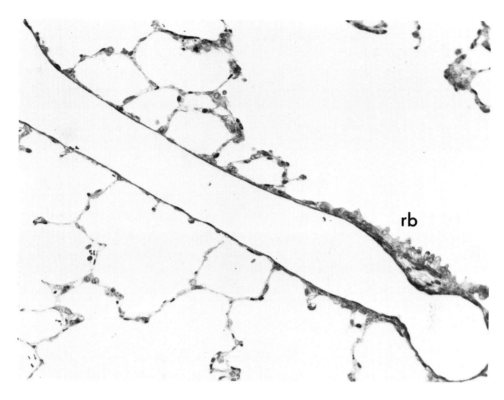

FIGURE 14A. A light micrograph from a plastic section showing a nonmuscular artery approximately 60 μm in external diameter and running with a respiratory bronchiole (rb). (Magnification × 240.) (From Meyrick, B. and Reid, L., *Anat. Rec.*, 193, 71, 1979. With permission.)

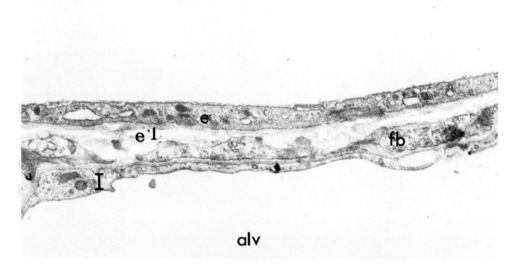

FIGURE 14B. This electron micrograph shows part of the wall of a nonmuscular region of the artery shown in 14A. The endothelial cell (e) lies internal to a single fragmented elastic lamina (el). A process from a fiberblasts (fb) is located between the artery and alveolus (alv) which is lined by Type 1 neumocyte (I). (Magnification × 17,500.) (From Meyrick, B. and Reid, L., *Anat. Rec.*, 193, 71, 1979. With permission.)

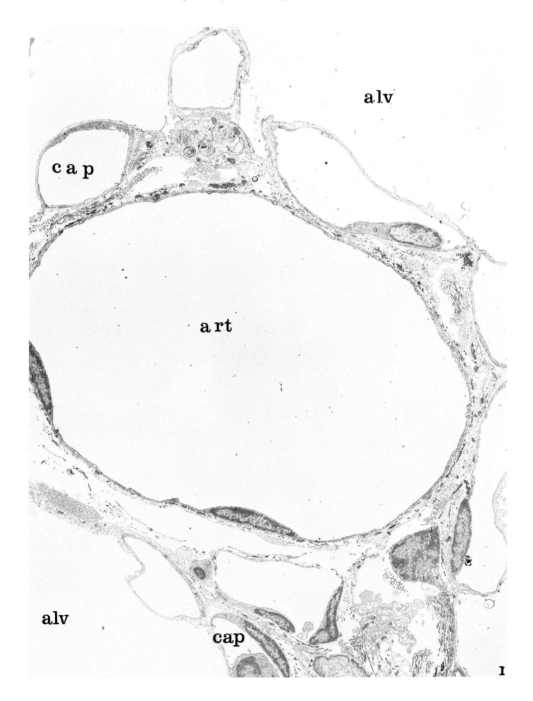

FIGURE 15.   A low power electron micrograph showing a small arteriole (art) which is surrounded by capillaries (cap) lying adjacent to the alveolar space (alv). (Magnification × 3000.)

Electron microscopic examination of the cardiovascular system has led to the recognition that endothelial cells lining the vascular wall form a continuous layer,[14,15,92,144,148] except in specialized segments of the vascular tree, where the endothelial cells may be extremely attenuated and contain fenestrae,[38,54,58,148,149,153,226,227] and in other specialized regions along various segments of the vascular wall there may be discontinuities.[46,75,140,223] Likewise, electron microscopic studies on pulmonary vessels have demonstrated ultrastructural features that are characteristic for a given segment of the arterial tree.[43,86,134,136,185,211] In addition, the continuity of endothelial cells lining the alveolar capillaries at the air-blood barrier was demonstrated in the 1950s[90,123] and is now well established.[155,173-176,218]

A. Ultrastructure of the Pulmonary Arterial Wall

A number of ultrastructural studies have been carried out to follow changes associated with various pathological conditions which involve and affect the blood vessels in the lung.[43,137,185,211] However, studies designed to outline the detailed structure within various segments of the normal pulmonary artery have only recently been undertaken.[134]

1. Tunica Intima

In man and large animals where the pulmonary trunk and large arteries exceed 3000 μm in diameter, such vessels are of the elastic type and extend about halfway along the axial pathway. Arising from the elastic segment of the pulmonary artery is a transitional segment that gives way to muscular arteries which accompany lobular, terminal, and respiratory bronchioles. In both elastic and muscular pulmonary arteries, the innermost layer of the vascular wall is formed by a single layer of endothelial cells. This layer is continuous and rests on a subendothelial layer of connective tissue with a prominent internal elastic lamina (see Figures 10 and 11A).

a. Endothelium

The luminal surface of the pulmonary arterial wall is lined by a simple squamous endothelium. The endothelial cells measure about 15 to 30 μm in length, with a thickness varying from 5 μm in the nuclear region to less than 1 μm in the more peripheral regions of the cell.[134] Scanning images of the luminal surfaces of pulmonary arteries also show the topography of squamous or oblong cells with prominent nuclear bulges occupying a central part of the cell (see Figure 19A). The nuclear bulges give a dome-shaped character which is relatively uniform over the luminal surface.

When lungs are perfused with a fixative at pressures close to systole, the lumen of the arteriole wall remains dilated and very few longitudinal folds are observed over the luminal surface.[1] However, when vessels are fixed by immersion, the luminal surfaces contain numerous folds which project into the lumen.[29,65,178,215] For the most part, the surface of pulmonary endothelial cells appear generally smooth, with occasional protoplasmic projections which give the appearance of short microvilli (see Figure 19B). These have been shown to increase with long exposure to saline perfusion prior to fixation. In scanning images, the intercellular junctions are recognized by the slightly elevated ridges produced by the overlapping of adjacent cell margins (see Figure 19B). Such marginal appendages are similar to the marginal folds observed in thin sections.[47] In thin sections of the pulmonary arterial wall, it is evident that the endothelial cells are held in close appositions at their margins by intercellular junctions which permit the formation of a continuous layer throughout the length of the vessels (see Figures 20 and 22). The cells contain elongate prominent nuclei located in the central cytoplasm which are oriented with their long axis parallel with the long axis of the vessel and also represent the direction of blood flow along the vascular wall.

The endothelial cytoplasm is surrounded by a plasmalemma which is characterized by the presence of numerous uniform infoldings of the cell membrane that measure 600 to 700 Å in diameter (pinocytolic vesicles or caveolae). These peripherally located plasmalemmal vesicles are located at both blood and tissue fronts of the endothelial cells and also lie free in the cytoplasm of the endothelial cells (see Figures 20 and 22). The population and density of vesicles varies from one vascular segment to another.

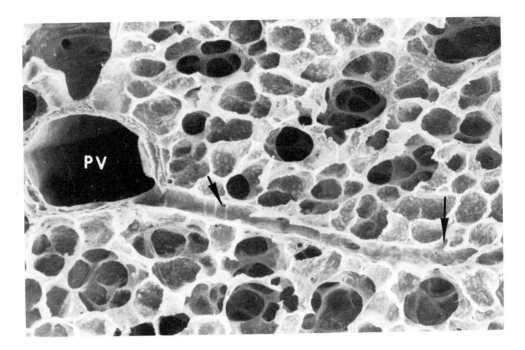

FIGURE 16A.   A low power scanning electron micrograph of rat lung that wis fixed by vascular perfursion. Venules (arrows) draining alveolar capillaries anastomose with muscular veins which are continuous with the interlobular pulmonary veins (PV). (Magnification × 80.)

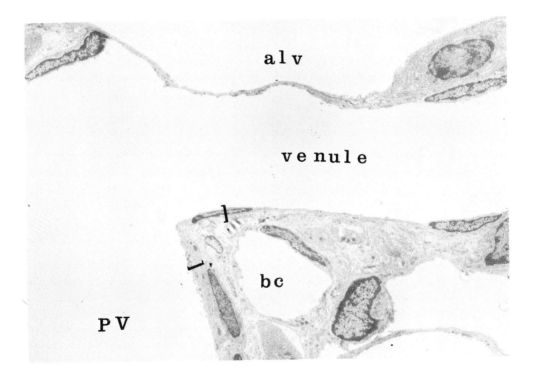

FIGURE 16B.   A low power electron micrograph showing a venule branching with muscular pulmonary vein (PV). Alveolar spaces (alv) and blood capillaries (bc) are as indicated. (Magnification × 2275.)

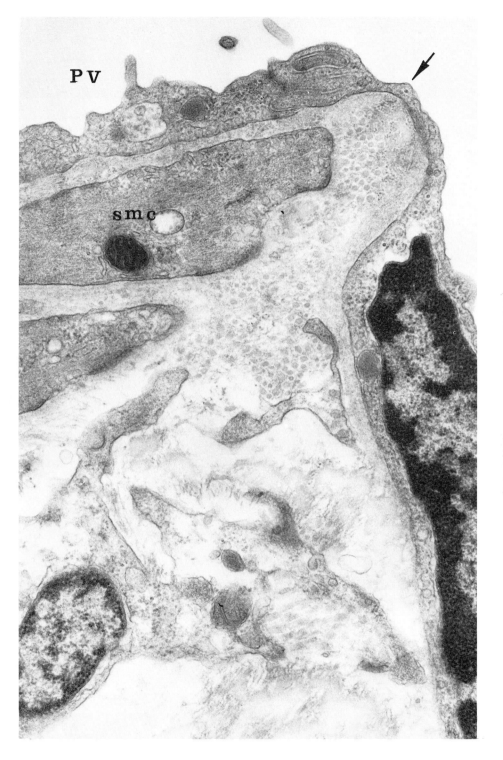

FIGURE 17. This electron micrograph shows an enlargement of the bracketed segment of venular wall from Figure 16B. At the site of branching (arrow) the wall of the pulmonary vein (PV) contains smooth muscle cells (smc), however, the venule wall lacks smooth muscle. (Magnification × 38,300.)

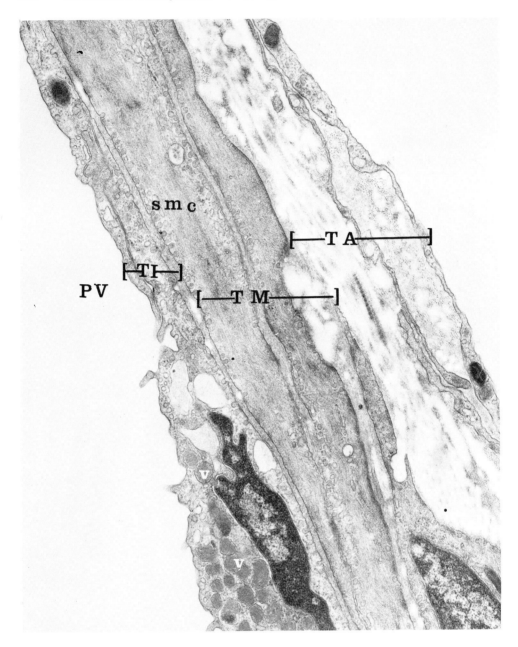

FIGURE 18. This micrograph illustrates a longitudinal section through the wall of a pulmonary vein (PV). The endothelial (e) cells contain numerous electron dense vesicles (v). Unlike pulmonary arteries of a similar wall thickness the pulmonary veins lack an internal elastic lamina. The tunica media contains one to two layers of smooth muscle cells (smc). (Magnification × 23,500.)

Simionescue[181] demonstrated that the population density of vesicles was two to three times higher in capillaries than in arterioles and venules, with the highest volume density of vesicles occurring in the endothelium of the venular segment of capillaries. The rapid uptake of water-soluble molecules from the lumen of blood vessels by plasmalemmal vesicles and the movement of vesicles filled with molecules across the endothelium to the connective tissue front provide evidence that these vesicles are indeed active in transendothelial transport.[176,181] The transendothelial movement of large molecules

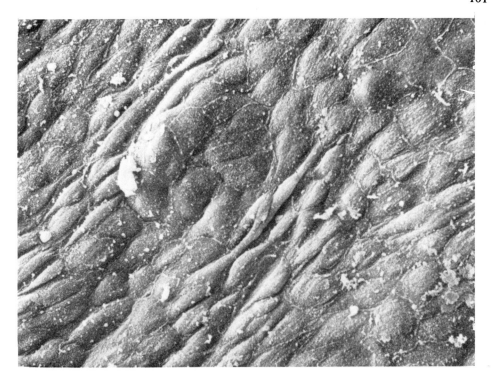

FIGURE 19A. Scanning electron micrograph showing the luminal surface of the pulmonary artery which is lined by squamous endothelial cells. (Magnification × 1260.)

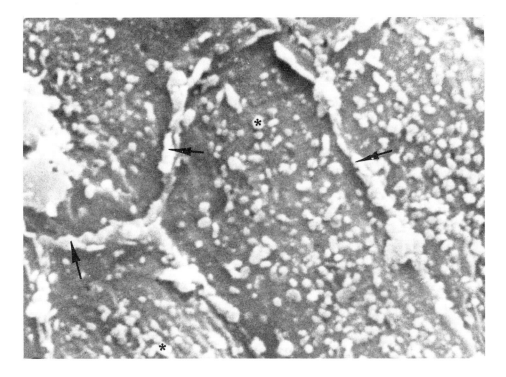

FIGURE 19B. The margins of adjacent endothelial cells overlap to form ridges (arrows) which mark the lateral border of cells. Short projections (*) are also seen on the apical surfaces of the endothelial cells. Since perfusion with saline was made prior to fixation, it is presumed that many of these microvillous-like projections may be a result of the saline perfusions. (Magnification × 12,000.)

across the arterial wall is supported by the recent studies of Florey and Sheppard,[56] who showed that i.v. injected protein (i.e., horseradish peroxidase) was rapidly removed from the arterial lumen within plasmalemmal vesicles as well as through the clefts of intercellular junctions. In addition to plasmalemmal vesicles, there are large vesicles and lysosomes in close proximity to the Golgi complex (see Figure 21).

The luminal surface of the plasmalemma is covered by a very thin surface coat, the endocapillary or endothelial layer.[125] This fuzzy coating measures 5 to 6 nm in thickness and also extends into plasmalemmal vesicles. The positive staining of this layer with ruthenium red suggests the presence of mucopolysacharides along the luminal surface of endothelial cells. In addition to the nucleus, the endothelial cells contain the usual complement of cytoplasmic organelles which include a Golgi complex and centriole which are located in the perinuclear region of the cell (see Figure 21).

Ribosomes appear free in the cytoplasm, and they are also attached to the endoplasmic reticulum (see Figure 20). Cysternae of the endoplasmic reticulum are also observed which lack ribosomes on their surface and represent endoplasmic reticulum of the smooth variety. Mitochondria appeared throughout the cytoplasm as round or oval-shaped structures. The internal structures, cristae, and matrix are common to those of mitochondria found in other organ systems (see Figure 22). Prominent in the endothelial cells of pulmonary vessels are elongated granules containing an electron-dense matrix (see Figure 20). These were described earlier by Weibel and Palade[221], and recent studies of Meyrick and Reid[134] suggest that these granules are most frequent in the endothelial cells of muscular arteries, while less frequent in partially muscular arteries and nonmuscular arteries and rare in alveolar capillaries. The findings of Meyrick and Reid[134] confirm the earlier findings of Fuchs and Weibel. Microtubules appear in close association with centrioles within the nuclear region and throughout the peripheral cytoplasm (see Figure 23). Filaments of about 6 nm in diameter also appear throughout the cytoplasm of endothelial cells (see Figure 22). There is now a wealth of information which provides both biochemical and morphological evidence for the presence of actin in endothelial cells as well as in the cytoplasm of a wide array of nonmuscular cells.[159,160] The observation of nuclear pinching and cellular shortening to provide intercellular gaps between adjacent endothelial cells following the application of certain stimuli suggests the presence of contractile components within the cytoplasm of endothelial cells.[127] In addition to the thin filaments, thick filaments which measure 10 to 11 nm in diameter are also found within the cytoplasm of endothelial cells.

b. Internal Elastic Lamina

The internal elastic lamina is a prominent structure of the subendothelial layer of the arterial wall (see Figures 11A and B; 13A and B; and 21, 22, and 24). Immediately adjacent to the basal surface of the endothelial cell there is an amorphous matrix of 30 to 50 nm wide which separates the endothelial cells from the remaining connective tissue components of the subendothelial layer. The internal elastic lamina and collagen fibers are organized into longitudinal bundles that for the most part run parallel with the long axis of the vessel. The width of the subendothelial layer is often bridged by basal endothelial projections that extend to make junctional contact with smooth muscle cells in the tunica media. In addition, lateral projections from smooth muscle cells also penetrate the internal elastic membrane to make intimate contact with endothelial cells to form myoendothelial junctions (see Figures 25A and B).

2. Tunica Media: Smooth Muscle Cells and Connective Tissue

Prominent in the media of large- and medium-sized arteries and veins are smooth muscle cells that are arranged circularly and in a helical fashion (see Figures 11B and

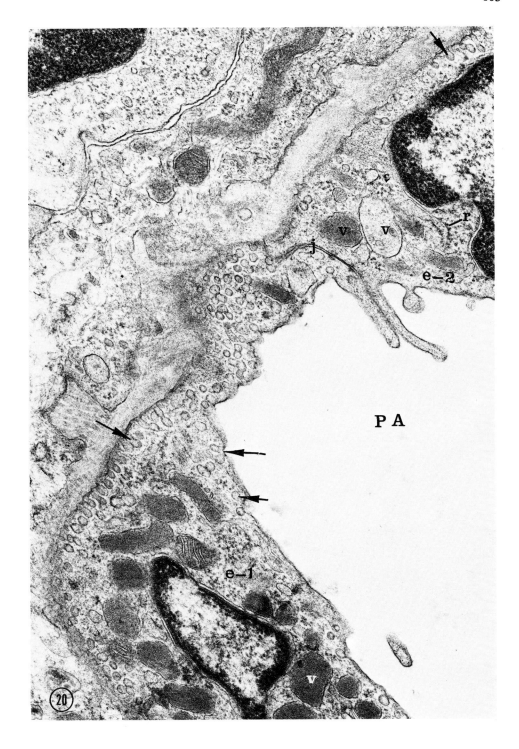

FIGURE 20. Electron micrograph of pulmonary artery (PA) showing portions of two endothelial (e-1 e-2) cells. The cytoplasm contains electron dense vesicles (v). There are also numerous plasmalemmal invaginations (arrows) on the connective tissue side as well as along the luminal surface. Adjacent cells are held together by intercellular junctions (J). (Magnification × 32,600.)

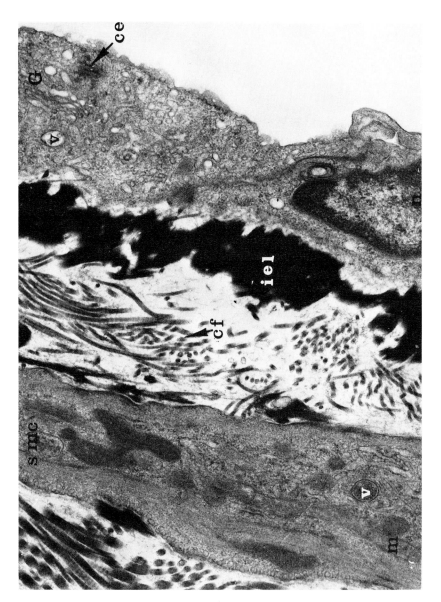

FIGURE 21. Portion of endothelial cells of pulmonary artery showing part of the Golgi apparatus (G) and centrioles (Ce). A portion of the nucleus (n) is shown at the bottom of the micrograph. The internal elastic lamina (iel) is separated from the smooth muscle cells (smc) by bundles of collagen fibers (cf). The smooth muscle cell contains numerous cytoplasmic filaments in the peripheral cytoplasm while cytoplasmic organelles such as mitochondria (m) and vesicles (v) are located in the central portion of the cell. (Magnification × 23,500.)

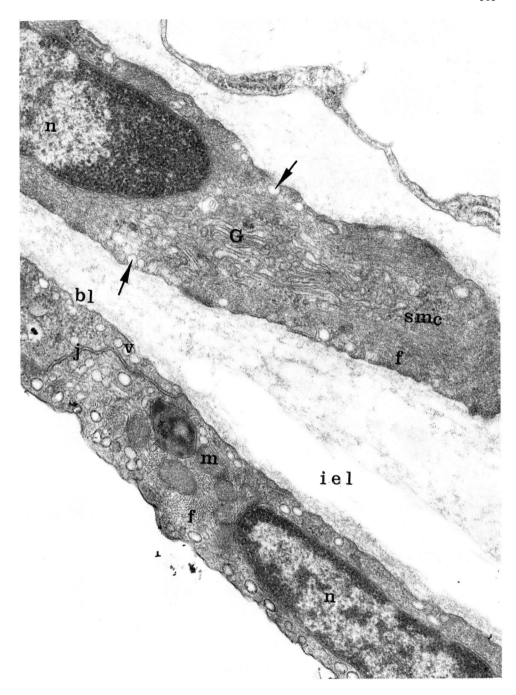

FIGURE 22. This electron micrograph illustrates numerous cytoplasmic filaments (f) in the perinuclear region of the endothelial cells of a pulmonary artery. Plasmalemmal vesicles (v), mitochondria (m), and intercellular junctions (j) are as indicated. The basal lamina (bl) separates the endothelium from the internal elastic lamina ground substance of the subendothelial layer. A portion of a smooth muscle cell (smc) shows the nucleus (n) and Golgi (G) apparatus. In addition, cytoplasmic filaments (f) are observed in the peripheral regions of the cell. (Magnification × 32,000.)

18). Each muscle cell is surrounded by a basal lamina except in regions of close apposition between adjacent cells which are held together by gap junctions (communicating junctions). Such areas have been shown to provide for the conduction of impulses and the transmission of materials of low molecular weight between adjacent cells.[32,124,180] The cells measure from 25 to 80 μm in length and are smaller than smooth muscle cells in other organs of the body.

The sarcolemma which surrounds the smooth muscle cells is characterized by the presence of numerous plasmalemmal invaginations which have been termed caveolae (see Figure 22). They are quite numerous over the surface of the cell and provide an increased surface area as well as bringing the membrane in close contact with the peripherally located myofilamentous components of the sarcoplasm (see Figure 22).

The nucleus occupies a centrally located position within the sarcoplasm and is surrounded by organelles of the sarcoplasm (see Figure 22). These organelles include a Golgi complex, with numerous vesicles at both forming and maturing faces, centrioles within the juxtanuclear area, and rough endoplasmic reticulum within the perinuclear sarcoplasm as well as distributed throughout various regions along the length of the cell. Mitochondria are spherical or elongated structures and are most numerous in the juxtanuclear region of the cell. They are also found throughout the sarcoplasm between myofilaments as well as the peripheral areas of the cell subjacent to the sarcolemma (see Figures 21 and 22).

A salient feature of the sarcoplasm includes myofilaments which occupy major areas of the sarcoplasm. They are arranged with their long axes coinciding with that of the cell and measure 6 to 8 nm in width (see Figures 21 and 22). Dense segments of myofilaments are also observed near the periphery of the cell and are presumed to serve as attachment areas for the myofilaments to the sarcolemma.[92,101,152,165,166] Both morphological and biochemical studies suggests that two types of myofilaments are present in the smooth muscle cell.[48,142,150,161]

In the tunica media of vessels which contain more than one layer of smooth muscle cells, intervening layers of elastic and collagen fibers are found between adjacent layers of smooth muscle cells. Very few neuromuscular junctions are observed in the tunica media, therefore, only a small portion of the smooth muscle cells are innervated.[166] It is suggested that excitation may spread between adjacent cells through gap junctions.[32,183]

3. Adventitia and Connective Tissue

Collagen fibers comprise a major fiber type of the tunica adventitia. They are loosely arranged into bundles and extend into the adjoining connective tissue. The elastic fibers are sparse, appearing as scattered or isolated fibrils within the adventitia (see Figures 12A, 35, and 36). Connective tissue cells include fibroblasts and mast cells which may be in close proximity to the wall of the vasa vasorum found in the walls of the larger vessels. Fibroblasts with extremely attenuated cytoplasmic processes also appear near the outer boundary of the tunica adventitia to provide a line of demarcation between the outer boundary of the vascular wall and adjoining connective tissue (see Figure 12B). These attenuated cell processes are similar to those observed in the vascular walls of veins and arteries by Majno[126] and Rhodin[166,167] and in the walls of larger lymphatic vessels by Leak.[114] Nerve axons completely or partially surrounded by Schwann cells and *vasa vasorum* are also found in the adventitial layer (see Figure 12B).

B. Nonmuscular Arteries (Arterioles)

With successive branching, the muscular pulmonary artery approaches the size range of the microvascular bed (i.e., 15 to 60 μm in diameter). At this level, the partially

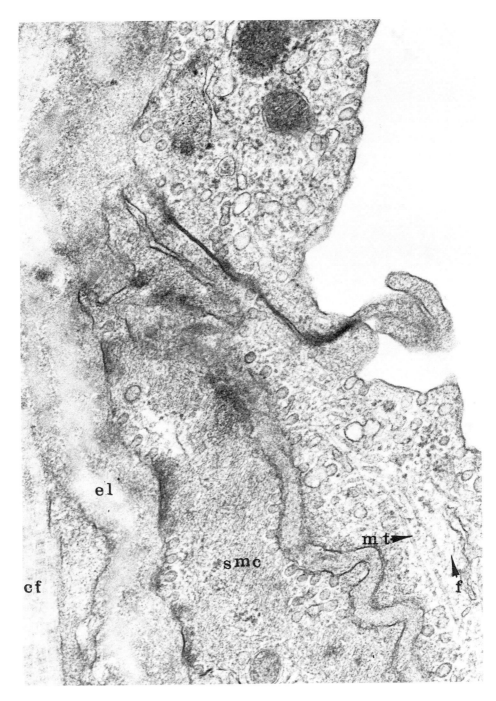

FIGURE 23. This electron micrograph shows the appearance of microtubules (mt) and cytoplasmic filaments (f) within the endothelium of a pulmonary artery. Part of a smooth muscle cell (smc) is in close apposition to the endothelial cells. Collagen fibers (cf) and elastic fibers (ef) are as indicated. (Magnification × 53,300.)

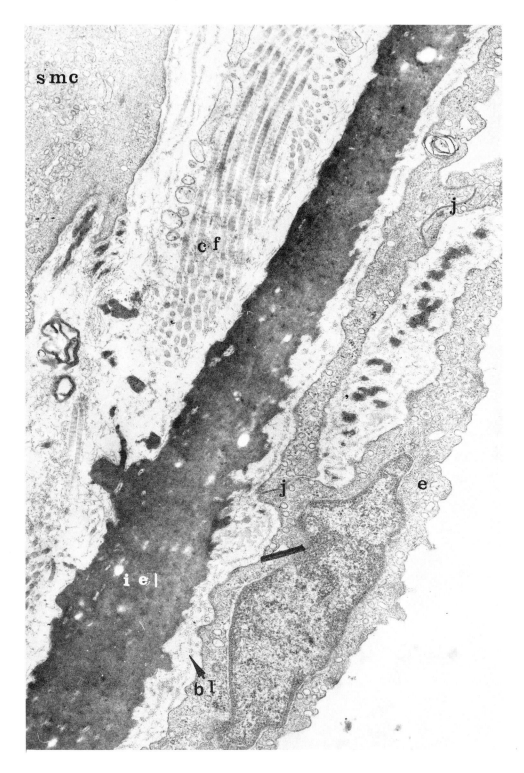

FIGURE 24.   The tunica intima of a pulmonary artery is illustrated in this electron micrograph. Endothelial (e) cells are held together by intercellular junctions (j) and rest on a basal lamina (bl) which is separated from a band of elastic fibers comprising the internal elastic lamina (iel). Bundles of collagen fibers (cf) and the elastic fibers comprise the subendothelial layer. A small portion of a smooth muscle cell (smc) is shown in the upper left hand corner of the micrograph. (Magnification × 26,300.)

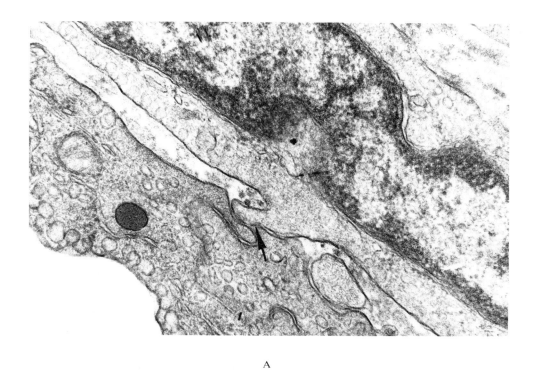

A

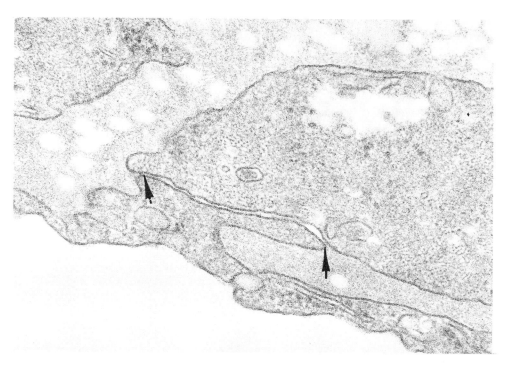

B

FIGURE 25. This electron micrograph shows a portion of the endothelial cell of a pulmonary artery which makes close contact with the smooth muscle cell to form a myoendothelial junction (arrow). (Magnification × 43,100.) The contact between endothelial cells and smooth muscles can be extensive (arrows) as illustrated in (B). (Magnification × 83,700.)

muscular arteries give way to arteries around which the smooth muscle cell is completely lacking (see Figures 14A and B). At this point, the wall consists of an intima and adventitia only. The intima is composed of an endothelial lining in which adjacent cells are held in close apposition by intercellular junctions. In freeze-fracture replicas of arteriolar junction (see Figure 32A), intramembrane particles (8 to 10 nm in diameter) are arranged into three to six rows which interconnect as low ridges on the PF face or in shallow grooves on the EF face.[174] Occasionally some areas of the junctional mesh-work are occupied by closely packed particles (PF face) or pits (EF face) which appear to be gap junctions (see Figure 32A). The endothelial cells rest on a basal lamina, and a fragmented internal elastic lamina with a sparse distribution of collagen fibers (see Figure 14B).

In the systemic circulation, the precapillary vessels with diameters of 100 μm and below are defined as arterioles.[50,98,166] The contraction and relaxation of the smooth muscle cells within the walls of these vessels serve to regulate blood pressure and the supply of blood to various organs of the systemic circulation. However, terminal vessels, within the pulmonary arterial tree below 100 μm in diameter were classified by Brenner[11] as arterioles. Unlike the arterioles in the systemic circulation, the medial coat of the smaller pulmonary arterioles lacks smooth muscle cells (see Figure 14B). Since no muscle is found in the wall of pulmonary arterioles in the size range of 50 μm in diameter, this segment of the terminal pulmonary arterial tree is not well suited as the site of intense vasoconstriction (precapillary sphincter area). On the otherhand, the somewhat larger arteries, in the size range of 100 μm and above, contain a well-formed media[51,134,199] and are located adjacent to the respiratory bronchioles. These vessels branch at right angles, giving rise to smaller vessels (see Figures 3 and 26). At the point of bifurcation, the smooth muscle cells around the orifice of the branching vessels are arranged to regulate the amount and flow of blood entering the precapillary vessels by contraction and relaxation.[36,51,73]

Sphincteric muscle bundles have been previously described in pulmonary arteries of the guinea pig,[207] in the cow[18] and the horse,[80] Likewise, sphincteric regions occurring at the orifice of peripheral vessels which originate by the right angle branching of arterioles were described in the lungs of rabbit and rat by Ferenez.[49] The corresponding precapillary sphincter segment in the systemic circulation takes place in vessels of 50 to 10 μm in diameter.[4,20,166,230,231]

In a detailed ultrastructural study of the pulmonary arterial tree in the rat, Meyrick and Reid[134] observed that the terminal segment contains squamous endothelial cells with a centrally placed nucleus and that the distribution of cytoplasmic organelles was similar to that of the endothelial cells in the larger arteries. The endothelial cells rest on a basal lamina which is occasionally shared by a pericyte that is located internal to a single fragmentary elastic lamina. In addition, the basal lamina is often shared by epithelial cells of the alveolar wall.

At this level of the microvascular bed, there is an occasional fibroblasts in close proximity to the arteriole and capillary walls. The adventitial layer of the arteriole contains a random distribution of collagen and elastic fibrils that are also a part of the alveolar wall.

C. Pulmonary Capillaries

In studies of the pulmonary microvascular bed, Irwin et al.[85] observed that if the terminal arterioles of the lungs in living animals (guinea pigs and rabbits) were constricted while blood flow was allowed to continue, a single arteriole was observed to taper as it joined a capillary. This arrangement was similar to the termination of arterioles in various organ systems of the systemic circulation (i.e., mesentery and muscle). In the case of dilated arterioles in the living animals, the arterioles terminated bluntly

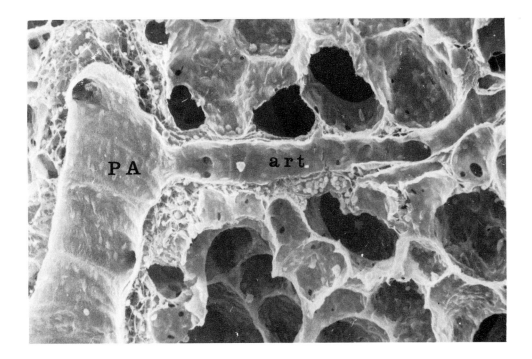

A

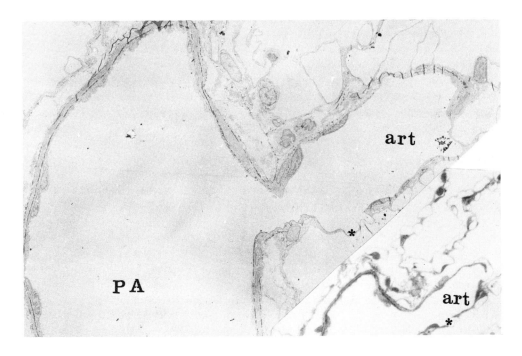

B

FIGURE 26.   The branching pattern of pulmonary ateries (Pa) into arterioles (art) and alveolar capillaries
(*) is illustrated in (A) scanning. (Magnification × 80.) (B) Transmission. (Magnification × 838.) (C) Light
micrographs. (Magnification × 400.)

to supply a number of capillaries which covered aveoli.[85] These authors also noted that a network of capillaries over an alveolar surface was supplied by several distinct terminal arterioles and each network of capillaries was in turn drained by several venules. Thus, several arterioles supply blood to a network of capillaries covering one to several aveoli which are in turn drained by several venules.

Between the pre- and postcapillary vessels, the capillaries are arranged as an interconnecting mesh of channels (see Figure 27A and B). In general, the systemic capillaries are composed of long thin tubes to form a loose mesh. In contrast, pulmonary aveolar capillaries form a dense network which is enclosed in the aveolar wall (see Figure 28). They form short segments which range from 9 to 13 μm in length and are about 8 μm in diameter (see Figures 27A and B).

1. Capillary Endothelium

The pulmonary capillary is lined by endothelial cells which rest on a continuous basal lamina (see Figure 29).[3,90,123,158,216,220] The glycoprotein basal lamina also surrounds perivascular cells (pericytes) (see Figures 31 and 34). The endothelium is extremely attenuated in those areas of the capillary which face the alveolar space (see Figures 29 and 30). The thicker area of the endothelium is occupied by the nucleus which lies adjacent to the central connective tissue septum of the alveolar wall (see Figures 29 and 30). Located in the perinuclear region are Golgi complex, centriole, mitochondria, and vesicles of various sizes, some of which contain electron-dense material (see Figure 29). A sparse distribution of mitochondria, free ribosomes, and cisternae of the endoplasmic reticulum are found in the thin sheets of endothelial cytoplasm. Microtubules and cytoplasmic filaments appear in the juxtanuclear region as well as within the attenuated regions of the endothelium (see Figure 29). Like the endothelium in the systemic circulation, the aveolar capillary endothelial surface is characterized by the presence of plasmalemmal invaginations (caveolae), over both blood and tissue fronts (see Figure 31). They are similar to the pinocytotic vesicles observed in skeletal and cardiac muscle capillaries.[144] Studies by a number of investigators have since demonstrated the passage of water-soluble molecules across the endothelium within pinocytotic vesicles[54,55,182] (*vide infra*).

Adjacent endothelial cells are held in close apposition along their lateral borders by intercellular tight junctions (see Figure 32). In ultrathin sections these areas appear as focal sites of fusion of the outer leaflets of adjacent plasmalemma. Other areas of the intercellular cleft lack these specializations, and the adjacent endothelial cells are separated by a space of approximately 4 to 6 nm in width (see Figure 31). In freeze-cleaved preparations, the junctions consist of one to several ridges or shallow grooves with discontinuities as shown in Figure 33A and B.[176,181,183]

2. Pericytes

In the systemic circulation, the pericyte is closely associated with the tissue surface of the endothelium. Scattered along the capillary wall, the pericyte is surrounded by a basal lamina which is jointly shared by the endothelium at points of close apposition between the two cells (see Figure 31). Recent studies[50,167,182] have shown highly branched pericytes within the transitional segment between capillaries and collecting venules.

In the lungs, pericytes are observed within the intimal layer in nonmuscular arteries (pulmonary arterioles) as well as the aveolar capillary wall and venules.[133,177,219] Like the pericyte in the systemic circulation, it is stellate in structure with numerous cytoplasmic projections (see Figures 31 and 34). It is surrounded by a basal lamina that is also continuous with the endothelial cell of the pulmonary vessel. The nucleus is centrally located and is surrounded by the usual compliment of cytoplasmic organelles as well as occasional filamentous components (see Figure 31).

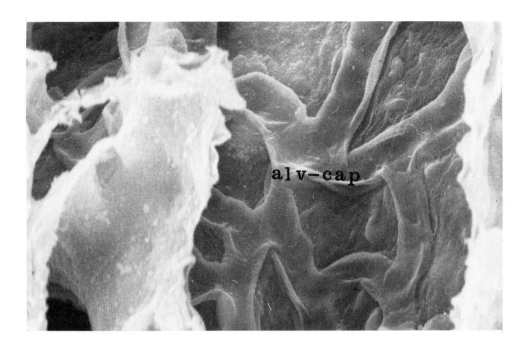

FIGURE 27A. A scanning electron micrograph illustrating the branching pattern of alveolar capillaries (alv-cap). (Magnification × 1400.)

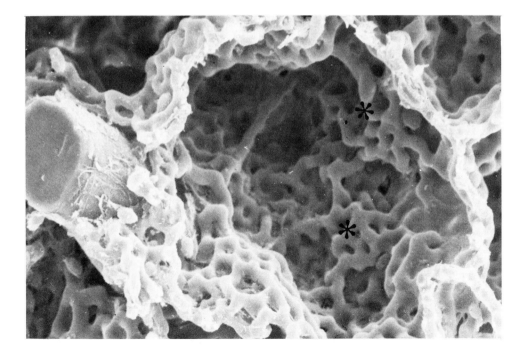

FIGURE 27B. The anastomosing of alveolar capillaries to form an elaborate network (*) within the alveolar wall is illustrated in this latex cast of the alveolar capillary network. (Magnification × 680.)

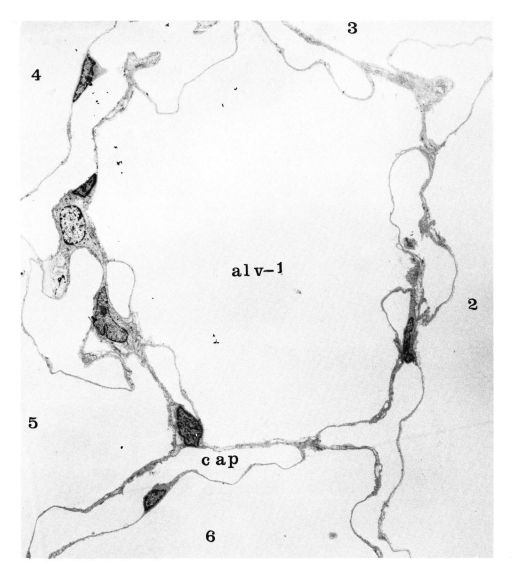

FIGURE 28.   This low-power electron micrograph shows a section through the walls of several pulmonary alveoli (alv), 1 to 6, which consists of capillary endothelial cells and epithelial cells which line the alveolar space. (Magnification × 1368.)

D. Pulmonary Venules and Veins

Receiving blood from several alveolar capillaries, pulmonary venules of about 10 μm (see Figure 16) may drain directly into muscular veins or they may increase to a vessel size of 150 μm in diameter after several anastomosis.[85] These proceed away from the bronchiole of their respiratory unit toward the interlobular septum to join the larger venous trunks.[139] The wall structure of venules and small veins is similar to the nonmuscular and smaller muscular arteries (see Figures 14B and 16B). However, their location away from the bronchial tree facilitates the identification of veins in this small size range.[11,72,209,210]

The venular wall is lined by endothelial cells which form a continuous layer (see Figure 17). The cells are flattened and folded to form a very thin tube, except at areas occupied by the nucleus which projects into the lumen. A basal lamina forms a contin-

115

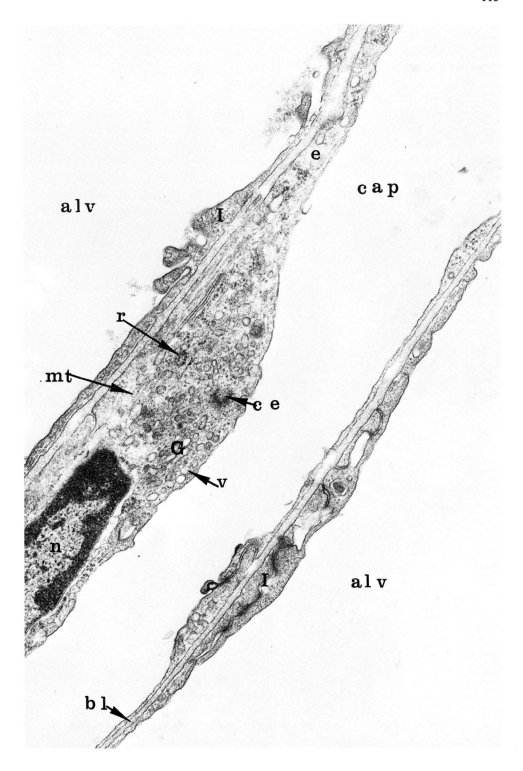

FIGURE 29. A longitudinal section of an alveolar capillary showing the accumulation of cytoplasmic organelles in the juxtanuclear region of the endothelial cells (e). Portion of Golgi apparatus (G), centriole (ce), vesicles (v), microtubules (mt) and free ribosomes (r) are illustrated. A thin basal lamina separates capillary endothelial cells from epithelial type I pneumocyte (I). (Magnification × 30,000).

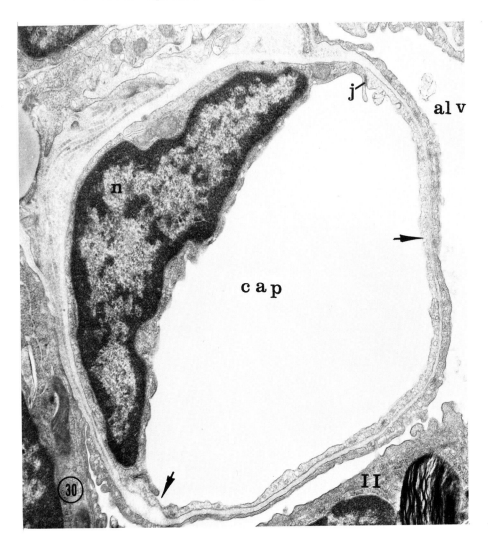

FIGURE 30.   Cross-section of alveolar capillary. The endothelial cells are held together by intercellular junctions (j) and are extremely attenuated (arrows) except in areas occupied by the nucleus (n). A small portion of a type II pneumocyte is seen in the lower part of the micrograph. (Magnification × 19,100.)

uous layer around the vessel wall. Pericytes may also be found along the connective tissue surface of the vessel and are also surrounded by a basal lamina which at some points are shared by the endothelial cell. The adventitia contains loosely arranged collagen and elastic fibers. Venules of the systemic circulation are characterized as being sensitive to a range of vasoactive substances such as histamine and serotonin.[25,83,127,222]

The intercellular junctions of systemic venules are loosely arranged as determined by the presence of discontinuities in the low-profile ridges and grooves seen in freeze-fracture replicas (see Figure 32B).[174,182] When stimulated to contract with vasoactive substances, adjacent endothelial cells of systemic venules will separate, permitting large amounts of fluids as well as large molecules and particulate substances to pass between cells and into the perivascular area.[129]

Bronchial venules in the walls of bronchi and terminal bronchioles have been shown to be selectively sensitive to vasoactive substances (i.e., histamine) which cause the bronchial venules to leak colloidal carbon into the extravascular spaces, however, bronchial tube capillaries and pulmonary small vessels were unaffected.[156,157]

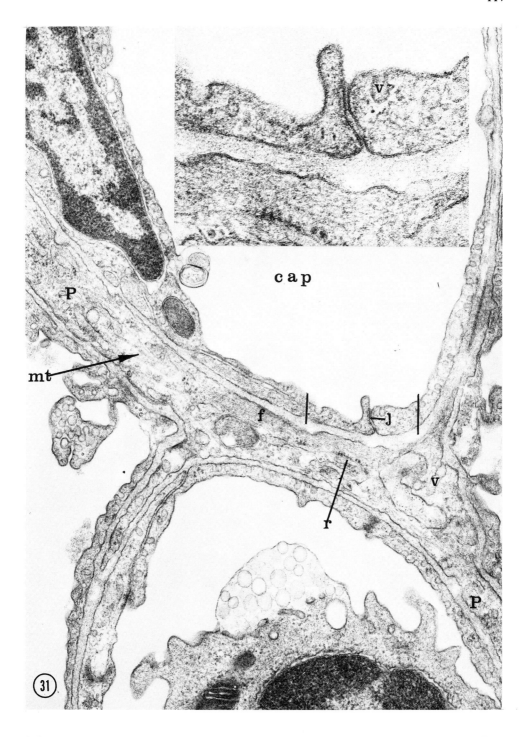

FIGURE 31.   The relationship between pericyte (P) and endothelial (e) cells of alveolar capillaries is illustrated in this electron micrograph. The cytoplasm of the pericyte contains microtubules (mt), cytoplasmic filaments (f), ribosomes attached to small segments of endoplasmic reticulum, and plasmalemmal vesicles (v). (Magnification × 36,366.) Inset in upper portion of micrograph shows enlargement of intercellular junction (j) between endothelial cells of the alveolar blood capillary wall. (Magnification × 112,860.)

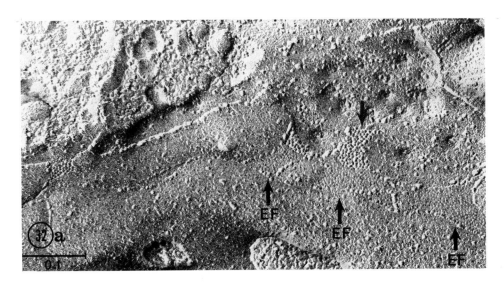

FIGURE 32A.   Tight junction and associated gap junctions in the presumed arteriolar segment of the pulmonary bed. The gap junctions appear as clusters of pits on the exoplasmic fracture (EF) face and particles on the protoplasmic fracture (PF) face between the network of tight junctions. (Magnification × 107,200.) (From Schneeberger, E. E. and Karnovsky, M. J., *Circ. Res.*, 38, 404, 1976. With permission.)

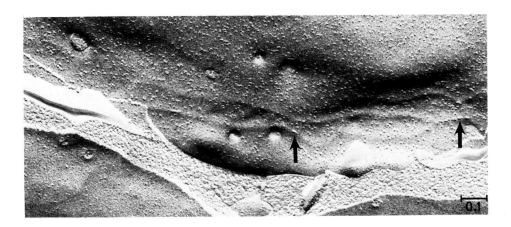

FIGURE 32B.   Endothelial junction in the presumed venular portion of the capillary bed. The junction is composed of low-profile creases on the apexes of which are few small segments of a fibril (arrow). (Magnification × 60,000.) (From Schneeberger, E. E. and Karnovsky, M. J., *Circ. Res.*, 38, 404, 1976. With permission.)

As the venules in the systemic circulation increase in diameter (beyond 100 μm in diameter), pericytes are replaced by cells that are intermediate in appearance between the pericyte and smooth muscle cells.[166] The cell is spindle in shape with a centrally placed nucleus, and the cytoplasm contains numerous filaments. Like the pericyte, the intermediate cell is also surrounded by a basal lamina which may fuse with areas in close proximity to the endothelial cells. Plasmalemmal invaginations similar to caveolae of the smooth muscle cells are also observed in the peripheral regions of the cell.

In the larger pulmonary veins, the wall also contains three basic tunics (see Figure 18). There is an intima, a media, and an adventitia. The tunica intima contains a con-

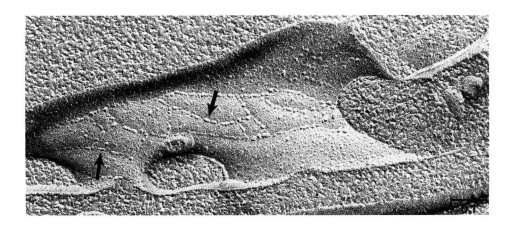

FIGURE 33A. Endothelial capillary junction in mouse lung fixed at 140 cm H_2O pressure. The junction is composed of three interconnected rows of particles. In several areas, the junctional particles appear as segments of a fibril (arrows). Several small areas of discontinuities are present. The capillary lumen is at the top and the extravascular space is at the bottom of the electron micrography (Magnification × 94,000.) (From Schneeberger, E. E. and Karnovsky, M. J., *Circ. Res.*, 38, 404, 1976. With permission.)

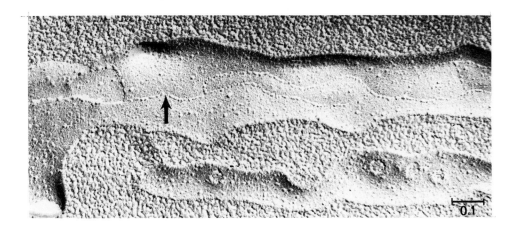

FIGURE 33B. Endothelial capillary junction composed of one and two parallel interconnected rows of particles showing a single discontinuity (arrow). (Magnification × 82,500.) (From Schneeberger, E. E. and Karnovsky, M. J., *Circ. Res.*, 38, 404, 1976. With permission.)

tinuous layer of polygonal endothelial cells which rest on a continuous basal lamina and are held together by intercellular junctions. Short cytoplasmic projections extend from the basal surfaces to form myoendothelial junctions with smooth muscle cells within the tunica media. In the main pulmonary vein, the subendothelial layer contains a mesh-work of collagen fibers and short segments of elastic fibers (see Figure 36). The tunica media is much thinner in the walls of veins than those of arteries of comparable external diameter (see Figure 18). It consists of one to several layers of smooth muscle cells that are separated by bundles of collagen fibers that are longitudinally arranged. Smooth muscle cells form gap junctions (communicating) at the terminal margins of adjacent cells. Like the smooth muscle cells in the tunica media of arteries, the close contact between adjacent smooth muscles in the form of gap junctions would also provide a means for the conduction of impulses from one cell to another within the same layer as well as between those cells in adjacent layers of the tunica media.

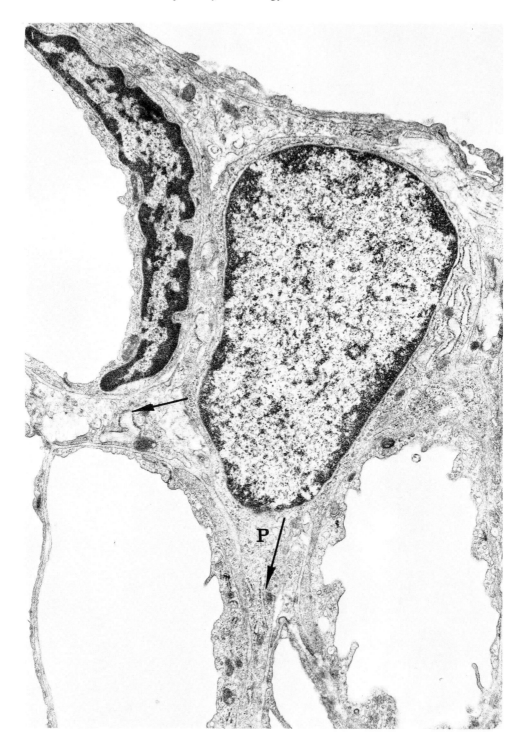

FIGURE 34.   Electron micrograph of the alveolar wall showing a pericyte (P) with cytoplasmic processes (arrows) associated with several alveolar capillaries. (Magnification × 14,730.)

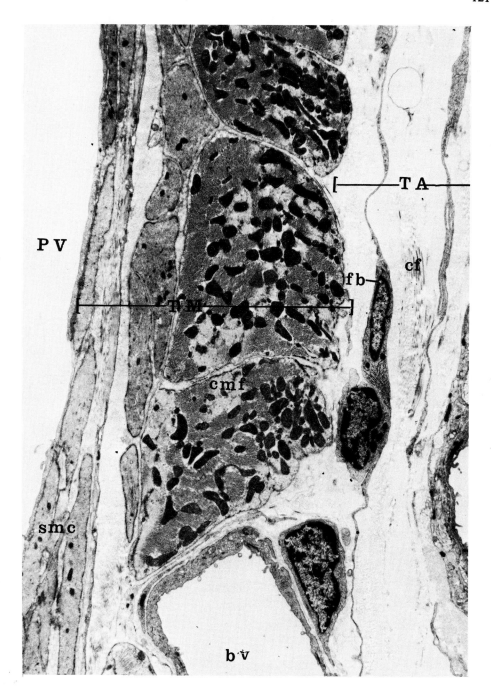

FIGURE 35.   Electron micrograph showing intrapulmonary vein (PV) whose wall contains smooth muscle cells (smc) as well as cardiac myofibers (cmf) in the tunica media (TM). A small blood vessel (bv) is interposed between two adjacent cardiac myofibers. The tunica adventitia (TA) contain fibroblast (fb) and collagen fibrils (cf). (Magnification × 7,300).

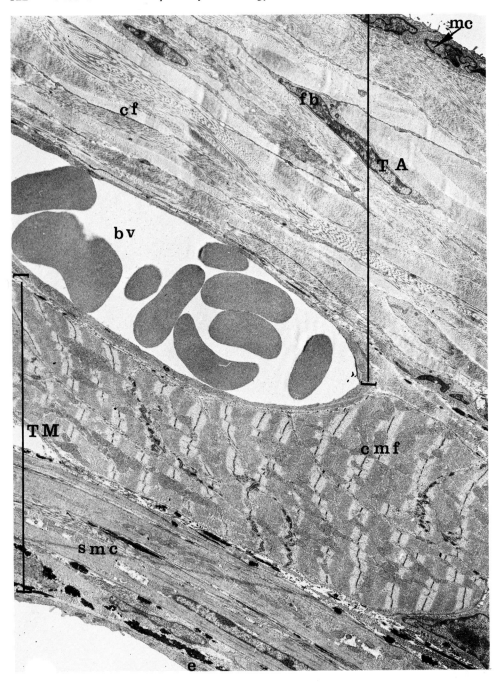

FIGURE 36.   A longitudinal section through the wall of the main pulmonary vein of the rat showing its general organization. The lumen is lined by endothelial cells (e). Both smooth muscle cells (smc) and cardiac myofibers (cm) make up the tunica media. A blood vessel (bv) is located between the tunica media and the tunica adventitia. The tunica adventitia contains bundles of collagen fibers (cf) interposed between fibroblasts (fb). Mesothelial cells (mc) line the surface of the pulmonary vein that is exposed to the mediastinum. (Magnification × 4900.)

Organelles within the smooth muscle cells share those features common to smooth muscle cells in the media of arteries and other regions of the body (see Figure 37). Like the adventitia of veins of the systemic circulation, there are large bundles of collagen fibers and a sparse distribution of elastic fibers between the bundles of collagen and fibroblasts.

In the wall of the large pulmonary veins, cardiac muscles continue from the left atrium for varying distances along its axis (see Figures 35 and 36). The cardiac muscle is separated from the tunica media by a layer of connective tissue consisting of fibroblast, collagen, and elastic fibers. Blood vessels and nerves are also found in the adventitia (see Figures 35 and 36).[11] In the major pulmonary vein, the external boundary of the adventitia is marked by a layer of mesothelial cells which contain microvilli that are exposed to the thoracic cavity (anterior mediastinum) (see Figures 36 and 38).

E. Ultrastructure of the Bronchial Vessel

A component of the systemic circulation, the bronchial vessels, reflect the high-pressure vascular system. Therefore the structural features and variations along its wall for the most part reflect those features seen in arteries, veins, and the microcirculation in other organ systems (see Figures 39 and 40).[72,194,209]

VI. PERMEABILITY OF THE PULMONARY VESSELS

Unlike other organ systems of the body, the lungs are provided with a dual blood vascular system. There is a pulmonary circulation of low pressure which delivers blood to a capillary bed that is closely exposed to alveolar air spaces. Located between blood and air spaces is an extremely thin barrier containing two attenuated cell layers (epithelial and endothelial) which are separated by a very thin connective tissue layer (see Figure 29). This arrangement provides for rapid gas exchange.[51] The bronchial circulation on the other hand has a relatively low volume of blood at systemic pressure and provides nutrients for the various pulmonary structures. This system delivers blood to a microcirculatory bed which is drained by systemic and pulmonary veins.[131,139,194]

Designed for rapid gaseous exchange over extensive areas of its length, oxygenation of blood within the macrovascular bed of the lung commences with blood vessels (arterioles) that are for the most part of a larger diameter than capillaries of other organ systems.[186] Located in the alveolar wall, the nonmuscular pulmonary artery is presumed to be capable of gaseous exchange at a speed comparable to that in the capillary wall.[133] Data from physiological studies have shown that the alveolar epithelium forms the main permeability barrier to water-soluble solutes.[37,99,191-193]

Recent studies of the intercellular junctions of alveolar epithelium have shown that tight junctions consist of continuous networks of interconnecting filaments on the protoplasmic (P), fracture face, with corresponding grooves on the complimentary particle free exoplasmic (E) fracture face.[84,174,175] The presence of several layers of ridges arranged in complex networks are considered to be characteristic of intercellular junctions which provide a tight seal between adjacent epithelial cells, while shallower bands of discontinuous ridges are correlated more with tissues that are more leaky.[21] In contrast to the alveolar epithelium, the alveolar capillary endothelium has been shown to be a highly permeable porous structure which permits the transport of various water-soluble molecules.[192,193]

Using large molecular weight substances, physiologists have been able to selectively demonstrate the movement of substances of differing molecular weights across the vascular wall.[61,66,100] Based on such physiological studies, it was suggested that the capillary endothelium is penetrated by uniform water-filled channels (i.e., pores).[100,146,147] While a number of studies have used physiological[192,193] and morpho-

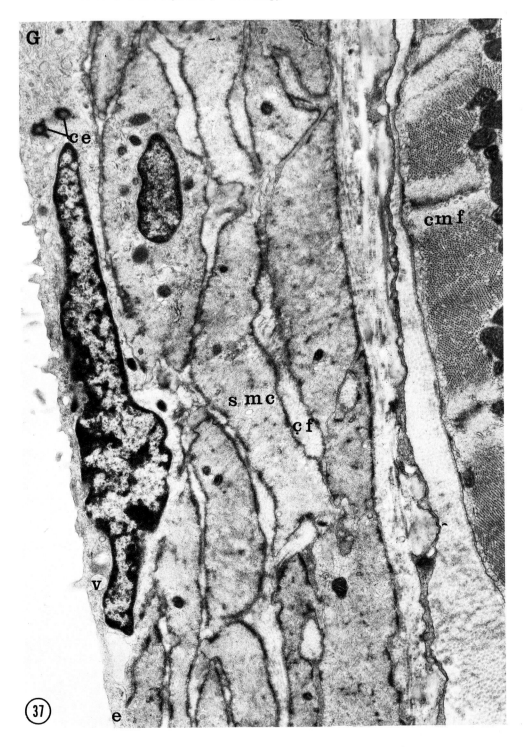

FIGURE 37.   Portion of pulmonary vein showing endothelial (e) cells whose perinuclear region contain centrioles (ce), Golgi (G) and vesicles (v) of varying sizes and densities. The smooth muscle cells of the tunica media are separated from each other by collagen fibrils (cf). A portion of a cardiac myofiber (cmf) is seen in the righthand side of the micrograph. (Magnification × 17,800.)

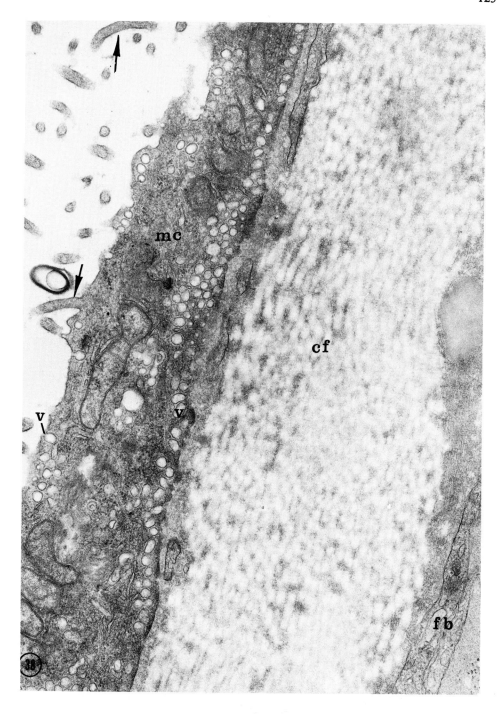

FIGURE 38. A portion of mesothelial cells (Mc) which covers the surface of the main pulmonary vein. The apical surface contains microvillus projections (arrows). Numerous plasmalemmal invaginations occur along both mediastinal and connective tissue surfaces. Bundles of collagen fibers (cf) and fibroblasts (fb) which lie underneath the mesothelial cells are continuous with the tunica adventitia of the pulmonary vein. (Magnification × 29,000.)

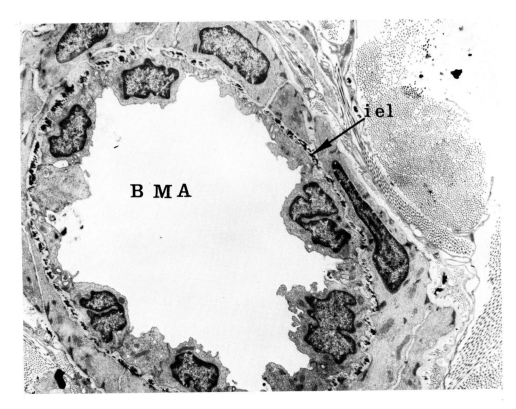

FIGURE 39.   Electron micrograph showing cross section of bronchial muscular artery (BMA). The wall structure and arrangement is similar to muscular arteries of the systemic circulation. There is a prominent internal elastic lamina (iel), but the external elastic lamina is missing. (Magnification × 4470.)

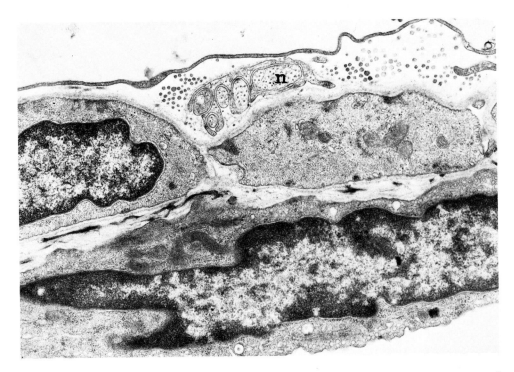

FIGURE 40.   A longitudinal section through the wall of bronchial muscular artery (BMA). A group of nerve (n) axons are located in the adventitia. (Magnification × 17,000.)

logical[13,22,89] methods to determine the structural counterpart of the small- and large-pore systems, there is still much debate as to the type of pores, their size, and distribution along the vascular wall. Electron-dense probe substances have also been used to identify the structural components of the alveolar capillary wall that are responsible for the exchange of water-soluble molecules. The results from these studies show that some endothelial junctions are permeable (see Figure 41B) to cytochrome c which has a mol wt of 12,000 daltons, while other junctions are not (see Figure 41A).[176] By increasing the hydrostatic pressure, larger tracer molecules such as horseradish peroxidase (40,000 daltons) are allowed to pass through the intercellular channels.[155]

In freeze-fracture studies of the alveolar capillary endothelium, the tight junctions between endothelial cells show one to two rows of particles with very few interconnections and rare discontinuities.[175,176] Differences have also been found in the structure of tight junctions according to various segments within the capillary bed, e.g., in the arteriolar end, up to five rows of particles are observed that are associated with gap junctions. However, at the venular end, very few junctional particles are found associated with the low P-face ridge.[176] Therefore the intercellular junctions have been identified as structures within the alveolar capillary endothelial wall whereby the exchange of water-soluble molecules can take place. In addition to permitting molecules of a size range of 1.5 nm to pass the intercellular clefts (see Figure 41B),[175] the junctions seem to be labile, since molecules of a larger molecular weight and size (40,000 daltons ae 3.0 nm) can escape through the intercellular channel when the hydrostatic pressure is increased.[155]

VII. PULMONARY LYMPHATIC VESSELS

Unlike the blood circulatory system, lymphatics provide a unidirectional drainage system which begins at the tissue lymph interface where fluids, proteins, and cells are taken up by thin-walled vessels, the lymphatic capillaries. These extend into the connective tissue spaces where they anastomose to form a rich plexus of blind-end tubes or saccules. From the capillaries, lymph is propelled into an extensive system of collecting vessels that contain specializations at strategic points in the form of lymph nodes. These structures serve as filtering devices for selectively removing antigens and other foreign substances from the lymph before it is returned to the systemic blood circulation.[33,63,70]

The lymphatic collecting vessels follow the course of arteries and veins, and the lymph that is drained from these channels enters the main lymphatic vessels of the body which are represented by the thoracic duct on the left side and one to several trunks on the right side. These open into the venous system near or at the union of the internal juglar and subclavian veins.

Earlier investigators[26,130] described pulmonary lymphatics as consisting of two categories of vessels, a superficial system which is distributed within the pulmonary pleura and a system of deep vessels located in the intrapulmonary tissues. In subsequent studies, Miller[139] classified pulmonary lymphatics according to their regional distribution (i.e., pleural, peribronchial, perivascular, and septal). Although significant information regarding pulmonary lymphatics was obtained during the first part of the 20th century, there was also disagreement regarding the normal direction of lymph flow within the interlobular septum and toward the periphery of the lung from the pleura to the hilus, or whether the lymph traveled over the surface of the lung within the pleural lymphatics directly to the hilus. There was also disagreement regarding the existence, number, and distribution of valves within pulmonary lymphatic vessels within the deeper portions of the lung. While a number of the earlier studies suggested the existence of alveolar lymphatic vessels,[42,195] more recent studies at the ultrastruc-

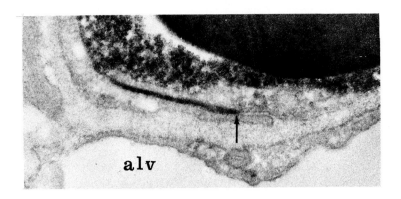

FIGURE 41A.   Alveolar capillary of mouse lung injected with cytochrome $\mathcal{C}$ in 0.05 mℓ saline 1 min before the animal was sacrificed. The reaction product occurs within the endothelial cleft but is prevented from entering into the basement membrane by a narrow area within the junction (arrow). (Magnification × 50,000.) (From Schneeberger, E. E., *Ultrastructural Basis for Alveolar Capillary Permeability to Protein in Lung Liquids,* Ciba Foundation Symposium, American Elsevier, New York, 1976, 38. With permission.)

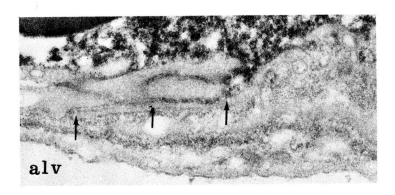

FIGURE 41B.   Alveolar capillary from the same animal as in 41A showing a small amount of reaction product throughout the length of the endothelial junction (arrows). In addition, the reaction product is also within the basal lamina. The alveolar space (alv) is at the bottom of the electron micrograph. (Magnification × 50,000.) (From Schneeberger, E. E., *Ultrastructural Basis for Alveolar Capillary Permeability to Protein in Lung Liquids,* Ciba Foundation Symposium, American Elsevier, New York, 1976, 38. With permission.)

tural level have failed to confirm their presence in the walls of alveoli, but have demonstrated lymphatics extending to the terminal bronchioles adjacent to alveoli.[102,103,105,107,115]

A. Organization and Distribution of Pulmonary Lymphatics

1. Pleural Lymphatics

In the earlier studies of pulmonary lymphatics, two major plexuses of lymphatics were described, a superficial layer and a deep one. The pleural lymphatic vessels were depicted as an elaborate plexus consisting of an irregular interconnecting meshwork of vessels located within the superficial layer of the lung.[170,172,224] Subsequent studies by Miller[138] showed that the pleura was composed of a thin mesothelial layer resting on an elastic layer and an underlying alveolar layer. In these studies, Miller[138,139] observed that the superficial lymphatics were located within the submesothelial connective tissue layer. In man and larger animals, this layer of connective tissue is very thick, with the lymphatics extending throughout its full thickness; thus, a superficial and a deep layer can be found in the pleural lymphatics in these animals. Using dyes to label pulmonary lymphatics, Cruikshank[26] observed that the pleural lymphatics were rapidly filled and communicated freely with each other over the surface of the lung. Using combined injection and serial section methods, Miller[138,139] demonstrated that the pleural lymphatics were organized into a wide mesh-work, with many of the interconnecting vessels sending out sidebranches which terminated as blind-end tubes or saccules.

Radiologic methods permit the visualization of both superficial and deep lymphatics in the intact lung (see Figure 42A). In addition, the three-dimensional topography and organization of both pleural and deep lymphatics provide useful information in clinical diagnosis involving disease of the lung.[28,93] For the larger lymphatics, this method also permits a delineation of the lymphatic valves (see Figure 42B) which are regularly spaced along the collecting lymphatics. Valves in the pleural vessels were observed to point in all directions, suggesting a "free circulation" of lymph within the confines of the pleura, precluding the drainage of lymph into the deeper lymphatics of the lung.[138] With improved radiologic methods, Trapnell[201] demonstrated that valves in the interlobular lymphatics pointed away from the pleura and toward the hilus in the normal and in cases of lymphangitis, carcinomatosis.

Although a back-and-forth movement of injected dyes has been shown to occur between the deep and the pleural lymphatics, convincing data are provided which indicate that the normal direction of lymph flow in the interlobular lymphatics is away from the pleura and toward the hilum.[77,88,154,179]

2. Interlobular Lymphatics

Closely associated with veins in the interlobular septum is an extensive plexus of lymphatics.[27,41,143,179,197,229] These lymphatic channels form an elaborate network which surrounds each secondary lobule that is demarcated by the connective tissue septum (see Figures 43A and B). Following the injection of colloidal carbon into pleural lymphatics of the fetal lung, the interlobular septa were shown to be spaced at regular intervals of about 1 mm from each other. The lymphatics within each septum drained carbon from the pleural network toward lymphatic vessels which surrounded blood vessels and the bronchial tree. A similar topographical arrangement between lymphatics and the pulmonary vein is retained in the adult lung.[141]

3. Intrapulmonary Lymphatics

Within the deeper regions of the lung and closely associated with the parenchyma, an elaborate network of lymphatics sprial around bronchi, arteries, and veins (see Figure 44A and B). In studies of the fetal lung, Cunningham[27] showed that the deep lymphatics were shared by bronchi and arteries, however, with postnatal development of the lung, two separate lymphatic plexuses become differentiated. One becomes closely associated with the bronchial tree, while the other becomes closely associated with arteries. Although forming two distinct plexuses, the vessels are connected at the branching of bronchi and also along the length of the bronchial tree.[139] In the large bronchial wall, a network of lymphatics occurs between the muscular and epithelial layer (see Figure 44). A second layer is found within the connective tissue of the adventitia and around the cartilagenous plates of the bronchi (see Figure 44A). These two layers of lymphatics are connected by means of anastomosing branches which bridge the connective tissue areas between the cartilagenous plates. As the walls of bronchi decrease in diameter, the two plexuses gradually merge to form one layer of lymphatics

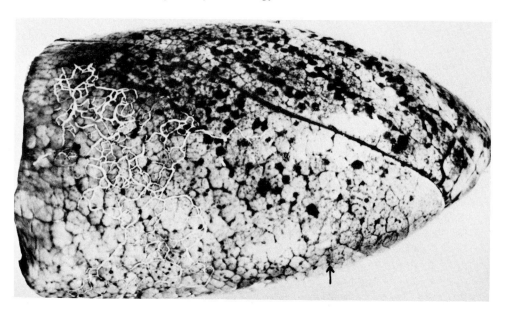

FIGURE 42A.   The distribution of pleural lymphatics over the lower lobe of the human lung is shown in this micrograph. (From Trapnell, D. H., *Br. J. Radiol.*, 36, 660, 1963. With permission.)

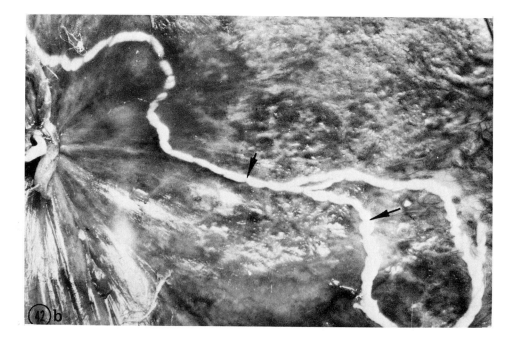

FIGURE 42B.   Pleural lymphatics showing the position of valves (arrows) as indicated by the constrictions along the length of the vessel. (From Trapnell, D. H., *Br. J. Radiol.*, 36, 660, 1963. With permission.)

(see Figure 44B). The reduction in wall diameter with repeated branching of bronchioles is also reflected in the size and distribution of the surrounding lymphatics.

Prior to the application of electron microscopy, the question regarding the extent to which pulmonary lymphatics extend to the peripheral lung still remained a subject of considerable debate. For example, extensive and detailed studies of Miller[139] suggested that lymphatics ended at the level of alveolar ducts, while Tobin[195] suggested that the pulmonary lymphatics which surround branches of arteries and venules extend to the alveolar wall. However, more recent studies have demonstrated that lymphatics are closely associated with the bronchial tree and pulmonary blood vessels down to the level of the respiratory bronchiole and its adjacent arterioles (see Figure 45).[73,103-105,107,115]

By using the combined methods of intravascular and intratracheal profusions, the distended state of pulmonary lymphatics and blood vessels is maintained.[115] In addition, the three-dimensional relationship of pulmonary interstitial components is also preserved. With the double prefusion technique, pulmonary lymphatic capillaries as well as lymphatic collection vessels are easily recognized in routine 1-μm-thick epon sections observed at the light optic level (see Figure 44A and B) and ultrathin sections observed in the transmission electron microscope (see Figure 45). Using such preparative techniques, the precise organization and morphology of lymphatics in the pleura, interlobular septum peribronchial, and perivascular areas can be identified and routinely observed.

In the light microscope, images of the lymphatic capillaries are recognized as vessels with an irregular caliber, a large lumen relative to the thickness of the endothelial wall, an extremely thin wall, and a lumen free of blood cells. In the prefused specimens, the presence of a protein precipitate within the vessel lumen provides an additional criterion for the identification of lymphatic vessels (see Figures 45 and 46).

Although lymphatic capillaries develop secondarily to major lymphatic trunks and collecting lymphatics, the functional activity begins with lymphatic capillaries. Indeed, it is the thin-walled lymphatic capillary which serves as the major site for the passage of interstitial fluids and large molecules into this one-way drainage system. While such terms as terminal, initial, and primary lymphatics have been used to describe this segment of the lymphatic vascular tree, the term capillary was used by both physiologists and morphologists to denote blood vessels whose walls provided for the rapid exchange of fluids and metabolites between the vessel and its adjoining connective tissue area.[5,20,95,97,230] Therefore, the term lymphatic capillary seems more appropriate as it reflects both the morphology and functional properties of this segment of the lymphatic system.

B. Morphology of the Lymphatic Capillary Wall

The lymphatic capillary is composed of endothelial cells. Although extremely attenuated over large areas of the vessel wall, the cells form a continuous lining (see Figures 45 and 46). The nucleus occupies a central position within the cell and produces a bulge which characteristically projects into the lumen (see Figure 45). The thin region of the cytoplasm measures 50 to 100 nm in thickness, while the thicker nuclear region measures up to 3 μm in width. The plasmalemma contains numerous invaginations (caveolae or pinocytotic vesicles) along its luminal and connective tissue fronts (See Figure 48A). In addition, vesicles also appear free in the thicker regions of the cytoplasm. The usual complement of cytoplasmic organelles are also present, many of which are organized around the nucleus and in close proximity to the golgi complex and centrioles (see Figure 48A).

Closely associated with the forming and mature faces of the golgi complex are vesicles of various sizes whose content exhibit varying degrees of electron densities. The

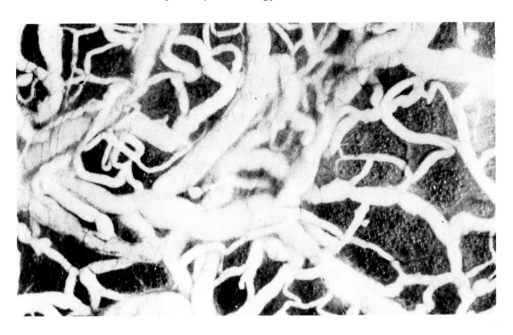

FIGURE 43A. This micrograph shows the rich supply of pulmonary lymphatic vessels obtained from a corrosion cast. (From Lauweryns, J. M., *Pathol. Annu.,* 4, 125, 1971. With permission.)

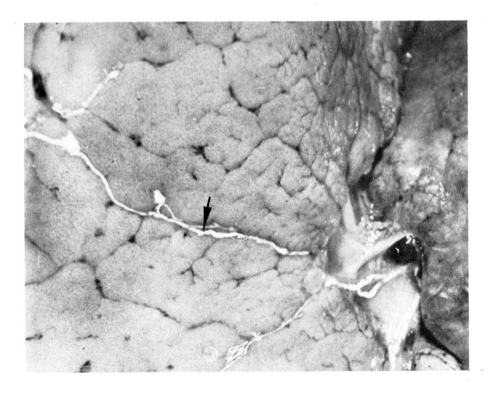

FIGURE 43B. The location of collecting lymphatics along the interlobular septum (arrow) is shown in this micrograph. (From Lauweryns, J. M., *Pathol. Annu.,* 4, 125, 1971. With permission.)

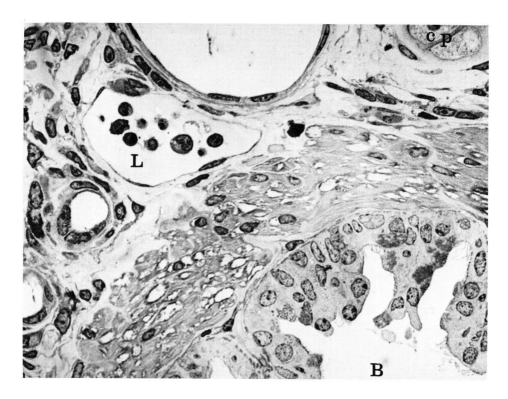

FIGURE 44A.   Light micrograph showing lymphatic vessels (L) in the adventitia of bronchus (B). The lumen of the lymphatic contains small and large lymphocytes. The lumen of the blood vessels are free of plasma and cells as the result of the perfusion fixation. A portion of a cartilage plate (cp) is seen in the upper right-hand corner of the micrograph. (Magnification × 302.) (From Leak, L. V., *Respiratory Defense Mechanisms,* Brain, J. D., Proctor, D. F., and Reid, L. M., Eds., Marcel Dekker, New York, 1977, 361. With permission.)

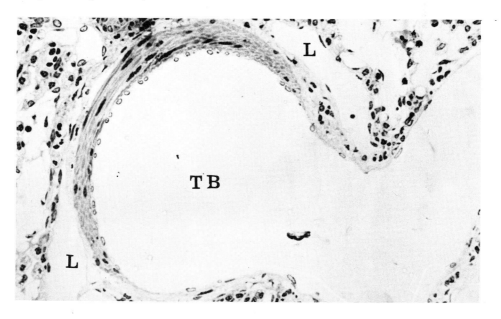

FIGURE 44B.   This micrograph shows the location of lymphatics (L) in relation to a terminal bronchiole (Tb) and adjacent alveoli. (Magnification × 188.) (From Leak, L. V., *Respiratory Defense Mechanisms,* Brain, J. D., Proctor, D. F., and Reid, L. M., Eds., Marcel Dekker, New York, 1977, 361. With permission.)

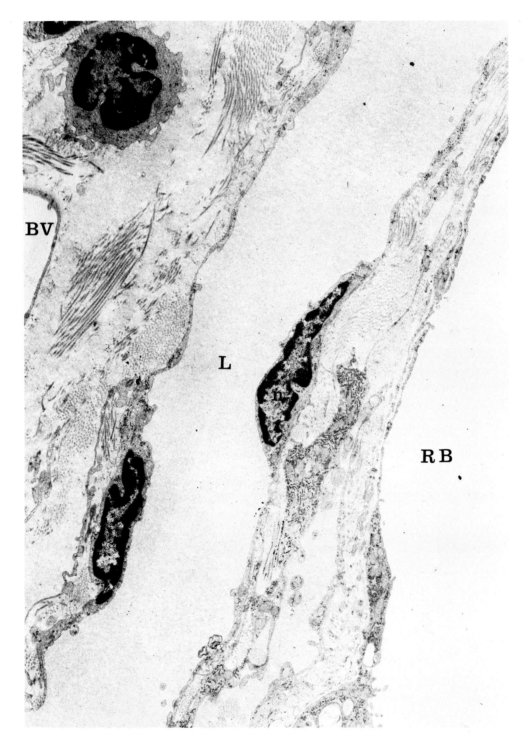

FIGURE 45.   An electron micrograph showing the relationship between pulmonary lymphatic (L) and a respiratory bronchiole (RB). The lymphatic lumen contains a gray flocculent percipitate and is lined by a continuous endothelium which is extremely attenuated except for areas occupied by the nuclear (n) regions. Small portion of a blood vessel (BV) is shown in the upper left-hand corner of the micrograph. (Magnification × 7980.) (From Leak, L. V., *Respiratory Defense Mechanisms*, Brain, J. D., Proctor, D. F., and Reid, L. M., Eds., Marcel Dekker, New York, 1977, 361. With permission.)

demonstration of acid phosphatase activity within vesicles in the vicinity of the Golgi confirms the presence of lysosomes in the lymphatic endothelial cells. Such vesicles have an electron-dense central core and have been shown to reach the size of autophagic vacuoles in the regressing tailfin of amphibians.[110] Studies of Weber[214] demonstrated that the occurrence of autophagic vacuoles coincided with an increase in soluble acid hydrolases in cytoplasmic particles of the regressing tailfin. It was suggested that these structures played an important role in the intracellular digestion of engulfed substances that were removed from the surrounding interstitium during tailfin resorption.[110]

The endoplasmic reticulum is represented by a few randomly dispersed cisternae with attached ribosomes (see Figure 46). These are generally seen in the perinuclear region, but may also be observed in the thin areas of the cytoplasm. Ribosomes are also free throughout the cytoplasm as clusters of polyribosomes (see Figure 48A). The paucity of endoplasmic reticulum would indicate that lymphatic endothelial cells like those of the blood vascular system are engaged in only a moderate production of synthetic activity which is mainly geared for maintenance of the cell.

Mitochondria occur throughout the juxtanuclear areas and small numbers populate the attenuated rim of cytoplasm. They present oval and elongated profiles and display an internal structural arrangement in common with the mitochondria of other cells. The outer membrane exhibits a smooth contour while the inner membrane is invaginated into the matrix to form cristae (see Figure 46).

Microtubules are found in the vicinity of the cell center, in close proximity to centrioles. They are approximately 25 nm in diameter and are also found in other areas of the cytoplasm generally aligned parallel to the long axis of the endothelial cell.

The endothelial cells are characterized by the presence of cytoplasmic filaments which measure 4 to 6 nm in diameter. They are usually arranged parallel to the long axis of the cell and appear in discrete bundles or fasicles throughout the cytoplasm (see Figure 48B).

Recent studies of Lauwyrens et al.[107,108] demonstrated that cytoplasmic filaments within the lymphatic endothelial cells in the lungs were capable of forming arrowhead complexes with heavy meromyosin, suggesting the presence of actin. Such a contractile system within the lymphatic capillary endothelial cells would provide a mechanism for the active regulation of the intercellular clefts between adjacent cells and thus play an active role in regulating the permeability of the lymphatic capillary wall.

The rhythmic contraction noted for the larger lymphatic collecting vessels can be attributed to smooth muscle cells within the tunica media of their walls.[53,71,81,94,212,213] and like the smooth muscle in the media of arteries and veins are also under neurological control, as indicated by the closely applied nerve axons.

In studies of lymphatic capillaries in other regions of the body using cinephotographic methods, lymphatic capillaries were observed to undergo rhythmic contractions.[112] Since the smooth muscle cells are absent from the walls of lymphatic capillaries, it is suggested that the cytoplasmic filaments represent the intrinsic contractile components responsible for the rhythmic contractions in these vessels.

Pulmonary lymphatic capillaries are also distinguished by the presence of numerous plasmalemmal invaginations that extend into the cytoplasm for varying distances along its luminal as well as abluminal surfaces (Figure 47A and 48A). Appearing in the periphery as well as the deeper regions of the cytoplasm, the vesicles often appear to be in transit across the lymphatic endothelium. These vesicles are of a similar dimension to the micropinocytotic vesicles (approximately 75 nm in diameter) that occur in the endothelial cells of blood vessels.[12,144,145,165]

In efforts to determine the role of these vesicles in the transendothelial movement of water-soluble molecules, various electron-dense trace substances have been used to

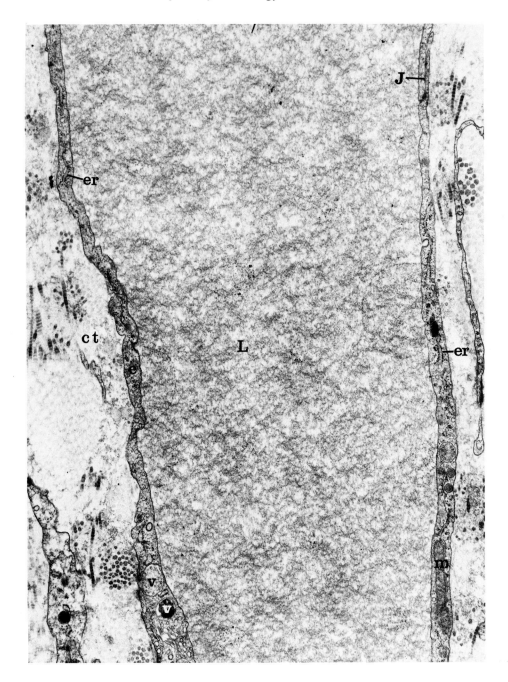

FIGURE 46.   Longitudinal section of pulmonary lymphatic capillaries showing the extremely attenuated endothelial (e) cells which contain mitochondria (m), endoplasmic reticulum (er), vesicles (v) of varying sizes and densities. An intercellular junction (J) is shown in the upper right-hand portion of micrograph. The endothelial cells are held in close apposition to the surrounding connective tissue area (Ct). (Magnification × 17,800.)

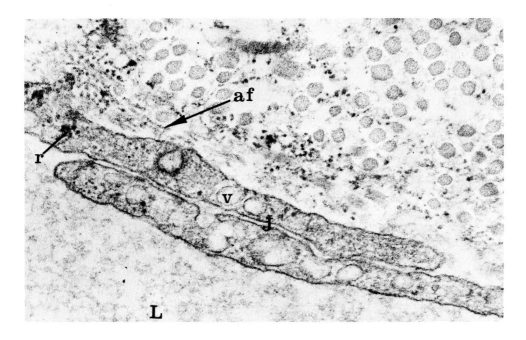

A

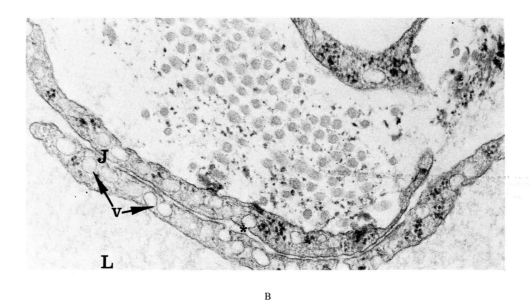

B

FIGURE 47. Adjacent endothelial cells overlap for long distances to form intercellular junctions (J), with a resulting intercellular cleft whose width may vary considerably over the length of the junction. While the endothelial cells lack a continuous basal lamina, filamentous elements which represent the anchoring filaments (af) can be seen along the abluminal surface of the endothelial cells. Plasmalemmal vesicles (v) are also seen in the cell margins. (A: Magnification × 70,200.) (B: Magnification × 50,160.) In (C) the intercellular junction is patent (*). (Magnification × 23,600.)

follow the movement of both water-soluble and inert substances across the lymphatic endothelial cells.[16,112,116] Such studies indicate that particles are removed from both luminal and connective tissue fronts within vesicles and may aggregate into large vacuoles within the endothelium. This is evidenced by the accumulation of inert particles such as carbon and thorium dioxide into aggregates within vacuoles that may reach several microns in diameter and can be observed up to 12 months following intercellular injections of the particles. These tracer experiments indicate that vesicular transport is not unidirectional in the lymphatic capillary endothelial cells, but that the transport of large molecules and proteins within vesicles proceeds from both luminal and connective tissue fronts toward the central cytoplasm.[112] Here the smaller vesicles become fused with lysosomal vacuoles that contain hydrolytic enzymes for intracellular digestion.[30,31] Exogenous protein, such as peroxidase and ferritin, that accumulate in large lysosomal vacuoles are broken down into smaller units within 18 to 24 hr, presumably for utilization by the cells.[13,57,62,164] This, however, is not the case for the inert substances, such as colloidal carbon, thorium, and latex spheres which are injected interstitially and accumulate into very large vacuoles which remain in the cells for an indefinite period.[112]

1. Intercellular Junctions of the Lymphatic Capillary

Lymphatic capillary endothelial cells are held in close apposition by intercellular junctions in which the adjacent cell margins are extensively overlapped (see Figures 47A and 47B). The adjacent cells may be separated by distances as great as several microns which may extend the total length of the intercellular cleft between the adjacent cells (see Figure 47C). Such openings represent patent intercellular junctions that are unique to this segment of the lymphatic vascular system (i.e., lymphatic capillaries). The intercellular cleft in these instances represent open passageways through which large molecules, particulate substances, and cells may enter the lymphatic lumen. However, there are also many areas along the length of the lymphatic capillary wall in which the adjacent plasma membranes are closely approximated. At such, regions, apposed membranes are held together by *maculae adherentes* or desmosomes, in which case, the distance between apposing cells may range from 10 to 25 nm in width. Occasionally, there are areas of close apposition in which short segments of the intercellular cleft are obliterated thus preventing the passage of tracer molecules such as lanthanum and peroxidase; these short segments appear as intermittent seals within the intercellular cleft that are formed by a fusion between the outer leaflets of adjacent cell membranes and are recognized as quintuple structures which represent *maculae occludentes*. While many of the adjacent cells may be loosely apposed to each other, the specialized sites (i.e., *maculae occludentes*) would serve to maintain a firm adhesion of adjacent cells without causing a complete obliteration along the total length of the intercellular cleft, providing instead, a spot-welled effect for maintaining a close continuity between cells along the total length of the lymphatic capillary wall. Therefore, many of the adjacent cell margins may remain loosely apposed to each other and are free to separate to form patent channels. Such areas would be readily available to accommodate the rapid and continuous passage of excess amounts of interstitial fluids and cells from the interstitium into the lymphatic capillary lumen.

2. Lymphatic Capillary Anchoring Filaments

The extracellular components of the lymphatic capillary wall consist of short segments of basal lamina interspersed between anchoring filaments. The anchoring filaments are in close association with elastic fibers and collagen fibers that are in intimate contact with the endothelial surface (see Figure 47A). The filaments range from 6 to 10 nm in diameter and insert within a densely staining substance on the external surface

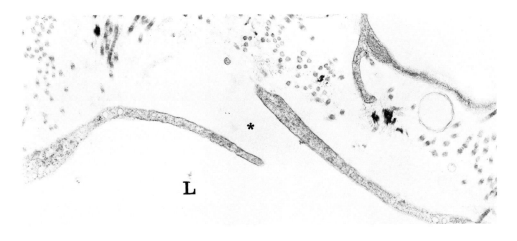

FIGURE 47C

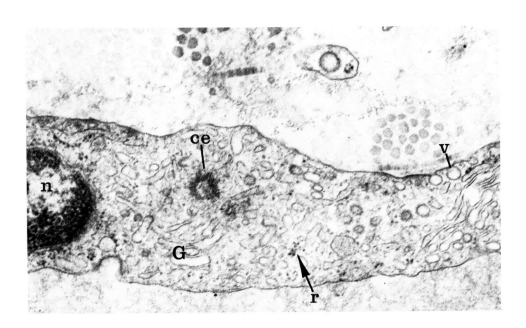

FIGURE 48A. Longitudinal section of lymphatic endothelial cell showing part of nucleus (n), ribosomes (r), portion of Golgi aparatus (G), and the closely associated centriole (ce). Vesicles (V) occur along lumen and connective tissue fronts. (Magnification × 38,350.)

of the unit membrane. They extend for various distances into the adjoining interstitium between collagen bundles and connective tissue cells (see Figure 48C).

The term lymphatic-anchoring filaments was used to describe these structures because of their topographical relationship to the lymphatic capillary wall and the surrounding connective tissue components.[117] Such an arrangement would prevent collapse of the lymphatic capillary wall by stabilizing and anchoring the lymphatic endothelial cells to the closely adjoining connective tissue areas in which the anchoring filaments are firmly embedded. Although not found in the alveolar wall or septum, the lymphatic capillaries are located within the interstitium in close topographical relation to the alveolar space (saccule) and are separated from the air spaces by the

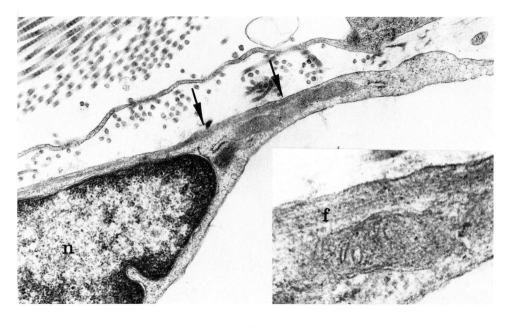

B

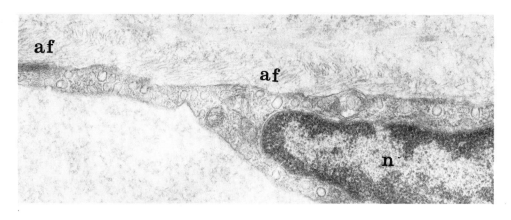

C

FIGURE 48 B and C.   Electron micrograph of lymphatic capillary endothelium showing distribution of cytoplasmic filaments (arrows). (Magnification × 18,800; inset × 75,240.) In (C) anchoring filaments (af) are shown along abluminal surface. (Magnification × 31,920.)

alveolar wall and a thin band of connective tissue. Occasionally small blood capillaries are interposed between lymphatic and alveolar saccules (see Figure 49). Lymphatic vessels situated in close proximity to the alveolar wall were described as juxtalveolar lymphatic capillaries,[103-105] and subsequent studies of lung lymphatics in our laboratory revealed a similar relationship between lymphatics and the alveolar space.[115]

C. Pulmonary Collecting Lymphatic Vessels

The lymphatic capillary drains into vessels of increasing diameter and wall thickness. Proximal to the terminal bronchioles, the thickness and complexity of the adjoining connective tissue sleeve around the peribronchial and perivascular lymphatics become more elaborate (see Figure 50).

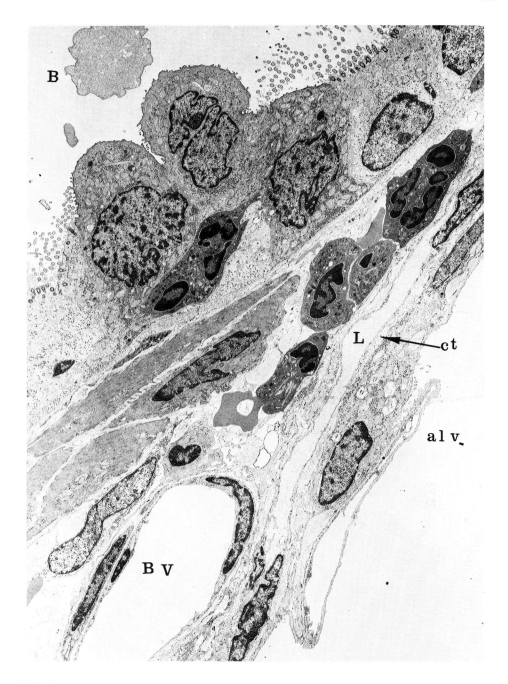

FIGURE 49. This electron micrograph shows a juxta-alveolar lymphatic vessel (L) that is separated from the alveolar space by a thin band of connective tissue (ct) and epithelial cells lining the alveolar space (alv). The lymphatic vessel lies in close proximity to a blood vessel (Bv) which is also in the connective tissue sleeve of the bronchiole (B). (Magnification × 4742.)

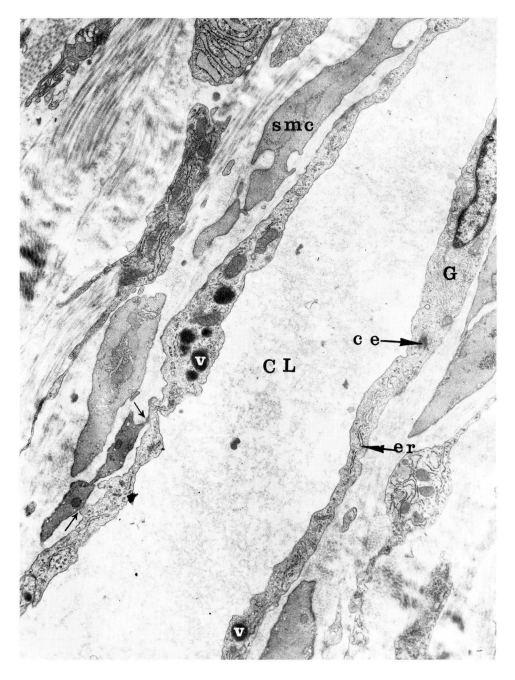

FIGURE 50.   A longitudinal section through a collecting lymphatic vessel (CL) — the endothelial cells
contain electron-dense vesicles (v) as well as the usual complement of cellular organelles such as endoplasmic
reticulum (er), centriole (ce), and Golgi (G) which lies in the perinuclear region. The wall contains an incomplete layer of smooth muscle cells (smc), several of which come in close contact with the connective tissue
surface of the endothelial cells (arrow) to form myoendothelial junctions. (Magnification × 10,500.) (From
Leak, L. V., *Respiratory Defense Mechanisms,* Brain, J. D., Proctor, D. F., and Reid, L. M., Eds., Marcel
Dekker, New York, 1977, 361. With permission.)

Similar to collecting lymphatic vessels in other organs, the pulmonary collecting lymphatic wall is characterized by the presence of three tunics: an intima, a media, and an adventitia. The collecting lymphatic is also distinguished by the presence of valves which appear to be more numerous than those in large veins of the extremities. In common with the valves of veins, they project into the lumen in the direction of fluid flow. This arrangement allows for free and rapid passage of lymph toward the major lymphatic trunks in a continuous and unidirectional flow.

1. Tunica Intima

With a large diameter and thicker wall, the collecting lymphatics are lined by endothelial cells which are held in close apposition by *maculae adherentes*. There are numerous plasmalemmal vesicles along the luminal and tissue surface of the vessel, and the unusual complement of organelles such as mitochondria, Golgi complex, and endoplasmic reticulum are also observed in the cytoplasm (see Figure 50). A population of cytoplasmic filaments and microtubules is also distributed throughout the cytoplasm.

In segments of collecting lymphatics that are in close proximity to the lymphatic capillary, short strands of basal lamina are observed. Since a continuous basal lamina is usually found underlying endothelial cells in collecting lymphatics, it is presumed that such areas represent a transitional zone between the lymphatic capillary and the larger lymphatic collection vessels. Closely apposed to the basal lamina are strands of elastic and collagen fibers that separate the endothelial cells from the adjoining layer of smooth muscles within the tunica media.

2. Tunica Media

The tunica media of collecting vessels consists of smooth muscle cells that may be arranged in a discontinuous layer of cells that are coiled around the vessel or there may be several complete layers of smooth muscle cells (see Figure 50). Like the smooth muscle cells in the media of large blood vessels, they are fusiform cylinders with tapering ends and are connected at their marginal ends by gap junctions. Cell processes extend from the lateral borders of smooth muscle cells to make contact with the endothelial cells of the lymphatic wall to form myoendothelial junctions (see Figure 51). The nucleus occupies a central portion of the cell which is also the area of its greatest dimension; located in the perinuclear region are the Golgi complex, centrioles, mitochondria, and cisternae of the endoplasmic reticulum and numerous vesicles that are closely associated with the Golgi complex.

3. Tunica Adventitia

The outermost layer surrounding the collecting vessels consists of fibroblasts that appear in close relation to bundles of collagen fibers that surround the smooth muscle cells. Occasionally, small blood vessels and nonmylenated nerve axons are also seen in the outermost layer of the wall of collecting lymphatic vessels.

D. Lymphatic Valves

In appropriate sections through the lymphatic collecting vessels, the valves appear as leaflets of endothelial cells which extend from the wall of the collecting vessels and project into the lumen as folds. The endothelial folds are separated by a narrow band of connective tissue (see Figure 51B). This narrow band consists of collagen and elastic fibers and an occasional fibroblast which may cause apposing endothelial cells to be widely separated from each other. The smooth muscle cells of the tunica media are excluded from this intervening band of connective tissue.

When appropriate areas of the lymphatic vessels are examined in the scanning elec-

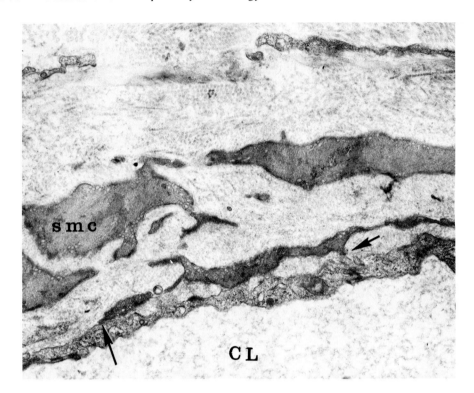

FIGURE 51A.   This electron micrograph shows a portion of wall from a collecting lymphatic (CL) vessel in which smooth muscle cells come in close contact with the lymphatic endothelial cells at several locations (arrows) to form myoendothelial junctions. (Magnification × 12,300.) (From Leak, L. V., *Respiratory Defense Mechanisms,* Brain, J. D., Proctor, D. F., and Reid, L. M., Eds., Marcel Dekker, New York, 1977, 361. With permission.)

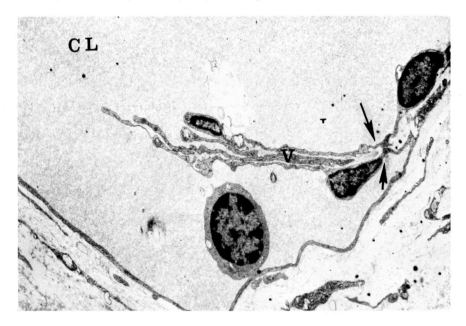

FIGURE 51B.   Electron micrograph showing a segment of a valve (v) from a lymphatic collecting vessel. (Magnification × 6380.) (From Leak, L. V., *Respiratory Defense Mechanisms,* Brain, J. D., Proctor, D. F., and Reid, L. M., Eds., Marcel Dekker, New York, 1977, 361. With permission.)

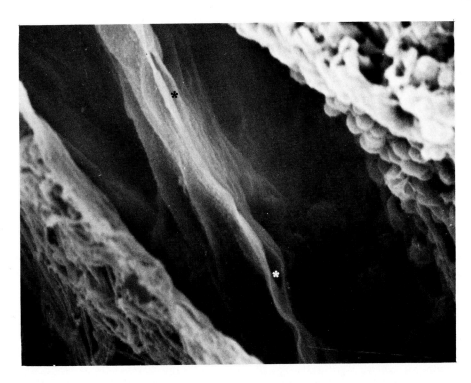

FIGURE 52A.   Scanning electron micrograph showing lymphatic valves of a collecting vessel in which the leaflets are partially separated (*). (Magnification × 1320.)

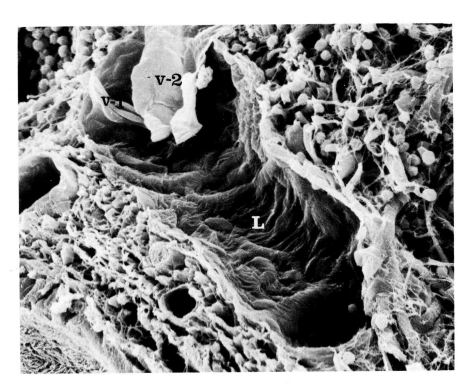

FIGURE 52B.   Scanning electron micrograph showing anastomosis of several lymphatic vessels and the position of valves at the junction of these vessels (arrow V1, V2). (Magnification × 720.) (om Leak, L. V., *Respiratory Defense Mechanisms,* Brain, J. D., Proctor, D. F., and Reid, L. M., Eds., Marcel Dekker, New York, 1977, 361. With permission.)

tron microscope, it is evident that the lining endothelium is reduplicated as a ring which encircles the lumen of the vessel to form paired leaflets (see Figure 52A). They consist of two thin cusps whose surfaces are lined with flattened endothelial cells. The medial borders of the adjacent leaflets are fused at the periphery for a short distance as they emerge from the vessel wall. Therefore the apposing leaflets are free to separate in the center of the vessel, allowing a free flow of fluids along the axis of the vessel. The free borders are covered with flattened endothelial cells. Both leaflets project into the lumen at an angle such that their free edges fit together as a miter joint without fusing with each other (see Figures 52A and B). Immediately adjacent to the point of insertion of the paired leaflets, the lymphatic wall of the collecting vessel is expanded into a sinuous or pouch. This bulging is responsible for the numerous outpouchings seen along the length of the vessel, giving the vessel a beaded appearance when it is fully dilated. The scanning electron microscopic image of the leaflet depicts endothelial cells that are uniformly distributed over its surfaces. The endothelial cells rest on a basal lamina that continues into the connective tissue around endothelial cells of the vessel wall. The cytoplasm of the endothelial cells which comprise the valve leaflet contain numerous filaments in contrast to the small amount of filaments noted in cells of the collecting lymphatic vessel wall. The presence of numerous cytoplasmic filaments within the endothelial cells of the valve leaflet suggest that these structures play an important contractile function, especially since an orifice must periodically open and close for a smooth and continuous flow of lymph and cells to the larger lymphatics upstream.

Lymphatic valves were described by Lauweryns and co-workers as a simple cone- or funnel-shaped structure which is longitudinally suspended in the lumen of the vessel with an opening at the deepest point of the funnel.[104,106] These workers also suggested that most of the pulmonary lymphatic valves appeared to be monocuspid instead of the biscuspid structure noted by other workers. Recent scanning electron microscopic studies of lymphatic valves in the lung and other regions of the body suggest that the valves are bileaflets (bicuspids) and in the shape of a miter joint which would maintain a unidirectional flow of lymph.

VIII. STRUCTURAL BASIS FOR LYMPHATIC CAPILLARY PERMEABILITY

In their studies on the permeability of lymphatics, Hudack and McMaster[82] demonstrated that the movement of interstitially injected vital dyes into lymphatics was shown to occur across the lymphatic capillary wall. However, the questions regarding lymphatic capillary permeability remain controversial because the resolution provided by light optics was inadequate to give specific information on the precise relationship between adjacent endothelial cells of the lymphatic capillary and the surrounding connective tissue components. With the advent of electron microscopy and the applications of tracer methods in studies of the lymphatic system, it was shown that the major uptake across the lymphatic wall occurs by way of intercellular junctions. In addition, it was also shown that lymphatic endothelial cells were able to engulf large molecules and particulate materials from the surrounding interstitium.[16,17,45,116] A similar condition has also been found for pulmonary lymphatic capillary endothelial cells.[91,105,109,115]

A. Tracer Experiments

The phagocytic property of the lymphatic capillary endothelium is used to advantage, not only to label pulmonary lymphatics for their positive identification at the ultrastructural level, but also to ascertain the mechanism involved in the transport of fluids, large molecules, and cells across the air tissue-lymph interface and the blood tissue-lymph interface.

1. Intratracheal Injections of Tracer Particles

In efforts to monitor the clearance and pathways for the movement of large molecules and particulate substances from the alveolar spaces, suspensions of electron-dense particles were instilled into the trachea of young adult rats. The particle size ranged from approximately 8 (colloidal ferritin) to 35 nm (colloidal carbon) in diameter. At various time periods following the intratracheal installation of suspensions of colloidal particles, the lungs were fixed by vascular profusion and processed for transmission electron microscopy. At short periods (15 to 30 min) after ferritin was injected into the trachea, large amounts of the tracer particles were seen in the lumen of the bronchial tree (see Figure 53A). Ferritin particles were also observed in alveolar macrophages as well as cells lining the alveolar space. Occasionally, ferritin particles were seen within the alveolar interstitium, but no ferritin particles were observed in lymphatic vessels at this early time period. However, at 2 hr and longer after intratracheal installation of ferritin, the tracer was seen in alveoli, the connective tissue area surrounding lymphatics, and vesicles of varying sizes within the lymphatic endothelial cells (see Figure 53B).

The size and electron density of colloidal carbon make this particle a very useful probe for use in following the clearance patterns in lung. It is easy to recognize at both light optical and electron microscopic levels. After 15 to 30 min following its installation, its distribution is very similar to that of ferritin (see Figure 54A). For time periods of up to 24 hr, the number and size of vesicles containing tracer particles are greatly increased in alveolar lining cells, alveolar macrophages, and lymphatic endothelial cells (see Figure 54B). This increase in size and number suggest that the tracer substances are continuously being removed from the alveolar space by alveolar macrophages as well as alveolar lining cells.

For the long-term tracer experiments (3 to 6 months after intratracheal instillations), the location of lymphoid tissue and lymph nodes were outlined by the concentration of entrapped carbon particles in these areas. Carbon particles are also retained in large autophagic vacuoles within the lymphatic endothelium for long periods of time and are seen up to 6 months after instillation of the tracer.

2. Intravascular Injection of Tracer Substances

While the interstitial injection of tracer particles provide a means for monitoring the egress of substances from the interstitium toward and into lymphatics, there still remains the problem for producing trauma due to excessive fluid pressures being created within the interstitium surrounding the injection site. Likewise, there is also the possibility of producing a mild inflammatory response as indicated by an increased immigration of neutrophils and macrophages to the site of instillation. Much of this difficulty, however, is overcome by the use of i.v. injections of a probe molecule which is compatible with physiological activities and can be rendered electron-dense for its subsequent visualization in the electron microscope.

By using the procedures of Simionescue and Palade,[184] dextran of varying molecular weights (60,000 to 300,000) was injected via the tail or saphenous veins in young adult rats. The extensive studies of Grotte[66] showed that intravascular-injected dextran passes across the blood capillary wall and is subsequently removed from the interstitium by the lymphatic vessels. In order to concentrate dextran in the interstitium and lymphatic lumina, the lungs were perfused for a short period with saline followed by fixation with a gluraldehyde formaldehyde mixture in phosphate buffered at pH 7.4 at 0° C.[184] With this procedure, dextran particles are preserved as a homogeneously distributed precipitate within the plasma that is retained in the interstitium and lumen of lymphatic vessels. This product is then rendered electron-dense which is considerably enhanced by postfixation in osmic acid in a phosphate buffer solution.

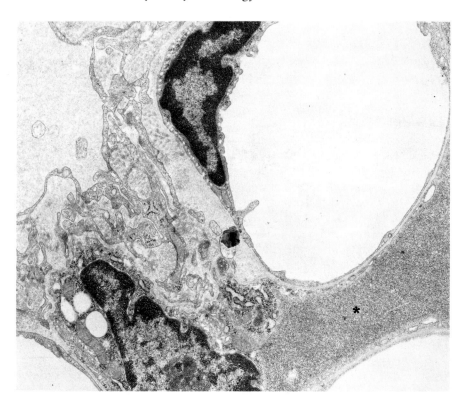

FIGURE 53A. Electron micrograph showing the occurrence of ferritin particles (*) within the alveoli at 30 min after intratracheal injections. (Magnification × 11,000.) (From Leak, L. V., *Respiratory Defense Mechanisms,* Brain, J. D., Proctor, D. F., and Reid, L. M., Eds., Marcel Dekker, New York, 1977, 361. With permission.)

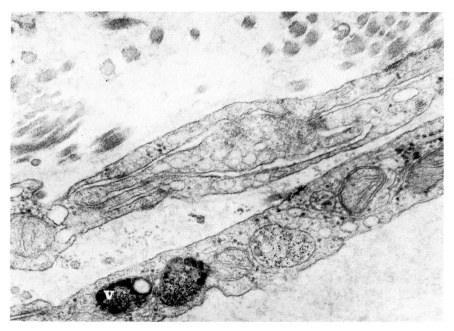

FIGURE 53B. For periods of up to 24 hr, intratracheally instilled colloidal ferritin is observed in vesicles within the lymphatic endothelial cells as shown in this electron micrograph. (Magnification × 50,160.) (From Leak, L. V., *Respiratory Defense Mechanisms,* Brain, J. D., Proctor, D. F., and Reid, L. M., Eds., Marcel Dekker, New York, 1977, 361. With permission.)

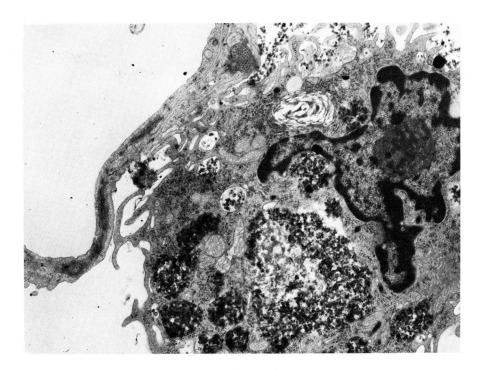

FIGURE 54A. This electron micrograph illustrates the appearance of colloidal carbon within the alveolar space as well as within alveolar macrophages at 30 min following its instillation into the trachea. (Magnification × 13,000.)

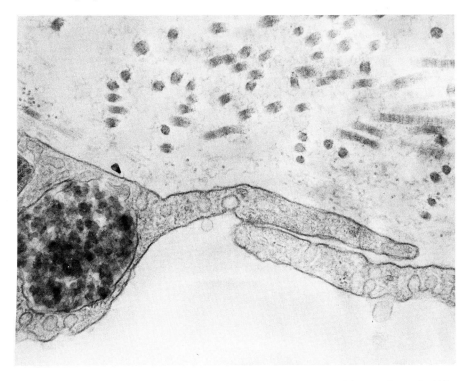

FIGURE 54B. For periods of 24 hr and longer, colloidal carbon particles are observed within large vesicles within the lymphatic endothelial cells as seen in this electron micrograph. (Magnification × 51,260.) (From Leak, L. V., *Respiratory Defense Mechanisms,* Brain, J. D., Proctor, D. F., and Reid, L. M., Eds., Marcel Dekker, New York, 1977, 361. With permission.)

For time periods of 5 to 15 min, the electron-dense product is seen throughout the interstitium and within the pulmonary lymphatic vessels (see Figure 55). The dense reaction product appears within the clefts of intercellular junctions as well as within vesicles in the lymphatic endothelial cells. The pattern of movement for dextran from blood vessels appears to be similar to peroxidase and stroma-free hemoglobin.[173,176]

B. Role of Pulmonary Lymphatics

Our studies with tracer particles instilled in the trachea of rats and those of Lauweryns and Bearet[105,109] demonstrated that both ferritin (8 nm in diameter) and carbon (35 nm in diameter) are transported across the alveolar epithelium into the alveolar interstitium. The particles are subsequently removed by pulmonary lymphatics. In studies of alveolar clearance of large molecules (i.e., bovine albumin and crystalline eggalbumin), Drinker and Hardenbergh[34] showed that there was no pulmonary absorption of homologous plasma albumin, while only a trace of egg albumin was detected in lymph fluid collected from the right lymphatic duct. Using similar methods, Courtice and Simmonds[23] confirmed the studies of Drinker and co-workers in addition to demonstrating an increase in protein absorption after anesthesia. Although it was generally agreed that large molecules (plasma proteins) and particulate materials absorbed from alveoli were removed by pulmonary lymphatics,[35] the volume of lymph drained from the lung was shown to be very small when compared to other viscera of the body.[24,202-204]

In spite of a relatively low rate of lymph drainage from the normal lung, pulmonary lymphatics are organized into an extensive plexus within the peribronchial and perivascular sleeves of connective tissue.

As in other organ systems, there is also a continuous outward flow of fluids from alveolar capillaries toward the interstitium in the lung.[187-189] If left to accumulate, this process would lead to the formation of interstitial edema.[128,187] However, under normal conditions, a state of equilibrium is maintained between the inflow of fluids into the interstitium and the constant outflow from the interstitium toward and into the pulmonary lymphatics.[67,68]

The alveolar blood capillaries are surrounded by an extremely thin band of connective tissue which forms a continuum with the interstitial space surrounding the bronchial and vascular trees. Embedded within this connective tissue sheet around the conducting airways and blood vessels, there is a rich supply of lymphatic capillaries, some of which are found closely apposed to air spaces in the juxtaalveolar regions.[103-105,109,115] The extension of lymphatic capillaries to the level of the terminal bronchioles and their location in close proximity to the alveolar spaces in the form of juxtaalveolar lymphatics place lymphatic capillaries at what appears to be a long distance from large areas of the alveolar interstitial space. However, the studies of Guyton and co-workers have indicated a probable presence of a negative pressure fluid within the normal pulmonary interstitium.[68] Thus, in the normal lung, the direction of fluid movement is from the positive pressure side (i.e., blood capillary) toward the negative fluid pressure areas of the interstitium and the lymphatic capillaries. Therefore the pulmonary lymphatic vessels subserve the lung by constantly removing pulmonary interstitial fluids and plasma proteins that are not returned across the blood vascular wall. Thus, the flow of fluid within the alveolar connective tissue septa continues without interruption toward the interstitial fluid sump of the connective tissue sleeve in which lymphatic capillaries are located.

The presence of tracer particles (ferritin and colloidal carbon) within alveolar macrophages and in vesicles of alveolar epithelial cells at short time intervals (15 to 30 min) and the subsequent appearance of the tracer particles in pulmonary lymphatic vessels provide morphological evidence at the ultrastructural level, demonstrating that

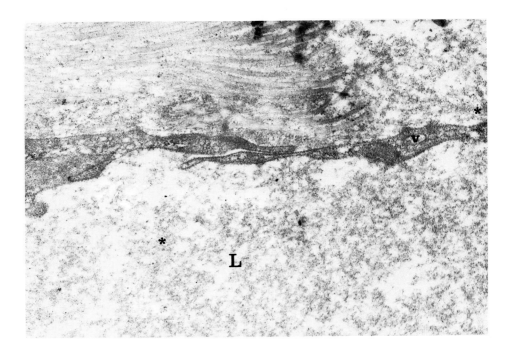

FIGURE 55. This electron micrograph shows part of the lymphatic vessels from an animal injected with dextran which appears as a very electron-dense percipitate (*) within both the connective tissue, vesicles (v) of the endothelium, and lumen (L) of the lymphatic vessel within 15 min after an injection of 10% solution of dextran via the saphenous vein. (Magnification × 29,000.) (From Leak, L. V., *Respiratory Defense Mechanisms,* Brain, J. D., Proctor, D. F., and Reid, L. M., Eds., Marcel Dekker, New York, 1977, 361. With permission.)

large particles are able to cross squamous epithelial cells within vesicles. There is also convincing evidence that large protein molecules, such as albumin and γ-globulin are transported from the interstitium into the alveolar lumen as well as a slow transport of protein from the alveolar space into the interstitium.[23,64]

Using the tracer horseradish peroxidase, a number of workers have demonstrated the passage of this probe molecule across the alveolar epithelium within pinocytotic vesicles.[173,174] Once in the connective tissue compartment which has a negative interstitial fluid pressure,[68,132] the particles move toward the lymphatics and are subsequently removed by these vessels in a fashion similar to that in other regions of the body.[111,113] Although the major pathway for the movement of interstitial fluids and large molecules is via the clefts of intercellular junction, lymphatic endothelial cells are also capable of removing fluids and large molecules from both the connective tissue and luminal fronts via vesicular uptake. From the information obtained from the studies carried out in our laboratory[112,113], as well as that from the work of others,[109] it is evident that large portions of molecules taken up by this process (pinocytosis or endocytosis) are packaged into phagocytic vacuoles for subsequent breakdown rather than transported directly across the lymphatic endothelium.

The efficiency of gas exchange in the lung is dependent on a rapid diffusion of gases between the alveolar air spaces and blood capillary surfaces. In order to maintain a short diffusion distance between the air and blood cavities, the fluid exchange from the alveolar interstitium must be constant to minimize the extracellular fluid space. Under normal conditions, the efficient draining of fluids away from the alveolar system and into the lymphatics prevents the accumulation of fluids and thus, providing a dry barrier between the air space and capillary blood over a wide surface.

REFERENCES

1. Albert, E. N. and Nayak, R. K., Surface morphology of human aorta as revealed by the scanning electron microscope, *Anat. Rec.,* 185, 223, 1976.
2. Bader, H., The anatomy and physiology of the vascular wall, in *Handbook of Physiology,* Section 2, Circulation, American Physiological Society, Bethesda, Md., 1965.
3. Bargmann, W. and Knoop, A., Vergleichende Elektronenmikroskopische Untersuchungen der Lungenkapillaren, *Z. Zellforsch.,* 44, 263, 1956.
4. Beachman, W. S., Koneski, A., and Hunt, C. C., Observations on the microcirculatory bed in rat mesocecum using differential interference contrast microscopy *in vitro* and electron microscopy, *Am. J. Anat.,* 146, 385, 1976.
5. Benninghoff, A., Blutgefasse und Herz, in *Handbook der Mikroskopischen Anatomic des Menschen,* Vol. 7, Part 1, Von Moolendorff, W., Ed., Springer-Verlag, Berlin, 1930.
6. Best, P. V. and Heath, D., Pulmonary thrombosis in cyanotic congenital heart disease without pulmonary hypertension, *J. Pathol. Bacteriol.,* 75, 281, 1958.
7. Bignon, J., Chahinian, P., Feldman, G., and Sapin, C., Ultrastructural immunoperoxidase demonstration of autologous albumin in the alveolar capillary membrane and in the alveolar lining material in normal rats, *J. Cell Biol.,* 64, 503, 1975.
8. Bignon, J., Iaurand, M. C., Pinchon, M. C., Sapin, C., and Warnet, J. M., Immunoelectron microscopic and immunochemical demonstrations of serum and proteins in the alveolar lining material of the rat lung, *Am. Rev. Respir. Dis.,* 113, 109, 1976.
9. Boyden, E. A., The intrahilar and related segmental anatomy of the lung, *Surgery,* 18, 706, 1945.
10. Braunwald, F., Fishman, A. P., Cournand, A., Time relationship of dynamic events in the cardiac chambers, pulmonary artery and aorta in man, *Circ. Res.,* 4, 100, 1956.
11. Brenner, O., Pathology of the vessels of the pulmonary circulation. I. *Arch. Intern. Med.,* 56, 211, 1935.
12. Bruns, R. R. and Palade, G. E., Studies on blood capillaries. I. General organization of blood capillaries in muscle, *J. Cell Biol.,* 37, 244, 1968.
13. Bruns, R. R. and Palade G. E., Studies on blood capillaries. II. Transport of ferritin molecules across the wall of muscle capillaries, *J. Cell Biol.,* 37, 277, 1968b.
14. Buck, R. C., The fine structure of endothelium of large arteries, *J. Biophys. Biochem. Cytol.,* 4, 187, 1958.
15. Buck, R. C., The fine structure of the aortic endothelial lesions in experimental cholesterol arterosclerosis of rabbits, *Am. J. Pathol.,* 34, 897, 1959.
16. Casley-Smith, J. R., An electron microscopic study of injured and abnormally permeable lymphatics, *Ann. N.Y. Acad. Sci.,* 116, 803, 1964.
17. Casley-Smith, J. R. and Florey, H. W., The structure of normal small lymphatics, *Q. J. Exp. Phys.,* 46, 101, 1961.
18. Castigli, G., Observazioni sui del Polmone, *Monit. Zool. Ital.,* 56, 112, 1947.
19. Cauldwell, E. W., Siekert, R. G., Leninger, R. E., and Anson, B. J., The bronchial arteries, an anatomic study of 150 human cadavers, *Surg. Gynecol. Obstet.,* 86, 395, 1948.
20. Chambers, R. and Zweifach, B. W., Topography and function of the mesenteric capillary circulation, *Am. J. Anat.,* 75, 173, 1944.
21. Claude, P. and Goodenough, D. A., Fracture faces of *zonulae occludentes* from "tight and leaky" epithelium, *J. Cell Biol.,* 58, 390, 1973.
22. Clementi, F. and Palade, G. E., Intestinal capillaries. I. Permeability to peroxidase and ferritin, *J. Cell Biol.,* 41, 33, 1969.
23. Courtice, F. C. and Simmond, W. J., Absorption from the lungs, *J. Physiol. (London),* 109, 103, 1949.
24. Courtice, F. C. and Simmond, W. J., Physiological significance of lymph drainage of the serous cavities and lungs, *Phys. Rev.,* 34, 419, 1954.
25. Cotran, R. and Majno, G., A light and electron microscopic analysis of vascular injury, *Ann. N.Y. Acad. Sci.,* 116, 750, 1964.
26. Cruikshank, W., The anatomy of the absorbing vessels of the human body, *Geschichte and Beschreibung der Einsaugendern Gefasse oder Saugadern des Menschlichen Korpers,* Leipzig, 1789.
27. Cunningham, R. S., On the development of the lymphatics in the lungs of the pig, *Contrib. Embryol.,* 4, 47, 1916.
28. Cureton, B. J. R. and Trapnell, D. H., Post-mortem radiography and gaseous fixation of the lung, *Thorax,* 16, 138, 1961.
29. Davis, P. F. and Bowyer, D. E., Scanning electron microscopy: arterial endothelial integrity after fixation at physiological pressure, *Atherosclerosis,* 21, 465, 1975.

30. DeDuve, C., General properties of lysosomes, the lysosome concept, in *Lysosomes,* Ciba Foundation Symposium, de Reuck, A. V. S., and Cameron, M. P., Eds., Little, Brown, Boston, 1963, 1.
31. DeDuve, C. and Wattiaux, R., Function of lysosomes, *Annu. Rev. Phys.,* 28, 435, 1966.
32. Dewey, M. M. and Barr, L., A study of structure and distribution of nexus, *J. Cell Biol.,* 23, 553, 1964.
33. Drinker, C. K., Field, M. E., and Ward, H. K., The filtering capacity of lymph nodes, *J. Exp. Med.,* 59, 393, 1934.
34. Drinker, C. K. and Hardenberg, E., Absorption from the pulmonary alveoli, *J. Exp. Med.,* 86, 7, 1947.
35. Drinker, C. K., The absorption of toxic and infectious material from the respiratory tract in *Virus and Rickettial Diseases,* Symposium, Harvard School of Public Health, Harvard University Press, Cambridge, Mass., 1940, 381.
36. Edwards, J. E., Functional pathology of the pulmonary vascular tree in congenital heart disease, *Circulation,* 15, 164, 1957.
37. Egan, E. A., Nelson, R. M., and Oliver, R., Lung inflation and alveolar permeability to nonelectrolytes in the adult sheep *in vivo, J. Physiol. (London),* 260, 409, 1976.
38. Ekholm, R. and Sjostrand, F. S., The ultrastructural organization of the mouse thyroid gland, *J. Ultrastruct. Res.,* 1, 178, 1957.
39. Elliott, F. M., The Pulmonary Artery System in Normal and Diseased Lungs. Structure in Relation to Pattern of Branching, Ph.D. thesis, University of London, 1964.
40. Elliott, F. M. and Reid, L., Some new facts about the pulmonary artery and its branching pattern, *Clin. Radiol.,* 16, 193, 1965.
41. Emery, J., Connective tissue and lymphatics, in *The Anatomy of the Developing Lung,* Emery, J., Ed., Lavenharm Press, London, 1969, 49.
42. Engle, S., The bronchial glands, in *Lung Structure,* Charles C Thomas, Springfield, Ill., 1980.
43. Esterly, J. A., Glagov, G., and Ferguson, D. J., Morphogenesis of intimal obliterative hyperplasia of small arteries in experimental pulmonary hypertension, *Am. J. Pathol.,* 52, 325, 1968.
44. Euler, U. S. and Lishajko, F., Catecholamines in the vascular wall, *Acta Phys. Scand.,* 42, 333, 1958.
45. Farley, E. E. and Weiss, L., An electron microscopic study of the lymphatic vessels in the penile skin of the rat, *Am. J. Anat.,* 109, 85, 1961.
46. Fawcett, D. W., Observations on the cytology and electron microscopy of hepatic cells, *J. Natl. Cancer Inst.,* 15, 1475, 1955.
47. Fawcett, D. W., Comparative observations on the fine structure of blood capillaries, in *The Peripheral Blood Vessels,* Orbison, J. L. and Smith, D., Eds., Williams & Wilkins, Baltimore, 1963, 17.
48. Fay, F. S. and Cooke, P. H., Reversible disaggregation of myofilaments in vertebrate smooth muscle, *J. Cell Biol.,* 56, 399, 1973.
49. Ferencz, C., Pulmonary arterial design in mammals. Morphologic variations and physiologic constancy, *Johns Hopkins Med. J.,* 125, 207, 1969.
50. Fernando, N. V. P. and Movat, H. Z., The fine structure of the terminal vascular bed. IV. The venules and their perivascular cells, *Exp. Mol. Pathol.,* 3, 98, 1964.
51. Fishman, A. P., Dynamics of the pulmonary circulation, in *Handbook of Physiology,* American Physiological Society, Bethesda, Md., 1963, 1667.
52. Florange, W., Anatomie and Pathologie der Arteria Bronchialis, *Erjeb. Allg. Pathol.,* 39, 152, 1960.
53. Florey, H. W., Reactions of and absorption by lymphatics with special reference to those of the diaphragm, *Br. J. Exp. Pathol.,* 8, 479, 1927.
54. Florey (Lord), H. W., The structure of normal and inflamed small blood vessels of the mouse colon, *J. Exp. Physiol.,* 46, 119, 1961.
55. Florey (Lord), H. W., The endothelial cell, *Br. Med. J.,* 2 (2512), 487, 1966.
56. Florey (Lord), H. W. and Sheppard, B. L., The permeability of arterial endothelium to horseradish peroxidase, *Proc. R. Soc. London Ser. B,* 174, 435, 1970.
57. Florey (Lord), H. W., The uptake of particulate matter by endothelial cells, *Proc. R. Soc. London Ser. B,* 166, 375, 1967.
58. Friederici, H. H., The three dimensional ultrastructure of fenestrated capillaries, *J. Ultatrastruct. Res.,* 23, 444, 1968.
59. Fuch, A. and Weibel, E. R., Morphometrische Untersuchung der Verteilung einer spezifischen Cytoplasmischen Organelle in Endothelzellen, der Ratte, *Z. Zellforsch.,* 73, 1, 1966.
60. Fulton, G. P., Microcirculatory terminology, *Angiology,* 8, 102, 1957.
61. Garlick, D. G. and Renkin, E. M., Transport of large molecules from plasma to interstitial fluid and lymph, *Am. J. Phys.,* 219, 1595, 1970.
62. Garnick, S., Ferritin, its properties and significance for ion metabolism, *Chem. Rev.,* 38, 379, 1946.
63. Good, R. A., Immunodeficiency in developmental perspective, *Harvey Lect.,* 67, 1, 1971.

64. Goodale, R. L., Goetzman, B., and Visscher, W. B., Hypoxia and iodoacetic acid and alveolocapillary barrier permeability to albumin, *Am. J. Phys.*, 219, 1226, 1970.

65. Groniowski, J. W., Biezyskowa, W., and Walski, M., Scanning electron microscopic observations on the surface of vascular endothelium, *Folia Histochem. Cytochem.*, 9, 243, 1971.

66. Grotte, G., Passage of dextran molecules across the blood lymph barrier, *Acta Chir. Scand. Suppl.*, 211, 84, 1956.

67. Guyton, A. C., Granger, H. J., and Taylor, A. E., Interstitial fluid pressure, *Physiol. Rev.*, 51, 527, 1971.

68. Guyton, A. C., Parker, J. C., Taylor, A. E., Jackson, T. E., and Moffatt, D. S., Forces governing water movement in the lung, in *Pulmonary Edema,* Fishman, A. P. and Renkin, E. M., Eds., Williams & Wilkins, Baltimore, Md., 1979, 65.

69. Hall, B. V., Studies of normal glomerular structure by electron microscopy, in *Proc. 5th Annu. Conf. of Nephrotic Syndrome,* New York National Nephrosis Fund, New York, 1953, 1.

70. Hall, J. G., The response of a node to stimulation with foreign tissue, *Congr. Colloq. Univ. Liege,* 45, 1, 1967.

71. Hall, J. G., Morris, B., and Woodley, G., Intrinsic rhythmic propulsion of lymph in the anesthetized sheep, *J. Physiol.*, 180, 336, 1965.

72. Harris, P. and Heath, D., *The Human Pulmonary Circulation,* 2nd ed., Churchill Livingstone, Edinburgh, 1977.

73. Von Hayek, H., *The Human Lung,* Hafner, New York, 1960.

74. Hamilton, W. F., Section on circulatory system lungs, in *Medical Physics,* Vol. 2, Glasser, O., Ed., Year Book Medical Publishing, Chicago, 1950, 207.

75. Hampton, J. C., An electron microscopic study of the hepatic uptake and excretion of submicroscopic particles injected into the blood stream and into the bile duct, *Acta Anat.*, 32, 262, 1958.

76. Harvey, W., *Movement of the Heart and Blood in Animals,* translated by Franklin, K. J., Charles C. Thomas, Springfield, Ill., 1957.

77. Harvey, D. and Zimmerman, H. M., Studies on the development of the human body. I. The pulmonary lymphatics, *Anat. Rec.*, 61, 1935.

78. Heath, D. and Edwards, J. E., Configuration of elastic tissue of aortic media in coarctation, *Am. Heart J.*, 57, 29, 1959.

79. Heath, D. and Best, P. V., The tunica media of the arteries of the lung in pulmonary hypertension, *Pathol. Bacteriol.*, 75, 165, 1958.

80. Heindenreich, J., Morphologische Studien am Blutkreislauf der Lunge des Pferdes, *Zentralb. Veterinarmed.*, 7, 794, 1960.

81. Hortsmann, E., Motor activity of lymphatics, *Eur. J. Physiol.*, 336, S-43, 1972.

82. Hudack, S. S. and McMaster, P. D., Permeability of wall of lymphatic capillary, *J. Exp. Med.*, 56, 223, 1932.

83. Hurley, J. V., *Acute Inflammation,* William & Wilkins, Baltimore, 1972, 15.

84. Inoue, S., Michel, R. P., and Hogg, J. C., *Zonulae occludentes* in alveolar epithelium and capillary endothelium of dog lungs studied with freeze fracture technique, *J. Ultrastruct. Res.*, 56, 215, 1976.

85. Irwin, J. W., Burrage, W. S., Aimar, C. E., and Chestnut, R. W., Jr., Microscopical observations of the pulmonary arterioles, capillaries, and venules of living guinea pigs and rabbits, *Anat. Rec.*, 119, 391, 1954.

86. Jaenke, R. S. and Alexander, A. F., Fine structural alteration of bovine peripheral pulmonary arteries in hypoxia-induced hypertension, *Am. J. Pathol.*, 73, 377, 1973.

87. Johnson, V., Hamilton, W. V., Katz, L. N., and Weinstein, W., Studies on the dynamics of the pulmonary circulation, *Am. J. Physiol.*, 120, 624, 1937.

88. Kampmeier, O. F., The distribution of valves and the first appearance of definite direction in the drainage of lymph in the human lung, *Tuberc. Pulm. Dis.*, 18, 360, 1928.

89. Karnovsky, M., The ultrastructural basis of capillary permeability studies with peroxidase as a tracer, *J. Cell Biol.*, 35, 213, 1967.

90. Karrer, H. E., An electron microscopic study of the fine structure of pulmonary capillaries and alveoli of the mouse, *Bull. Johns Hopkins Hosp.*, 98, 65, 1956.

91. Kato, F., The fine structure of the lymphatics and the passage of ink particles through their walls, *Nagoya Med. J.*, 12, 221, 1966.

92. Keech, M. K., Electron microscope study of the normal rat aorta, *J. Biophys. Biochem. Cytol.*, 7, 533, 1960.

93. Kinmonth, J. B., *The Lymphatics: Diseases Lymphography and Surgery,* Arnold, London, 1972.

94. Kinmonth, J. B. and Taylor, G. W., Spontaneous rhythmic contractility in human lymphatics, *J. Physiol. London,* 133, 3, 1956.

95. Kolleker, A., *Handbuch der Gewebelehre des Menschen,* 1867.

96. Krogh, A., *The Comparative Physiology of Respiratory Mechanism,* University of Pennsylvania Press, Philadelphia, 1941.

97. Krogh, A., *The Anatomy and Physiology of Capillaries,* Hafner, New York, 1959.

98. Krogh, A. and Vimtrup, B., in *Special Cytology,* Vol. 1, 2nd ed., Crowdry, E. V., Ed., Harper (Hoeber), New York, 1932, 475.

99. Kylstra, J. A., Simplified technique of lavage of the lung, *Acta Physiol. Pharmacol. Neerl.,* 9, 225, 1960.

100. Landis, E. M. and Pappenheimer, J. R., Exchange of substances through capillary walls, in *Handbook of Physiology,* Vol. 2, Section 2, American Phys. Society, Washington, D.C., 1963, 961.

101. Lane, B. P. and Rhodin, J. A. G., Cellular interrelationships and electrical activity in two types of smooth muscle, *J. Ultrastruct. Res.,* 10, 470, 1964.

102. Lauweryns, J. M., The lymphatic vessels of the neonatal rabbit lung, *Acta Anat.,* 63, 427, 1966.

103. Lauweryns, J. M., The juxta-alveolar lymphatics in the human adult lung. Histological studies in 15 cases of drowning, *Am. Rev. Respir. Dis.,* 102, 877, 1970.

104. Lauweryns, J. M., The Blood and Lymphatic Microcirculation of the Lung, Somers, S. C., Ed., Appleton-Century-Crofts, New York, 1971, 365.

105. Lauweryns, J. M. and Baert, J. H., The role of the pulmonary lymphatics in the defenses of the diseased lung: morphological and experimental studies of the transport mechanism of intratracheally instilled particles, *Ann. N.Y. Acad. Sci.,* 221, 244, 1974.

106. Lauweryns, J. M. and Boussauw, L., The ultrastructure of lymphatic values in the adult rabbit lung, *Z. Zellforsch.,* 143, 149, 1973.

107. Lauweryns, J. M., Baert, J. H., and DeLoecker, W., Fine filaments in lymphatic endothelial cells, *J. Cell Biol.,* 68, 163, 1976.

108. Lauweryns, J. M., Baert, J. H., and DeLoecker, W., Intracytoplasmic filaments in pulmonary lymphatics endothelial cells: fine structure and reaction after heavy meromyosin incubation, *Cell Tissue Res.,* 163, 111, 1975.

109. Lauweryns, J. M. and Baert, J. H., State of the art: alveolar clearance and the role of the pulmonary lymphatics, *Am. Rev. Respir. Dis.,* 115, 625, 1977.

110. Leak, L. V., Lymphatic capillaries in tailfin of amphibian larva, an electron microscopic study, *J. Morphol.,* 125, 419, 1968.

111. Leak, L. V., Electron microscopic observation of lymphatic capillaries and the structural components of the connective tissue lymph interface, *Microvasc. Res.,* 2, 361, 1970.

112. Leak, L. V., Studies on the permeability of lymphatic capillaries, *J. Cell Biol.,* 50, 300, 1971.

113. Leak, L. V., The transport of exogenous peroxidase across the blood-tissue lymph interface, *J. Ultrastruct. Res.,* 39, 24, 1972a.

114. Leak, L. V., The fine structure of the lymphatic system, in *Handbuch der Allgermeinen Pathologie,* Messen, H., Ed., Springer-Verlag, Berlin, 1972b, 149.

115. Leak, L. V., Pulmonary lymphatics and their role in the removal of interstitial fluids and particulate matter, in *Respiratory Defense Mechanisms,* Part 2, Brain, J. D., Proctor, D. F., and Reid, L. M., Eds., Marcel Dekker, New York, 1977, 361.

116. Leak, L. V. and Burke, J. F., Fine structure of the lymphatic capillary and the adjoining connective tissue area, *Am. J. Anat.,* 118, 785, 1966.

117. Leak, L. V. and Burke, J. F., Ultrastructural studies on the lymphatic anchoring filaments, *J. Cell Biol.,* 36, 129, 1968.

118. Leibow, A. A., Hales, M. R., and Lindskag, G. E., Enlargement of the bronchial arteries and their anastomoses with pulmonary arteries in bronchiectasis, *Am. J. Pathol.,* 25, 211, 1949.

119. Leibow, A. A., The bronchopulmonary venous collateral circulation with special reference to emphysema, *Am. J. Pathol.,* 29, 251, 1953.

120. Leibow, A. A., Hales, R., and Bloomer, W. E., Relation of bronchial to pulmonary vascular tree, in *Pulmonary Circulation,* Adams, W. and Ueith, I., Eds., Grune & Stratton, New York, 1959, 70.

121. Leibow, A. A., Hales, M. R., Harrison, W., Bloomer, W., and Lindskog, G. E., The genesis and functional implications of collateral circulation of the lungs, *Yale J. Biol. Med.,* 22, 637, 1950.

122. Lendrum, A. C., Staining of erythrocyte in tissue sections; new methods and observations on some modified mallory connective tissue stains, *J. Pathol. Bacteriol.,* 61, 443, 1949.

123. Low, F. N., Electron microscopy of the rat lung, *Anat. Rec.,* 113, 437, 1952.

124. Lowenstein, W. R., Permeability of the junctional membrane, in *International Cell Biology,* Brinkley, B. R. and Porter, K. R., Eds., Rockefeller University Press, New York, 1976, 70.

125. Luft, J. H., Ruthenium red and violet II fine structural localization in animal tissues, *Anat. Rec.,* 171, 396, 1971.

126. Majno, G., Ultrastructure of the vascular membrane, in *Handbook of Physiology,* Vol. 3, Section 2, Hamilton, W. F. and Down, P., Eds., American Phys. Society, Washington, D.C., 1965, 1299.

127. Majno, G., Shea, S. M., and Leventhal, M., Endothelial contraction induced by histamine type mediators, *J. Cell Biol.*, 42, 647, 1969.
128. Mayerson, H. S., The physiologic importance of lymph, in *Handbook of Physiology*, Vol. 2, Section 2, 1963, 1035.
129. Majno, G., Palade, G. E., and Schoefl, G. I., Studies on inflammation. II. The site of action of histamine and serotonin along the vascular tree: a topographic study, *J. Biophys. Biochem. Cytol.*, 2, 607, 1961.
130. Mascagni, P., Vasorum Lymphaticorum, Corporis Humani Descriptio et Iconographia, Siena, 1787.
131. Mathis, M. E., Holman, E., and Reichert, F. L., A study of the bronchial, pulmonary and lymphatic circulations of the lung under various pathological conditions experimentally produced, *J. Thorac. Surg.*, 1, 339, 1932.
132. Meyer, E. C., Domengriez, E. A. M., and Bensch, K. G., Pulmonary lymphatics and blood absorption of albumin from alveoli. A quantitative comparison, *Lab. Invest.*, 20, 1, 1969.
133. Meyrick, B. and Reid, L., The alveolar wall, *Br. J. Dis. Chest.*, 64, 121, 1970.
134. Meyrick, B. and Reid, L., Ultrastructural features of the distended pulmonary arteries of the normal rat, *Anat. Rec.*, 193, 71, 1979.
135. Meyrick, B. and Reid, L., The effect of continued hypoxia on rat pulmonary arterial circulation, an ultrastructural study, *Lab. Invest.*, 38, 188, 1978.
136. Meyrick, B., Hislop, A., and Reid, L., Pulmonary arteries of the normal rat — thick walled oblique muscle segment, *J. Anat.*, 125, 209, 1978.
137. Merkow, L. and Kleinerman, J., An electron microscopic study of pulmonary vasculitis induced by monocrotaline, *Lab. Invest.*, 15, 547, 1966.
138. Miller, W. S., Studies on tuberculous infection. II. The lymphatics and lymph flow in the human lung, *Am. Rev. Tuberc.*, 3, 193, 1919.
139. Miller, W. S., *The Lung*, 2nd ed., Charles C Thomas, Springfield, Ill., 1947.
140. Motta, P., Muto, X., and Fujita, F., *The Liver, an Atlas of Scanning Electron Microscopy*, Igaka-Shoin, Tokyo, 1978.
141. Nagaishi, C., Pulmonary lymph vessels, in *Functional Anatomy and Histology of the Lung*, University Park Press, Baltimore, 1972, 102.
142. Namura, Y., Myofilaments in smooth muscle of guinea pig taenia coli, *J. Cell Biol.*, 39, 741, 1968.
143. Ottaviano, G., Ricerche Anat sui Vasi Linfatici del Pulmoney Umono, *Morphol. Jb.*, 82, 453, 1938.
144. Palade, G. E., Fine structure of blood capillaries, *J. Appl. Phys.*, 24, 1424, 1953.
145. Palade, G. E., Transport in quanta across the endothelium of blood capillaries, *Anat. Rec.*, 136, 254, 1960.
146. Pappenheimer, J. R., Passage of molecules through capillary walls, *Physiol. Rev.*, 33, 387, 1953.
147. Pappenheimer, J. R., Renkin, E. M., and Borrero, L. M., Filtration diffusion and molecular sieving through peripheral capillary membranes: a contribution to the pore theory of capillary permeability, *Am. J. Physiol.*, 167, 13, 1951.
148. Pease, D. C., Electron microscopy of the vascular bed of the kidney cortex, *Anat. Rec.*, 121, 701, 1955.
149. Pease, D. C., An electron microscopic study of red bond marrow, *Blood*, 2, 501, 1956.
150. Pease, D. C., Structural features of unfixed mammalian smooth and striated muscle prepared by glycol dehydration, *J. Ultrastruct. Res.*, 23, 280, 1968.
151. Pease, D. C. and Paule, W. J., Electron microscopy of elastic arteries; the thoracic aorta of the rat, *J. Ultrastruct. Res.*, 3, 469, 1960.
152. Pease, D. C. and Molenari, S., Electron microscopy of muscular arteries, pial vessels of the cat and monkey, *J. Ultrastruct. Res.*, 3, 477, 1960.
153. Parker, F., An electron microscope study of coronary arteries, *Am. J. Anat.*, 103, 247, 1958.
154. Pennell, T. C., Anatomical study of the peripheral pulmonary lymphatics, *J. Thorac. Cardiovasc. Surg.*, 52, 629, 1966.
155. Pietra, G. G., Szidon, J. P., Leventhal, M. M., and Fishman, A. P., Hemoglobin as a tracer in hemodynamic pulmonary edema, *Science*, 166, 1643, 1969.
156. Pietra, G. G., Szidon, J. P., Carpenter, H. A., and Fishman, A. P., Bronchial venular leakage during endotoxin shock, *Am. J. Pathol.*, 77, 387, 1974.
157. Pietra, G. G., Magno, M., Johns, L., and Fishman, A. P., Bronchial venular leakage during endotoxin veins and pulmonary edema, in *Pulmonary Edema*, Fishman, A. P. and Renkin, E. M., Eds., Clinical Physiology Series, American Phys. Society, Bethesda, Md., 1979, 195.
158. Policard, A., Collet, A., and Giltaire Ralyte, L., Etude au Microscope Electronique des Capillaries Pulmonaries chez les Mammiféres, *C. R. Acad. Sci.*, 239, 687, 1954.
159. Pollard, T. D. and Weihing, R. R., Cytoplasmic actin and myosin and cell motility, *Annu. Rev. Biochem.*, 1974.

160. Pollard, T. D., Shelton, E., Werhing, R., and Korn, E. D., Ultrastructural characterization of F. actin isolated from acanthamoeba castellanii and identification of cytoplasmic filaments as F. actin by reaction with heavy meromyosin, *J. Mol. Biol.*, 50, 91, 1970.

161. Prosser, C. L., Burnstock, G., and Kahn, J., Conduction in smooth muscles, comparative electrical properties, *Am. J. Phys.*, 199, 553, 1960.

162. Reid, L., *The Pathology of Emphysema*, Lloyd-Luke London, 1967.

163. Reid, L., Structural and functional reappraisal of the pulmonary artery system, in *The Scientific Basis of Medicine Annual Review*, Athlone Press, Atlantic Highlands, N.J., 1968, 289.

164. Richter, G. W., Electron microscopy of hemosiderin: presence of ferritin and occurrence of crystalline lattice in hemosiderin deposits, *J. Biochem. Biophys. Cytol.*, 4, 55, 1958.

165. Rhodin, J. A. G., The fine structure of vascular walls in mammals with special reference to smooth muscle components, *Phys. Rev.*, 42, 48, 1962.

166. Rhodin, J. A. G., The ultrastructure of mammalian arterioles and precapillary sphincters, *J. Ultrastruct, Res.*, 18, 181, 1967.

167. Rhodin, J. A. G., Ultrastructure of mammalian venous capillaries, venules and small collecting veins, *J. Ultrastruct. Res.*, 25, 452, 1968.

168. Robb, G. P. and Steinberg, I., Visualization of the chambers of the heart, the pulmonary circulation, and the great blood vessels in man, *Am. J. Roentgen Radium Ther.*, 41, 1, 1939.

169. Robb, G. P., *An Atlas of Angiocardiography*, American Registry of Pathology, 1951.

170. Rudbeck, O., Nova Exercitatid Anatomica Exhibens Ductus Hepaticos Aquosos et Vasa Glandalorum Serosa, Arosiae Uppsals, 1653.

171. Sanders, D. A., Delarue, N. C., and Silerberg, S. A., Combined angiography and mediastinoscopy in bronchogenic carcinoma, *Radiology*, 97, 331, 1970.

172. Sappey, P. C., Anatomie Physiologic Pathologic de Vaisseaux Lymphatiques Consideres chez Homme et les Vertebres, Paris, 1874.

173. Schneeberger, E. E. and Karnovsky, M. J., The ultrastructural basis of alveolar capillary membrane permeability to peroxidase used as a tracer, *J. Cell Biol.*, 37, 781, 1968.

174. Schneeberger, E. E. and Karnovsky, M. J., Substructure of intercellular junctions in freeze-fractured alveolar capillary membranes of mouse lung, *Circ. Res.*, 38, 404, 1976.

175. Schneeberger, E. E., *Ultrastructural Basis for Alveolar Capillary Permeability to Protein in Lung Liquids*, Ciba Foundation Symposium, Elsevier, New York, 1976, 38.

176. Schneeberger, E. E., Barrier function of intercellular functions in adult and fetal lungs, in *Pulmonary Edema*, Fishman, A. P. and Renkin, E. M., Eds., American Physiology Society, Bethesda, 1979, 21.

177. Schultz, H., *The Submicroscopic Anatomy and Pathology of the Lung*, Springer-Verlag, Berlin, 1959, 86.

178. Shimamoto, T., Yamoshito, Y., and Sunaga, T., Scanning electron microscopic observation of endothelial surface of heart and blood vessels, *Proc. Jpn. Acad.*, 45, 507, 1969.

179. Simer, P. H., Drainage of pleural lymphatics, *Anat. Rec.*, 113, 269, 1952.

180. Simionescu, M., The organization of cell junctions in the peritoneal mesothelium, *Anat. Rec.*, 187, 713, 1977.

181. Simionescu, M., Transendothelial movement of large molecules in the microvasculature, in *Pulmonary Edema*, Fishman, A. P. and Renkin, E. M., Eds., American Phys. Society, Bethesda, 1979, 39.

182. Simionescu, N. M., Simionescu, M., and Palade, G. E., Permeability of muscle capillaries to small heme-peptides evidence for the existence of patent transendothelial channels, *J. Cell Biol.*, 64, 586, 1975a.

183. Simionescu, M., Simionescu, N., and Palade, G. E., Segmental differentiations of cell junctions in the vascular endothelium. The microvasculature, *J. Cell Biol.*, 67, 863, 1975b.

184. Simionescu, N. and Palade, G. E., Dextrans and glycogens as particulate tracers for studying capillary permeability, *J. Cell Biol.*, 50, 616, 1971.

185. Smith, P. and Heath, D., Ultrastructure of hypoxic hypertensive pulmonary vascular disease, *J. Pathol.*, 121, 93, 1977.

186. Staub, N. C., Gas exchange vessels in the cat lung, *Fed. Proc. Fed. Am. Soc.*, 20, 107, 1961.

187. Staub, N. C., State of the art review, pathogenesis of pulmonary edema, *Rev. Respir. Dis.*, 109, 358, 1974a.

188. Staub, N. C., Pulmonary edema, *Phys. Rev.*, 54, 678, 1974b.

189. Staub, N. C., Pathways for fluids and solutes fluxes in pulmonary edema, in *Pulmonary Edema*, Fishman, A. P. and Renkin, E. M., Eds., American Physiological Society Bethesda, Md., 1979, 113.

190. Steinberg, I. and Finby, N., Clinical and angiocardiographic features of congenital anomalies of the pulmonary circulation: a classification and review, *Angiology*, 7, 378, 1956.

191. Swann, H. C. and Spafford, N. R., Body salt and water changes during fresh and sea water drowning, *Tex. Rep. Biol. Med.*, 9, 356, 1951.

192. Taylor, A. E., Guyton, A. C., and Bishop, V.S.,Permeability of the alveolar membrane to solutes, *Circ. Res.*, 14, 353, 1965.

193. Taylor, A. E. and Gaar, K. A., Jr., Estimation of equivalent pore radii of pulmonary capillary and alveolar membranes, *Am. J. Phys.*, 218, 1133, 1970.

194. Tobin, C. E., The bronchial arteries and their connections with other vessels in the human lung, *Surg. Gynecol. Obstet.*, 95, 741, 1952.

195. Tobin, C. E., Lymphatic of the pulmonary alveoli, *Anat. Rec.*, 120, 625, 1954.

196. Tobin, C. E., Human pulmonic lymphatics, an antomic study, *Anat. Rec.*, 127, 611, 1957.

197. Tobin, C. E., Pulmonary lymphatics, *Am. Rev. Respir. Dis.*, 80, 50, 1959.

198. Tondury, G. and Weibel, E., Uber das Vorkommen von Blutegefassanastomosen in der Menschlichen Lunge, *Schweiz. Med. Wochenschr.*, 86, 265, 1956.

199. Tondury, G. and Weibel, E., Anatomie der Lungengefasse, in *Erg. Ges Tuberkulos und Lungenforschung*, Vol. 14, Engel, S., Heilmeyer, L., Heim, J., and Uehlinger, E., Eds., Thieme, Stuttgart, 1958, 59.

200. Trapnell, D. H., The peripheral lymphatics of the lung, *Br. J. Radiol.*, 36, 660, 1963.

201. Trapnell, D. H., Radiological appearances of lymphagitis carcinomatosis of the lung, *Thorax*, 19, 251, 1964.

202. Uhley, H., Leeds, S. E., Sampson, J. J., and Friedman, M., A technique for collection of right duct lymph flow in unanesthetized dogs, *Proc. Soc. Exp. Biol. Med.*, 112, 684, 1963.

203. Uhley, H., Leeds, S. E., Sampson, J. J., Rudo, W., and Freedman, M., The temporal sequence of lymph flow in the right lymphatic duct in experimental chronic pulmonary edema, *Am. Heart J.*, 72, 124, 1966.

204. Vaughan, T. R., Jr., Erdmann, A. J., III, Brigham, K. L., Woolverton, W. C., and Staub, N. C., Total lung lymph flow and interstitial albumin distribution, *Clin. Res.*, 20, 583, 1972.

206. Verloop, M. C., The arteriae bronchiales and their anastomising with the arteria pulmonalis in the human lung, a micro-anatomical study, *Acta Anat.*, 5, 171, 1948.

207. Verloop, M. C., The arteriae bronchiales and their anastomosing with the arteria pulmonalis in some rodents, a micro-anatomical study, *Acta Anat.*, 7, 1, 1949.

208. Wagenvoort, C. A., Vasoconstriction and medial hypertrophy in pulmonary hypertension, *Circulation*, 22, 535, 1960.

209. Wagenvoort, C. A., Heath, D., and Edwards, J. E., in *Pathology of the Pulmonary Vasculature*, Charles C Thomas, Springfield, Ill., 1964, 1.

210. Wagenvoort, C. A. and Wagenvoort, N., Pulmonary venous changes in chronic hypoxia, *Virchows Arch. Pathol. Anat. Histol.*, 373, 57, 1976.

211. Wagenvoort, C. A., Dingemans, K. P., and Lolgering, G. G., Electron microscopy of pulmonary vasculature after application of fulvine, *Thorax*, 29, 511, 1974.

212. Webb, R. L. and Nichol, P. A., Behavior of lymphatic vessels in the living rat, *Anat. Rec.*, 88, 351, 1944.

213. Webb, R. L. and Starzl, T. E., The effect of blood vessel pulsations on lymph pressure in large lymphatics, *Bull. J. Hopkins Hosp.*, 93, 401, 1953.

214. Weber, R., Behavior and properties of acid hydrolase in regressing tail of tadpoles during spontaneous and induced metamorphosis in vitro, in *Lysosomes*, Ciba Foundation Symposium, de Reuck, A. V. S. and Cameron, M. P., Eds., Little Brown, Boston, 1963, 281.

215. Weber, G. and Tosi, P., Observations with scanning electron microscope on the development of cholestrol aortic atherosclerosis in the guinea pig, *Virchows Arch. Pathol. A.*, 353, 325, 1971.

216. Weibel, E. R., *Morphometry of the Lung*, Academic Press, New York, 1963.

217. Weibel, E. R., Architecture of the human lung, *Science*, 137, 577, 1962.

218. Weibel, E. R., Morphological bases of alveolar capillary gas exchange, *Physiol. Rev.*, 53, 419, 1973.

219. Weibel, E. R., On pericytes, particularly their existence on lung capillaries, *Microvasc. Res.*, 8, 218, 1974.

220. Weibel, E. R. and Bachofen, H., Structural design of the alveolar septum and fluid exchange, in *Pulomary Edema.*, Fishman, A. P. and Renkin, E. M., Eds., American Phys. Society, Bethesda, 1979, 1.

221. Weibel, E. R. and Palade, G. E., New cytoplasmic components in arterial endothelium, *J. Cell Biol.*, 23, 101, 1964.

222. Weihelm, D. L., Chemical mediators, in *The Inflammatory Process*, Vol. 2, 2nd ed., Zweifach, B. W., Grant, L., and McClusky, R. I., Eds., Academic Press, New York, 1973, 251.

223. Weiss, L., An electron microscopic study of the vascular sinuses of the bone marrow of the rabbit, *Bull. Johns Hopkins Hosp.*, 108, 171, 1961.

224. Willis, T., Pharmaceutics rationalis, in *Opera Omnia*, 1681, translated into english in *The Operation of Medicines in Human Bodies*, Part 2, 1684, 13, London, 1675.

225. **Wolf, J. and Merker, H. J.,** Ultrastruktur und Bildung von Poren im Endothel von porosen und Geschlossenen Kapillaren, *Z. Zellforsch.,* 13, 174, 1966.

226. **Yamada, E.,** The fine structure of the renal glomerulus of the mouse, *J. Biophys. Biochem. Cytol.,* 1, 551, 1955.

227. **Zelander, T.,** The ultrastructure of the adrenal cortex of the mouse, *Z. Zellforsch, Mikrosk. Anat.,* 46, 710, 1957.

228. **Zimmerman, K. W.,** Der Feinere Bau der Blutkapillaren, *Z. Anat. Enwicklungagesch.,* 68, 29, 1923.

229. **Zurrch, S. K.,** Lung lymphatics, in *Progress in Lymphology,* Vol. 2, Viamonte, M., Koehler, P. R., Witte, M., and Witts, C., Eds., Thieme, Stuttgart, 1970.

230. **Sweifach, B. W.,** General principles governing behavior of the microcirculation, *Am. J. Med.,* 23, 684, 1957.

231. **Sweifach, B. W.,** Introduction: prespectives in microcirculation, in *Microcirculation,* Vol. 1, Kaley, G., and Altura, B. M., Eds., University Park Press, Baltimore, 1977, 1.

Chapter 4

TOXICOKINETICS OF UPTAKE, ACCUMULATION, AND METABOLISM OF CHEMICALS BY THE LUNG

Alan G. E. Wilson

TABLE OF CONTENTS

I. INTRODUCTION

Pharmacokinetic studies of drugs and chemicals have often overlooked or underestimated the lung as an organ of importance. However, there is now considerable evidence to indicate that the lung plays an important role in the removal, synthesis, release, and metabolism of a variety of endogenous substances.[1,2] In addition recent studies have shown that the lungs can modify the biological activities of certain inhaled and circulating xenobiotics.[3-5] These chemicals may be metabolically degraded by the pulmonary mixed-function oxidase (mfo) system and other enzyme pathways which are similar, in many ways, to the extensively studied hepatic enzyme system.[6] Although the lung may not contribute significantly to the total body clearance of most foreign chemicals, the uptake and subsequent metabolism of chemicals by the lung may be a prerequisite to the formation of lung carcinomas, development of some forms of chronic respiratory disease, and onset of other environmentally induced pulmonary disorders. In addition to metabolizing foreign chemicals, the lung can also accumulate and store chemicals.[7-9] However, it is only in recent years that this latter ability of the lung has been recognized and received attention. In this article, the mechanisms involved in the uptake and accumulation of chemicals by the lung are discussed, and the possible toxicological implications of such processes considered. Only uptake from the circulation is discussed, since disposition of airborne agents is considered in a separate chapter. Discussion of xenobiotic metabolism by the lung is limited to consideration of its role as a determinant in pulmonary clearance and the interrelationship with pulmonary toxicity and carcinogenesis. For a more comprehensive discussion of the metabolism of foreign chemicals by the lung, the reader is referred to several recent reviews.[3-5]

II. PULMONARY CLEARANCE OF ENDOGENOUS COMPOUNDS

A. Uptake and Metabolism

The ability of the lung to alter the biological activity of a variety of endogenous substances present in the pulmonary circulation is now well recognized and has been extensively documented.[1,2,10-12] The initial reports from Vane and co-workers (summarized in Reference 10) on the role of the lungs in the metabolism of circulating vasoactive substances have been followed by studies of the mechanism and cellular localization of these processes. There is now considerable evidence to indicate that the endothelial cell, lining the vascular wall, is the major site for the metabolism of a number of substances transversing the lung.[13,14] It is likely that the metabolic capabilities of the pulmonary capillary endothelium may be similar to that in other vascular beds. However, the extensiveness of the pulmonary vasculature provides this organ with the potential to modify inspired and circulating chemicals. That the lung receives the entire cardiac output merely augments its overall metabolic contribution. A variety of compounds, such as peptides, amines, nucleotides, and lipids, are hydrolyzed, oxidized, and/or taken up by the lungs (see Table 1). Pulmonary removal and metabolism is often quantitatively important enough to markedly modify the concentration of some circulating substances, creating considerable arterial-venous differences. Discussion of the mechanisms involved in the uptake and metabolism of such compounds is deliberately brief, since several extensive reviews have appeared in recent years.[1,2,10,16]

It is now apparent that the lung has the ability to remove and metabolize a considerable diversity of circulating vasoactive agents. The uptake of several of these endogenous compounds apparently involves energy-dependent mechanisms, e.g., the pulmonary clearance of 5-hydroxytryptamine (5-HT) and norepinephrine (NE) involves transcellular uptake, intracellular metabolism, and subsequent release. The removal of

Table 1

FATE OF VASOACTIVE SUBSTANCES IN LUNG

Class of substance	Metabolic fate and uptake processes	Ref.
Amines		
5-Hydroxytryptamine, L-norepinephrine	Inactivated, carrier-mediated transport, metabolized intracellularly by COMT and/or MAO	
Phenylethylamine, tyramine	Inactivated, passive diffusion, metabolized by MAO	
Epinephrine, dopamine, histamine	Largely unchanged, although some metabolism in rabbit IPL	17—30
Peptides		
Angiotensin I	Activated, metabolized by converting enzyme at endothelial surface and its caveolae	48,49
Bradykinin	Inactivated, metabolized by converting enzyme at endothelial surface and its caveolae	50
Lipids		
Prostaglandins E and F type	Inactivated, carrier-mediated transport, metabolized by prostaglandin dehydrogenase	34—42
Prostaglandins A type	Unaffected	
Adenine nucleotides		
Adenosine mono-, di-, and triphosphates	Inactivated, metabolized at endothelial surface	51—54

these two amines involves functionally distinct carrier-mediated transport systems that are sodium-dependent, saturable, and temperature- and energy-dependent.[17-23] In contrast histamine, dopamine, L-dopa, and epinephrine are apparently not significantly degraded or retained by the lungs of most species. Accumulated 5-HT and NE are rapidly metabolized by monoamine oxidases (MAO) and/or catechol-O-methyl transferases (COMT)[18,19,21,23] and released back into the circulation.[18,19,21,23] The nature and specificity of these enzymes, especially MAO, have been extensively studied.[24-29]

The extraction ratio for the first-pass clearance of 5-HT by isolated perfused lung preparations has been reported to be in the region of 0.2 to greater than 0.9, depending on the species[30] (see Table 2). These differences have been attributed to the inherent disparity between the species, however, differences in the experimental conditions employed in the various studies could also be a contributing factor. Pickett et al.[20] have shown that the extraction ratio for 5-HT under nonflow limited conditions is a function of the rate of removal and the rate of supply. Thus, when the rate of supply is significantly greater than the removal rate, the extraction ratio will be inversely proportional to flow rate. However, when the potential removal rate exceeds the flow-rate (i.e., flow-limited conditions), the extraction ratio will approach unity.[20,26,27,31,32] The differences observed in the extraction ratio of 5-HT for the different species, and within the same species, could also arise from variations in experimental conditions, especially when measured under flow-limited conditions. This is consistent with the data in Table 2 where markedly different clearance rates are obtained for 5-HT in the same species. Evidently many of these studies were performed under flow-limited conditions, and thus perfusion rate was the major determinant of clearance. It is apparent that experimental conditions must be carefully considered in determinations of pulmonary clearance and caution exercised in conclusions derived from studies performed at flow rates considerably lower than the cardiac output. The clearance of phenylethyleylamine (PHE) is apparently greater than either 5-HT or NE in both rat and rabbit lung. However, whereas for 5-HT and NE uptake is rate limiting, for PHE its subsequent metabolism by MAO is limiting.[28] The uptake of PHE into the lung apparently involves passive diffusion rather than an active transport process.[28,29,33]

Table 2

PHARMACOKINETIC PARAMETERS FOR ENDOGENOUS COMPOUNDS
IN IPL

Compound	Species	Dose (nmol/ml)[a]	Flow rate (ml/min)	Clearance (ml/min)[b]	Extraction ratio (ER)[c]	Ref.
Biogenic amines						
5HT	Rabbit	<0.17	∿220	105	0.48	20
		1.3	10	5.6	0.56	56
	Rat	0.025—0.05	8	7.4	0.92	17
		0.1	10	2.8—7.1	0.28—0.71	18,60,61
		0.2	13—14	11	0.79	57
	Guinea pig	0.006—5.7	20	10—12	0.5—0.6	58
		0.25	10	5.7	0.57	59
NE	Rabbit	0.59—2.96	10	3.9—2.9	0.39—0.29	56
	Rat	0.1	10	2—3.8	0.2—0.38	60,70
		0.1	14—15	9.4	0.63	61
Prostaglandins						
PG E$_1$	Rabbit	0.003	100	52.6	0.526	41
A$_1$	Rabbit	0.003	100	7	0.07	41
F$_{2\alpha}$	Rabbit	0.68	200—300	175—212	0.7—0.85	62
E$_1$	Guinea pig	0.003	30	23.7	0.79	41
A$_1$	Guinea pig	0.003	30	2.1	0.079	41
E$_1$	Rat	≤0.32	30	2.4	0.81	38
A$_1$	Rat	≤0.32	30	1.2	0.04	41
E$_2$	Rat	0.005—70	14	13—0.6	0.93—0.04	63
E$_2$	Rat	100 ng/ml	5	3.7	0.73	64
F$_{2\alpha}$	Rat	100 ng/ml	5	3	0.61	64
Nucleotides						
AMP	Rat	0.1	10	5.8	0.58	61
ADP	Rat	0.1—1.0	30	28.8—28.5	0.99—0.95	55
Peptides						
HHL[d]	Rat	500	10	0.42	0.042	61
Angiotensin I	Rabbit	300 ng/ml	200—300	125	0.37—0.63	62

[a] Nanomoles of chemical added to perfusate divided by perfusate volume.
[b] Clearance values were calculated either by the method of Rowland et al.[32] or from single-pass studies.
[c] Clearance rate divided by flow rate.
[d] Hippuryl histidyl leucine.

The lungs are known to play an important role in the metabolism and presumably the inactivation of circulating prostaglandins (PGs). Prior to metabolism by the intracellular enzymes, 15-hydroxy-PG-dehydrogenase (PGDH) or Δ^{13}-PG-reductase,[34-37] some PGs are removed from the circulation by carrier-mediated transport systems.[38,39] The substrate specificity for the inactivation of circulating PGs apparently resides with the transport systems.[38-40] However, other factors such as plasma protein binding have also been shown to affect the pulmonary uptake of PGs.[41] Eling et al.[42] have recently characterized the structural requirements necessary for a PG to be a substrate for the PG transport system. Pulmonary removal of PGs has been shown to increase in the order of PGA$_1$, < PGF$_{1\alpha}$, < PGE$_2$, = PGE$_1$, = PGF$_{2\alpha}$.[42]

The lung can also be regarded as an organ with endocrine functions.[1,43] In response to a variety of stimuli, both chemical and physical, and in anaphylaxis, the lungs release a variety of substances into the circulation, including prostaglandins, thromboxanes, slow-reacting substance of anaphylaxis, histamine, kinins, and eosinophilic chemotactic factor.[1,44-46] The ability of the lung to synthesize a range of products from arachidonic acid, including PGs, endoperoxides, and thromboxanes, has also been demonstrated.[47] Substances, such as angiotensin I,[14,48,49] bradykinin,[14,50] adenosine mono-, di-, and triphosphates,[14,15,51-55] are modified chemically at the endothelial surface without being taken up into the endothelial cells. The site of localization of angiotensin converting enzyme has been shown to be in caveolae on the surface of the endothelium.[15] Inactive angiotensin I is converted by this enzyme to the potent vasoconstrictor angiotensin II, whereas for bradykinin and adenosine diphosphate biological activity is lost.

The uptake and metabolic fate of endogenous agents in the pulmonary circulation has been summarized in Table 1. The pharmacokinetic parameters for the overall removal and metabolism of these compounds were determined in the most part with isolated perfused lung preparations (IPL) and are listed in Table 2. These values are of interest as a basis for comparison of the various compounds and for different species. However, the pharmacokinetic limitations inherent in these values must be considered when extrapolating to in vivo conditions or discussing the relative contributions of uptake and metabolic processes to the overall clearance by the lung. The significance and role of these uptake and metabolic systems in the functions of the pulmonary system is still uncertain. However, it is interesting to speculate that such systems may play important roles in vasopressor control and prevention of platelet aggregation.

B. Effect of Toxic Agents on Pulmonary Clearance of Endogenous Compounds

The effect that pharmacological agents may have on the pulmonary removal and metabolism of biogenic amines is well documented.[2,59,65,66] However, it is only in recent years that the effect of toxic agents and lung damage on these pulmonary clearance mechanisms has been investigated. Such an approach may provide a useful and early index of lung damage and give insight into the cellular location of injury. Most of the emphasis to date has been on the changes induced in the pulmonary clearance of biogenic amines by toxicants known to affect endothelial structure. However, this approach is now being extended, and other systems such as PG and angiotensin clearance are being studied.

Block and Fisher[67,68] utilized the pulmonary clearance of 5-HT as an index to assess lung damage resulting from hyperbaric oxygen (O_2) exposure. The ability of the lung to clear 5-HT from the circulation was shown to be depressed during the early stages of O_2 toxicity and appeared to be due to an impairment of the 5-HT transport system rather than an effect on 5-HT metabolism. The effect of O_2 on 5-HT clearance was reversible, potentiated by vitamin E deficiency, and partially preventable by superoxide dismutase.[57,69] The pulmonary clearance of NE and prostaglandins has also been shown to be decreased in lungs from rats exposed to high partial pressures of O_2.[70-72] The effect of O_2 is apparently on the metabolism of PGs by PGDH rather than on their transport into the cell.[73] Exposure of guinea pigs to nitrogen dioxide (49 ppm) has also been shown to inhibit pulmonary PG metabolism.[73] Exposure of rats for 18 hr to 100% O_2 at 1 atmosphere significantly reduced 5-HT clearance, however, the effect on PGE_2 inactivation was not seen until 36 hr of exposure.[72] This may suggest that 5-HT clearance is a more sensitive index of early O_2-induced lung damage than PG removal and metabolism.

Exposure of rats to the herbicide paraquat results in gross morphological changes in the lung.[74-76] Roth et al.[77] found a significant decrease in 5-HT clearance by the lung 3 days after treatment of rats with paraquat (25 mg/kg, i.p.). A decrease in pulmonary MAO was also evident; however, the decrease in 5-HT removal resulted from an impairment of its carrier-mediated transport into the lung. In contrast, Smith et al.[78] found no change in the pulmonary clearance of 5-HT 16 hr after an i.v. injection of paraquat into rats (21 mg/kg). The apparent discrepancy between these studies may be due to either a dosage or time effect. However, it may be that the pharmacokinetics of pulmonary 5-HT clearance is only a useful index in severely damaged lungs. A study, correlating the effects on 5-HT pulmonary kinetics with morphological and biochemical changes as a result of paraquat treatment would test this point. Lungs from paraquat-treated rats have decreased levels of angiotensin-converting enzyme; however, the pulmonary clearance of angiotensin I is unaffected.[77]

Monocrotaline is a pyrrolizidine alkaloid isolated from the seeds of the *Crotalaria spectabilis*. It produces a range of toxic effects, including pulmonary arterial hypertension which may progress to right ventricular hypertrophy and cor pulmonale.[79,80] The pulmonary clearance of 5-HT, NE, 5′-nucleotidase, and angiotensin-converting enzyme have been studied in IPL from monocrotaline-treated rats. Of these parameters, only 5-HT transport was specifically and markedly impaired, clearance being inhibited by up to 60%.[61] In a similar study, some effect on the NE transport system was also found.[60] MAO levels were unaffected which suggests that the effect on clearance resulted from damage to the endothelial transport system. The pulmonary damage produced by monocrotaline is suggested to result from the slow release of monocrotaline metabolites, probably dehydromonocrotaline and dehydroretronecine, from the liver. These metabolites are suggested to produce specific inhibition of the functional ability of the pulmonary endothelial cell.[61]

Measurement of the normal pharmacokinetic functions of the lung, i.e., its ability to remove and metabolize circulating endogenous agents, may therefore provide a useful index by which to assess pulmonary damage. However, more systematic and detailed studies are required, correlating clearance measurements with morphological and biochemical changes, before the usefulness of this approach can be established. It is apparent that the pharmacokinetic functions of the lung in both normal and disease states will continue to be an area of considerable research interest.

III. METABOLISM OF FOREIGN COMPOUNDS BY THE LUNG

It is now recognized that a wide diversity of exogenous chemicals, including drugs, steroids, herbicides, pesticides, and environmental carcinogens, are taken up by the lung.[3,5,9,81,82] In addition, it is now apparent that the lung has the capability to metabolize a considerable variety of foreign chemicals. Such compounds may then be either metabolically activated to toxic intermediates or detoxified by the pulmonary xenobiotic metabolizing enzyme system.[3-5] For detailed accounts of the drug-metabolizing enzymes identified in various preparations of pulmonary tissue, the reader should consult the reviews by Brown,[3] Hook and Bend,[4] and Philpot et al.[5]

The pulmonary system for metabolizing xenobiotics appears similar, in many respects, to that found in the liver. Both systems are localized in the subcellular fraction obtained by centrifugation of the postmitochondrial supernatant fraction at 100,000 g for 1 hr, both require NADPH and O_2 for optimal activity, both utilize the enzymes NADPH-cytochrome *C* reductase and cytochrome P-450, and both metabolize a wide range of substrates. The overall pathway of electron transfer from NADPH to cytochrome P-450 and the subsequent oxidation of the substrate appear to be the same in liver and lung. The microsomal mfo system is significantly more abundant in the liver than in the lung. This is reflected in the relative concentrations of cytochrome P-450 found in the two tissues, the ratio of hepatic to pulmonary cytochrome P-450 varying from 3 to 30, depending on the species examined. Differences in the substrate specificity between the pulmonary and hepatic systems exist and are probably due to differences in the cytochrome system. As with the hepatic system, the pulmonary system contains more than one form of cytochrome P-450. The similarity of the pulmonary cytochrome P-450s to the various forms identified and solubilized in the liver is now under intense investigation. The hepatic mfo system, with the possible exception of BP hydroxylase, is considerably more responsive to inducers than the pulmonary system. Total organ mfo activity in the lung is less than that of the liver for most chemicals.

In addition to oxidative metabolism by the mfo system, the lung contains other enzyme systems capable of degrading chemicals.[3,4,83,84] The hepatic and pulmonary epoxide hydrase and glutathione s-transferase systems are not as susceptible to inducers as the mfo. Thus, profound imbalances in the toxification detoxification pathways in the lung, and overall pulmonary clearance could arise from exposure to xenobiotics.

A number of studies have investigated the metabolism of a variety of chemicals by IPL preparations from a number of species.[5,9,81,82] The IPL is an ideal preparation for pharmacokinetic determinations of the metabolic clearance of chemicals by the lung.[32] Such studies also permit delineation of the contribution of the lungs to the whole body clearance of chemicals. However, in such extrapolative studies, the relevance of the experimental conditions to the in vivo situation must be carefully considered. A number of different IPL preparations and experimental conditions have been employed.[81] It cannot be overstated that the experimental conditions employed can profoundly affect the results obtained. Factors, such as the composition of the perfusate, perfusion rates, ventilation conditions, and temperature, may profoundly affect the kinetics of removal and metabolism of chemicals by lung. A summary of the results obtained for the metabolic clearance of exogenous chemicals by IPL preparations is presented in Table 3.

It would appear likely that the pulmonary uptake and metabolism of chemicals is only of minor quantitative importance, as compared to the liver, in the total body clearance of most foreign compounds. However, in the case of 5-HT, for example, it is probable that the lung contributes more to the total body clearance of 5-HT than does the liver.[26] In addition, stimulation of the pulmonary mfo system by cigarette smoke and other agents may enhance the contribution of the lung to the total body clearance of a chemical.

It is now realized that many chemicals require metabolic activation to reactive intermediates before their toxic or carcinogenic effect can be manifested. Thus, the balance between the metabolic activation and detoxification of chemical by the lung is likely to be of major importance in determining the susceptibility of the lung to chemical-induced toxicity and carcinogenesis. This is probably the case with the ubiquitous environmental carcinogens, the polycyclic aromatic hydrocarbons. Polycyclic hydrocarbons, such as benzo [a]pyrene (BP), produce a wide variety of biological effects, including tumor formation in experimental animals and mutagenesis and malignant transformation of cultured cells.[97] They represent one of the most important classes of carcinogenic chemicals in the etiology of lung cancer.[97-100]

Polycyclic aromatic hydrocarbons are metabolized to arene oxides by the cytochrome P-450 mfo system. These epoxides can then be further metabolized to dihydrodiols by epoxide hydrase, or to glutathione conjugates by glutathione s-transferase or converted nonenzymatically to phenols[101] which may subsequently form glucuronide or sulfate conjugates.[102-104] 6-Hydroxybenzo [α]pyrene, a major metabolite of BP in rats, is rapidly oxidized nonenzymatically to quinones.[105] Some dihydrodiols can be conjugated with UDP glucuronic acid[104] or metabolized further by the mfo system to diol-epoxides which are highly mutagenic and the probable ultimate carcinogenic forms of the polycyclic aromatic hydrocarbons.[106-108] In the case of BP, a likely candidate for the ultimate carcinogenic metabolite of BP is (+-BP-7β, 8α-diol-9α, 10α-epoxide (diol-epoxide I). This is based on the high mutagenicity of the diol-epoxide I in bacteria and mammalian cells, a high degree of malignant transformation in mammalian cells, and a high rate of carcinogenicity in rodents.[108-114] Furthermore, Buening

Table 3

PHARMACOKINETIC PARAMETERS FOR CLEARANCE OF
EXOGENOUS CHEMICALS BY IPL

Compound	Species	Dose (nmol/ml)[a]	Flow rate (ml/min)	Clearance (ml/min)[b]	Extraction ratio (ER)[c]	Ref.
Pesticides						
Aldrin	Rabbit	10	61	10.9	0.18	85
Parathion	Rabbit	3.2	147	22	0.15	86
Nicotine	Rabbit	667	155	3.1	0.02	87
Carbaryl	Rabbit	0.4	75	4.9	0.065	88
α-Naphthol	Rabbit	0.1—100	100	56—1.0	0.56—0.01	89
Narcotic/analgesics						
Methadone	Rabbit	30	150	12.0	0.08	90
Mescaline	Rabbit	0.1—10	10	6—4.9	0.6—0.49	91
Δ⁹-Tetrahydro- cannabinol	Rabbit	3.5	120	5.7	0.05	92
Aromatic hydrocarbons						
Benzo[a]pyrene (BP)	Rabbit	100	188	1.5	0.008	93
BP-4,5-oxide	Rabbit	25	140	12.7	0.09	180
Styrene oxide	Rabbit	200	180	7.0	0.039	94
Bronchodilators						
Ibuterol	Rat	0.1	13	5.4	0.41	94
	Guinea pig	0.1	13	4.8	0.36	
Terbutaline	Rat	0.1	13	0.17	0.013	94
	Guinea pig	0.1	13	0.28	0.021	
Miscellaneous						
Testosterone	Rat	0.037	10	0.35	0.035	95
Propranolol	Rabbit	1.68	40	22.4	0.56	96
Pentobarbital	Rabbit	667	175	0.07	0.04	86

[a] Nanomoles of chemical added to perfusate divided by perfusate volume.
[b] Clearance values were calculated either by the method of Rowland et al.[32] or from single-pass studies.
[c] Clearance rate divided by flow rate.

and co-workers[113] have suggested that diol-epoxide I may be the most potent compound ever tested for the induction of pulmonary tumors in mice.

One of the most intriguing problems has been the intracellular target site(s) with which the carcinogen interacts to induce malignant transformation. Although there is no unequivocal evidence that carcinogenesis is a mutagenic event and epigenetic mechanisms are theoretically feasible, considerable interest has centered on DNA and chemicals which bind covalently to DNA as the critical event in the initiation of tumors.[115,116] A good correlation has been found to exist for a series of polycyclic aromatic hydrocarbons of differing carcinogenicities between carcinogenic potency and binding to DNA, but not to RNA or protein.[115] It should not be overlooked, however, that RNA or protein might be the critical intracellular target at which chemical carcinogenesis is initiated.

Considerable emphasis has been directed at determining which polycyclic derivatives are most efficiently bound to DNA, the nature of the chemical bond, and which bases on DNA are involved. Much of the work in this area has been with BP which has become the prototype polycyclic aromatic hydrocarbon carcinogen. BP incubated in the presence of microsomal preparations and DNA results in BP metabolites becoming covalently bound to DNA. Analysis of the products of this reaction show that several

BP metabolite-DNA adducts are formed.[117,118] In contrast the nature of the BP-DNA adducts formed by intact cell models, such as hamster or mouse embryo cells, human or bovine bronchial explants, and mouse skin in vivo, suggest only one predominant adduct.[119,120] This adduct appears to result from an interaction between the C-10 position of diol-epoxide I and mainly the exocyclic amino group (N-2) of guanine.[121] This adduct is formed in the lung following i.v. administration of BP to 3-methylcholanthrene (3MC)-treated mice and when BP is incubated with lung slices from 3MC-treated genetically responsive C57BL/6N mice, but not in genetically nonresponsive DBA/2N mice.[122,123] It is also formed when BP is metabolized by IPL from 3MC-treated, but not untreated rats.[124] In a similar study with β-naphthoflavone-treated rats, an additional adduct due to a recycled phenol was also seen.[125] We have also observed an adduct apparently due to a recycled phenol in lungs from control rats administered BP.[126] It should not be overlooked, however, that the binding of other activated intermediates of BP to DNA may also be important in the initiation of tumorigenesis.

The increases seen in covalent binding upon pretreatment with compounds such as 3MC appears to be correlated with their ability to induce aryl hydrocarbon hydroxylase (AHH).[127] Pulmonary AHH has been shown to be highly inducible by a number of chemicals such as polycyclic aromatic hydrocarbons, flavones, and phenylbenzothiazoles (for detailed listing see Reference 5). In contrast, phenobarbital and steroids have little effect on pulmonary AHH activity.[5] Inducer compounds appear to play a major, if not absolute, role in the control of rat pulmonary AHH.[128] Cigarette smoke has also been shown to contain powerful inducers of this enzyme, and the level of this enzyme in alveolar macrophages from smokers has been shown to be considerably higher than from nonsmokers.[129,130] Such studies imply that the increased levels of pulmonary AHH may be of considerable significance in the higher incidence of lung cancer in smokers. However, other studies have also postulated that induction of pulmonary AHH may play a protective role against formation of pulmonary tumors. For example, β-naphthoflavone, a potent inducer of AHH, significantly protects against the formation of pulmonary adenomas in mice treated with BP or 7,12-dimethylbenzanthracene.[131,132] In addition, we have shown that the amount of BP diol-epoxide I-DNA adduct formed in the lung following oral administration of BP is significantly decreased in β-naphthoflavone treated mice.[133] However, other studies have found no correlation between AHH induction and polycyclic aromatic hydrocarbon-induced carcinogenesis.

Many of these apparent anomalies may be related to the predominant role of the liver in the fate of the carcinogen. Clearly inducers may affect both the rate at which the carcinogen is cleared by the liver and the metabolic profile. This would then profoundly affect the amount of carcinogen and its metabolites released into the circulation and reaching a target organ such as the lung. The active intermediate or its precursor could be formed in the liver and transported to the lung, or the liver could exert a detoxification function by reducing the amount of carcinogen available to the circulation. It is apparent that studies attempting to relate parameters, such as AHH activity and DNA adduct formation to tumor formation, must take into account the toxification/detoxification capabilities of nontarget tissues. There exists a need for detailed consideration of the pharmacokinetic interrelationships between target and nontarget tissue drug-metabolizing enzymes, the formation of specific carcinogen-DNA adducts, and the initiation of tumorigenesis.

IV. UPTAKE, ACCUMULATION, AND STORAGE OF FOREIGN COMPOUNDS BY THE LUNG

A. Basic Amines

A number of foreign compounds of diverse chemical structure have been shown to

Table 4
PULMONARY ACCUMULATION OF EXOGENOUS CHEMICALS

	Lung/blood ratio	Species	Ref.
Amphetamines			
Amphetamine	33(1)[a]	Rat	135
β-Monofluoramphetamine	20(1)	Rat	135
β,β-Difluoramphetamine	4(1)	Rat	135
Chloramphetamine	30(1)	Rat	136
Anorectic drugs			
Chlorphentermine	53(1),30(24)	Rat	137
Phentermine	49(1),3(24)	Rat	137
Antihistamines			
Cyclizine	112(4)	Rat	138
Chlorcyclizine	107(3)	Rat	138
Diphenhydramine	100(1)	Guinea pig	139
Tripelennamine	17(1)	Rat	140
Antipsychotics			
Fluphenazine	100(19)	Dog	141
Clozapine	49(1),47(6)	Rat	142
Tricyclic antidepressants			
Imipramine	150(10),10(24)	Rabbit	143
Desimipramine	400(10),20(24)	Rabbit	143
Desimipramine	400(2),150(12)	Rat	144
Analgesics and narcotics			
Methadone	100(3)	Rat	145
Morphine	2(0.5)	Rat	146
Δ⁹-Tetrahydrocannabinol	5(2),2(72)	Rabbit	147
β-Adrenergic blocking agents			
Propranolol	25(1/2)	Monkey	148
Propranolol	125(1)	Rabbit	149
KO 592	44(2)	Rat	150
Herbicides and pesticides			
Paraquat	4(1),14(32)	Rat	151
Nicotine	2(0.5)	Cat	152

[a]   Numbers in parentheses are hours after injection.

accumulate preferentially in the lung, resulting in high tissue-to-blood concentration ratios (see Table 4). Although exhibiting a diversity in both pharmacological and toxicological action many of these compounds are highly lipophilic basic amines, with pk_as in excess of 8. In contrast to the endogenous amines 5-HT and NE, basic amines, such as imipramine, methadone, propranolol, and nicotine, diffuse into the lung and accumulate as a result of binding.[7-9,87,90] For methadone and imipramine, the unidirectional flux of the compound into the lung is equal to the rate of supply of chemical.[90] In contrast, one component of amphetamine uptake is saturable with respect to perfusate concentration, suggesting the possible presence of carrier-mediated transport.[7,8] This view was also supported in studies of the uptake of amphetamine by guinea pig lung slices.[153] Amphetamine is structurally similar to NE and thus may utilize this transport system for uptake. There is now good evidence that uptake of the herbicide paraquat involves a carrier-mediated process (see section on paraquat). Studies with lung slices have also suggested that phenol red may be transported into the lung.[154] In general, however, it appears that for the majority of chemicals, uptake is by diffusion.[5,9]

The steady-state accumulation of basic amines, determined in the recirculating rabbit IPL, were shown to be considerably greater than for nonbasic amines.[7,8] The accumulation of nonbasic amines, imidazole, promazine, and aniline, was linearly related to perfusate concentration. In contrast, a nonlinear relationship between the accumulation of the basic amines, imipramine, methadone, amphetamine, and chlorcyclizine, and perfusate concentration was observed.[7] The steady-state accumulation of the basic amines as a function of perfusate concentration could be resolved into a saturable and nonsaturable component. The amount accumulated by the nonsaturable (linear) component of uptake was too large to be accounted for by diffusion alone.

The accumulation of basic amines has been further examined by using the single-pass or nonrecirculating rabbit IPL; this system permits an examination of the rates of efflux of accumulated chemical into chemical-free perfusate.[90,155] The rate of efflux of accumulated amines such as imipramine and methadone was resolvable into the sum of three exponential components, implying at least three distinct pools of accumulated chemical.[90,155] The linear component of accumulation from the recirculation studies correlated with the two components of efflux having the shorter half-lives. The efflux component with the longest half-life was found to be included in the saturable component and consisted of at least two types of binding sites. The linear component of accumulation is thought to represent partitioning of the amine into cellular membranes bathed by extracellular fluids, whereas the efflux pool with the longest half-life is the result of intracellular binding. Methadone was metabolized to a small extent by the IPL to its mono- and di-demethylated metabolites. These metabolites appeared to efflux at the rate corresponding to the longest half-life and may suggest that the intracellular binding sites are the same as metabolic sites. However, this view is not supported by studies with imipramine. Although imipramine exhibits similar efflux kinetics as methadone and is metabolized by rabbit lung subcellular fractions, it is not metabolized by the rabbit IPL.[90,155]

Summation of the amounts accumulated by the three pools of efflux did not account for all of the accumulated imipramine or methadone.[90,155] Rather, the amounts of these chemicals remaining in the lung during efflux approached a constant value.[90,155] This implied that the amine was localized in a pool not exhibiting decay during the perfusion period (noneffluxable or slowly effluxing pool, SEP).[90,143,155] This pool was shown not to be due to covalent binding and extractable by pulmonary lavage. Examination of the formation of this pool in vivo showed that it was formed by both imipramine and its demethylated metabolites and that the SEPs formed by these compounds decayed at comparable rates ($t\frac{1}{2}$ approximately 4 hr).[143] Other more polar metabolites were also associated with this pool and accounted for a significant fraction after 24 hr. The SEP accounted for greater than 90% of the total lung radioactivity 20 hr following injection. Thus, this pool would appear to make the major pharmacokinetic contribution to the observed persistence of lipophilic basic amines in the lung.

In contrast to the IPL studies, the lung-to-blood ratio for the SEP in vivo was found to decline with time.[143] This suggested that the pool was not in equilibrium with the blood. In addition, imipramine and its demethylated metabolites were removed at a faster rate from the lungs than from the blood. This pool may result from an interaction between the cationic form of the amine and a negatively charged group on a phospholipid; one type of interaction may be an amine-surfactant complex. It is thought that the phospholipid surfactant complex undergoes macrophage digestion and subsequent mucociliary clearance.[143] Therefore, if the assumption about the nature of the SEP is correct, the amine located in the SEP may be removed by the mucociliary clearance mechanism. If this is the case, then the decay in concentration of the SEP may be a reflection of the mucociliary clearance rate of imipramine and metabolites incorporated into alveolar macrophages. In the IPL, the mucociliary clearance mechanism may either be inoperative or the time frame of perfusion in the studies too short to detect a decay in the SEP. The ability of macrophages to accumulate basic drugs

The summary of the fate of methadone in the lung.

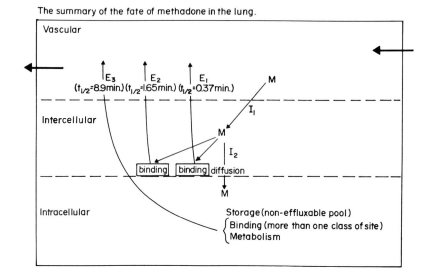

FIGURE 1.   Summary of pharmacokinetic model to describe uptake and release of methadone by IPL.

(1) Methadone is accumulated by diffusion and/or binding at rates I_1 and I_2 of uptake into four kinetically distinct pools.

(2) Two of these pools are suggested to represent partitioning with the intercellular space (Pools 1 and 2, $t^{1/2}$ of efflux = 0.37 and 1.65 min, respectively).

(3) A third pool is suggested to be intracellular probably representing methadone bound to intracellular binding sites (Pool 3, $t^{1/2}$ = 8.9 min).

(4) An additional pool (noneffluxable or slowly effluxing, SEP) exhibited higher affinity than the other three pools (Pools 1, 2, and 3). No significant efflux of this pool from IPL could be detected. Some metabolism of methadone by IPL was apparent to mono- and di-demethylated metabolites. These metabolites effluxed at the same rate as for Pool 3.

(Data from Wilson, A. G. E., Law, F. C. P., Eling, T. E., and Anderson, M. W., *J. Pharmacol. Exp. Ther.*, 199, 360, 1976. With permission.)

and other compounds has been recognized.[96,156] In addition, autoradiography and studies with isolated macrophages were consistent with incorporation of imipramine into macrophages.[157] A pharmacokinetic model summarizing the pulmonary uptake, metabolism, and release of methadone by the IPL is shown (see Figure 1). The model for imipramine is essentially the same with the exception that imipramine is not metabolized by the IPL.

1. Significance of Pulmonary Accumulation of Basic Amines
a. Drug-Induced Phospholipidosis

Animals fed or chronically injected with a number of basic amphiphilic amine drugs develop a condition, most notably in the lung, termed drug-induced phospholipidosis.[158] This condition is characterized by an increase in lung phospholipids and the appearance of "foam-cells" in the lung. A list of some of the chemicals known to induce phospholipidosis in the lung is presented in Table 5. Of these, chlorphentermine has been the most widely studied. Pharmacokinetic studies have shown that chlorphentermine persists in the lung and that the lung tissue-to-blood concentration ratio increases with duration of chronic treatment[159] (see Figure 2). It has been suggested that this increase is due to an increase in the number of binding sites in the lung for chlor-

Table 5
CHEMICALS KNOWN TO INDUCE
PHOSPHOLIPIDOSIS-TYPE CHANGES[158]

Anorectics
   Chlorphentermine
   Fenfluramine
   cis-7-Fluoro-1-phenyl 3-isochromanmethylamine (R 800)
Cholesterol biosynthesis inhibitors
   Triparanol
   trans-1,4-Bis-(chlorobenzyl amino methyl)-cyclohexane (AY 9944)
   Azacosterol
Antidepressants
   Iprindole
   Amitriptyline
   1-Chloroamitriptyline
   1-Chloro-10,11-dehydroamitriptyline
   Noxiptiline
   Imipramine
   Clomipramine
Neuroleptics
   Chlorpromazine
   Thioridazine
Antimalarial
   Chloroquine
   4-Cyano-5-chlorophenyl amidinourea
Miscellaneous
   4,4'-Diethylethoxyhexestrol
   2-*N*-Methyl piperazinomethyl 1,3-diazafluoro-anthen-1-oxide, (AC 3579)

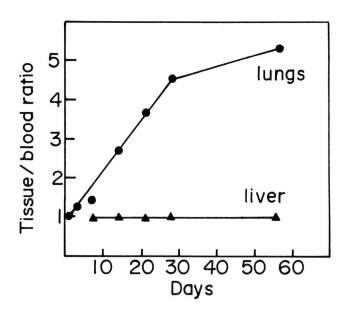

FIGURE 2. Tissue accumulation of chlorphentermine following chronic treatment (20 mg/kg i.p./day) ordinate is the multiples of tissue/blood ratio found 1 day after a single dose. (Data from Lullman, H., Lüllman-Rauch, R., and Wasserman, O., *CRC Crit. Rev. Toxicol.*, 4, 185, 1975. With permission.)

lung for chlorphentermine.[159] The persistence of chlorphentermine in the lung is thought to be related to the increase in lung phospholipids and the onset of phospholipidosis. Phentermine, a structurally related chemical, does not persist in lung tissue and does not induce lipidosis. Chlorphentermine, but not phentermine, has been shown to interact with lecithin by NMR spectroscopy.[160] The increased pulmonary phospholipid content was in the form of lamellar inclusion bodies in vascular endothelial cells, alveolar epithelial cells, smooth muscle cells, bronchiolar epithelium, and in alveolar macrophages. No significant increase in the lamellar inclusion bodies in the Type II alveolar epithelial cell could be detected.[161] The total lung phospholipid content was increased by threefold, and that in the alveolar macrophage was increased by 75% in chlorphentermine-treated rats.[162] The mechanisms involved in the observed accumulation of phospholipid and the onset of phospholipidosis remain unclear.

It is possible that there might be a relationship between the formation of an SEP in the lung, the increase in lung tissue-to-blood concentration ratio, and the induction of phospholipidosis. This possibility was investigated in the IPL for a series of compounds which do and do not induce lipidosis. Chlorphentermine, metadone, and imipramine formed a considerably larger SEP than phentermine or amphetamine.[143] The effect of chlorine substitution into the phentermine molecule (i.e., chlorphentermine) produced a dramatic increase in the size of the SEP. This would appear to be consistent with the observation of Lüllman et al.[137] that the lung tissue-to-blood ratio, 24 hr after oral dosing, was tenfold higher for chlorphentermine than for phentermine. Clearly these studies are at present tentative and must await more extensive investigations, however, they do suggest a possible relationship between compounds that induce phospholipidosis and their ability to form an SEP. It is tempting to speculate that the formation of an SEP by basic amines may be a prerequisite to the induction of phospholipidosis. If this is the case, then methadone may also induce phospholipidosis which may be of concern in chronic methadone use. It is apparent that the compounds shown to form SEPs are basic amphiphilic amines, a point also true for the compounds inducing lipidosis.

The in vivo half-life of the SEP in the lung, following a single i.v. dose, was approximately 4 hr for imipramine and its demethylated metabolites.[143] Evidently profound changes in the pharmacokinetics of elimination of the SEP during chronic exposure must occur to produce the increase in lung-to-blood concentration ratio observed by Lüllman et al.[158] Such a pharmacokinetic consequence would occur from an impairment of the mucociliary clearance mechanism. Chronic exposure to high doses may result in high concentrations of imipramine in the lung sufficient to impair the clearance mechanism for the SEP. The supposition that the SEP may be associated with the phospholipidosis produced by some basic amines appears to be consistent with the available evidence. However, further studies are clearly required to fully understand and evaluate the relationship between the persistence of basic amines in the lung and the onset of phospholipidosis.

b. Effect on Pulmonary Clearance of Vasoactive Agents

There are now a number of reports showing that the accumulation of basic amines by the lung alters the pulmonary clearance of vasoactive substances, such as NE, 5-HT, PGs, angiotensin, and brandykinin[1,5,9,81] (see also section on pulmonary clearance of endogenous compounds.) Alteration of these clearance processes would alter the circulating concentrations of these vasoactive agents with possible physiological and toxicological consequences. An example of the potentially serious clinical implications resulting from alteration of pulmonary clearance of endogenous amines was observed in Europe during 1967 to 1968. A rapid increase in the incidence of primary vascular hypertension was observed during this period.[163] Early clinical evaluation indicated the anorectic drug, aminorex, as the causative agent. Subsequent studies by Mielke et al.[164] have indicated a correlation between the pulmonary hypertension produced by anorectic drugs and impairment of 5-HT pulmonary clearance. Drugs, such as aminorex, chlorphentermine, imipramine, and iprindole, have been shown to impair the pulmonary clearance of vasoactive substances, such as 5-HT or NE, by effects on their carrier-mediated transport systems and/or metabolic degradation.[163-165]

Various tricyclic antidepressants have been reported to produce cardiovascular complications and toxicities.[166] The effect that accumulated amines may have on nonrespiratory functions has received comparatively little attention. However, it is likely that the effect on these functions will occur at considerably lower doses than those required to induce phospholipidosis and therefore of potentially greater significance.

B. Paraquat

The important role that pharmacokinetic processes can play in the onset of pulmonary toxicity is demonstrated in the case of paraquat. The closely related herbicides paraquat (1,1'-dimethyl-4,4'-bipyridilium) and diquat (1,1'-ethylene-2,2'-bipyridilium) have similar chemical and physical properties. However, they have very different toxic effects in mammals, paraquat producing a characteristic lung lesion, whereas diquat does not.[167,168] Sharp et al.[169] first demonstrated that i.v. administration resulted in higher concentrations of paraquat in the lung compared with other organs. Paraquat also appeared to persist in the lungs after the blood concentration had fallen to low levels, resulting in high lung tissue-to-blood concentration ratios. Rose et al.[170] have subsequently investigated the distribution of paraquat and diquat following oral administration. Apart from the lung, the kidney was the only other organ which showed significant accumulation of paraquat.

Rose and co-workers[170-173] have investigated the mechanisms involved in this apparent selective uptake of paraquat by the lung. Studies were performed in which rat lung slices were incubated with media containing either ^{14}C-diquat or ^{14}C-paraquat. The amount of diquat accumulated by the lung slices remained constant as a function of time of incubation and the tissue slice-to-medium ratio (T/M) was always less than unity. In contrast the T/M ratio of paraquat increased linearly with time and after 2 hr of incubation was in excess of 8. Uptake of parquat by the lung slices was inhibited by potassium cyanide, iodoacetate, rotenone, and nitrogen. The rate of uptake of paraquat by lung slices was dependent on the concentration of paraquat in the medium and was saturable at high concentration.[171] These observations led to the view that paraquat was accumulated by rat lung slices by an energy-dependent transport mechanism. Examination of the uptake of paraquat by slices from other rat tissues showed that the brain was the only other tissue that significantly accumulated paraquat. This uptake was shown to be linear with time and energy dependent. However, the uptake of paraquat by brain slices was less than one tenth that observed for lung.[170] These studies have also shown that lung slices from dog, monkey, rabbit, and man also accumulated paraquat in a manner that obeyed saturation kinetics.[170]

In their studies with lung slices, Rose et al. could not conclude whether the accumulation of paraquat resulted from uptake via the airways or vasculature. However, in studies with both the rat and rabbit IPL, we have shown that accumulation of paraquat, but not diquat, from the circulation is linear with respect to time and obeys saturation kinetics (see Figure 3 and Reference 174). This data is supportive of an energy-dependent mechanism of uptake of paraquat from the circulation. However, in both the rat and rabbit lung, less than 0.1% of the amount of paraquat supplied was accumulated by the lung. Nevertheless, in vivo considerable accumulation of paraquat does result in the lung and is likely to be even greater in situations where the dose of paraquat is sufficient to impair the elimination of paraquat by the kidney.[169,170]

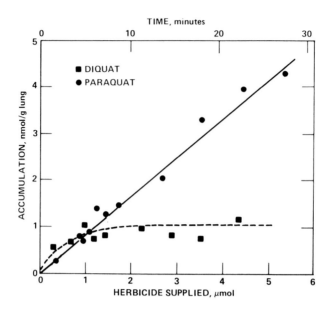

FIGURE 3.   Paraquat and diquat accumulation by the isolated
perfused rat lung. The perfusate contained 6.45 μM paraquat or
diquat (specific activity 0.8 μCi per milligram). Total radioactivity
in the lung was determined after various times of perfusion.

A number of compounds, including the vasoactive agents 5-HT and NE, as well as
several drugs, including propranolol, imipramine, betazole, burimimide, and chlor-
pheniramine, have been shown to inhibit paraquat accumulation by rat lung
slices.[172,175] Maling et al.[176] have also studied the effect of a series of β-adrenergic
agents on the pulmonary accumulation of paraquat. They concluded that there was
no correlation between the effect on paraquat uptake and the effect on paraquat induced mortality. Even though compounds such as 5-HT can inhibit paraquat uptake,
it does not appear that paraquat is accumulated by the 5-HT transport system. Furthermore, Rose and Smith have concluded that the system responsible for the accumulation of paraquat is probably located in the Type I and Type II alveolar epithelial
cells. They speculate that high cytoplasmic concentrations of paraquat will result in
these cells, leading to oxidation of NADPH, production of toxic oxygen radicals, and
cell death.[173]

C. Effect of Toxic Agents on Pulmonary Clearance of Foreign Compounds

Pharmacokinetic models for the pulmonary clearance of endogenous agents are
being increasingly used to assess lung damage resulting from exposure to toxic agents.
However, until recently the kinetic models for the handling of exogenous chemicals
by the lung were not sufficiently well defined to permit their use as indexes of pulmonary toxicity. However, we have recently been studying the effect of exposure to environmental toxicants on the pulmonary pharmacokinetics of imipramine.

Morpholine (tetrahydro-2H-1,4-oxazine) is a widely used industrial solvent for res-
ins, waxes, and dyes. Shea[177] has shown that exposure of animals to morpholine results
in pulmonary damage. More recent studies have shown that preexposure of rabbits to
morpholine results in marked changes in pulmonary function. In addition, morpholine
produces alterations in the activity of a number of enzymes associated with alveolar
macrophages. We have recently shown that the pulmonary accumulation and persistence of imipramine is reduced in rabbits exposed to morpholine.[178] Rabbits were ex-

posed to vaporized morpholine at 250 ppm, 6 hr/day for periods up to 8 weeks. Lungs were then removed and imipramine uptake into the IPLs studied.[178] A significant effect on the SEP of imipramine accumulation was observed, whereas no effect on any of the other pools of imipramine accumulation was apparent. This effect on the amount of imipramine accumulated into the SEP was related to, and dependent on, the length of exposure to morpholine. The phagocytic ability of the alveolar macrophages towards latex beads was also found to be reduced. This result would support our previous observation on the morphological location of the SEP as being the alveolar macrophage.

Mehendale[179] has also shown that the steady-state accumulation of imipramine is increased in animals preexposed to piperonyl butoxide or bisolvon. The increase in the pulmonary uptake induced by bisolvon was also accompanied by enlarged and more numerous concentric lamellae bodies in the Type II pneumocyte. The relationship between the enhanced drug uptake and induced pulmonary changes is at present unclear. However, it would be consistent with the altered lung-to-blood ratio seen for chlorphentermine in phospholipidotic states, where large increases in both size and number of concentric lamellar organelles are also seen.[158] In contrast to the effect of hyperoxia on 5HT pulmonary clearance in the rat, no effect on the pulmonary accumulation of imipramine was demonstrated.[70]

Modulation of the pharmacokinetics of uptake, accumulation, and metabolism of exogenous chemicals may provide a useful basis for the assessment of pulmonary damage resulting from exposure to toxic agents.

V. SUMMARY

This review has focused on the role of the lungs in the removal and metabolism of chemicals present in the circulation. It is apparent that the pulmonary system exhibits a considerable diversity in its ability to remove, metabolize, synthesize, and release a variety of endogenous compounds. Relatively little is known about the role and significance of such processes in normal lung function. However, it is apparent that their function is considerably more complex than simply a mechanism of vasopressor control. It is now recognized that potent agents, such as thromboxanes, prostacyclic, and prostaglandins, formed during the metabolism of arachidonic acid, play a vital role in the prevention of platelet adhesion and aggregation. However, the function of the variety of other mediators released in situations such as stress and anaphylaxis is unclear. It is apparent that more fundamental research is required before we can fully understand the significance of such normal pulmonary functions. Consequently, the physiological significances due to alteration of these processes induced by toxic agents is difficult to ascertain. However, it is apparent that modulation of such homeostatic control mechanisms has the potential for serious physiological, biochemical, and toxicological consequences. The appropriateness of this latter statement must, however, await verification.

The discussion on the pharmacokinetics of pulmonary clearance of exogenous chemicals and the relationship to carcinogenicity and toxicity has been deliberately brief. It is impossible in an article of this nature to give credit to the vast amount of information on the metabolism of foreign compounds by the lung. For detailed discussion, the reader should consult the references cited in the text. In contrast, relatively few studies have been performed which have systematically evaluated the role of the lungs in the whole body clearance of chemicals. From the data presented, it is apparent that for the majority of chemicals the lungs would appear to be of relatively minor quantitative significance to total body clearance. However, exceptions do exist, and it should not be overlooked that for certain chemicals, the lung may significantly contribute to total body clearance.

It is apparent that an intricate balance between metabolic aviation and detoxification pathways is a fundamental determinant in the susceptibility to pulmonary toxicity. Delineation of metabolic pathways and identification of toxic intermediates is essential in our understanding of the mechanisms of toxicity. Unfortunately, it is often impossible to accurately determine the relevant kinetic parameters for these pathways. In recent years, however, it has become evident that reactive intermediates of many toxic chemicals and carcinogens express their toxicity by interaction with critical cellular macromolecules, such as protein, RNA, and DNA. Studies on the kinetics of formation of such complexes have given considerable insight into mechanisms of toxicity; this has been especially true in the area of the formation of specific carcinogen adducts with DNA. The DNA damage resulting from such DNA-carcinogen adduct formation is suggested to be an essential event in the initiation of carcinogenesis. However, such damage does not in itself usually lead to cancerous transformation, and additional factors are necessary to promote the chain of cellular events culminating in transformation. It is essential to our understanding of the mechanism of carcinogenesis that the relevance of such DNA damage, resulting from covalent attachment of carcinogen to DNA, in the initiation and expression of carcinogenesis be explored.

Pharmacokinetic consideration of the relationships between the clearance of chemicals by target and nontarget tissue, the balance between toxification and detoxification pathways, and the expression of toxicity should play a major factor in our understanding of the mechanisms involved in toxicity and carcinogenicity. Clearly as more is learned about the detailed mechanisms of toxicity and carcinogenicity, it may be possible to define certain critical rate-limiting steps and thereby permit prediction of likely dose-response relationships at dosage levels too low to feasibly determine by animal bioassay.

ACKNOWLEDGMENT

The author would like to acknowledge the assistance of Ms. Frances Holloway in the typing of this manuscript.

REFERENCES

1. **Bakhle, Y. S. and Vane, J. R.,** Pharmacokinetic function of the pulmonary circulation, *Physiol. Rev.,* 54, 1007, 1974.
2. **Junod, A. F.,** Metabolism, production and release of hormones and mediators in the lung, *Am. Rev. Respir. Dis.,* 112, 93, 1975.
3. **Brown, E. A. B.,** The localization, metabolism, and effects of drugs and toxicants in lung, *Drug Metab. Rev.,* 3, 33, 1974.
4. **Hook, G. E. R. and Bend, J. R.,** Pulmonary metabolism of xenobiotics, *Life Sci.,* 18, 279, 1975.
5. **Philpot, R. M., Anderson, M. W., and Eling, T. E.,** Uptake, accumulation and metabolism of chemicals by the lung, in *Metabolic Functions of the Lung,* Vol. 4, Bakhle, Y. S. and Vane, J. R., Eds., Marcel Dekker, New York, 1977, 123.
6. **Bend, J. R. and Hook, G. E. R.,** Hepatic and extrahepatic mixed-function oxidases, in *Handbook of Physiology-Reactions to Environmental Agents,* Section 9, Lee, D. H. K., Falk, H. L., Murphy, S. D., and Geiger, S. R., Eds., American Physiology Society, Bethesda, Md., 1977, 419.
7. **Orton, T. C., Anderson, M. W., Pickett, R. D., Eling, T. E., and Fouts, J. R.,** Xenobiotic accumulation and metabolism by isolated perfused rabbit lungs, *J. Pharmacol. Exp. Ther.,* 186, 482, 1973.
8. **Anderson, M. W., Orton, T. C., Pickett, R. D., and Eling, T. E.,** Accumulation of amines in the isolated perfused rabbit lung, *J. Pharmacol. Exp. Ther.,* 189, 456, 1974.

9. Anderson, M. W., Philpot, R. M., Bend, J. R., Wilson, A. G. E., and Eling, T. E., Pulmonary uptake and metabolism of chemicals by the lung, in *Clinical Toxicology*, Duncan, W. A. M. and Leonard, B. J., Eds., Excerpta Medica, Amsterdam, 1977, 85.

10. Vane, J. R., The role of the lungs in the metabolism of vasoactive substances, in *Pharmacology and Pharmacokinetics*, Fogarty International Center Proceedings, No. 20, Teorell, T., Dedrick, R. L., and Condliffe, P. G., Eds., Plenum Press, New York, 1974, 195.

11. Gillis, C. N., Metabolism of vasoactive hormones by the lung, *Anesthesiology*, 39, 626, 1973.

12. Strum, J. M. and Junod, A. F., Radioautographic demonstration of 5-hydroxytryptamine-³H uptake by pulmonary endothelial cells, *J. Cell. Biol.*, 54, 456, 1972.

13. Junod, A. F., Metabolic activity of the pulmonary endothelium, in *Lung Cells in Disease*, Bouhuys, A., Ed., Elsevier/North-Holland, Amsterdam, 1976, 285.

14. Smith, U. S. and Ryan, J. W., Pulmonary endothelial cells and the metabolism of adenine nucleotides kinins and angiotensin I, *Adv. Exp. Med. Biol.*, 21, 267, 1972.

15. Ryan, J. W. and Ryan, U. S., Pulmonary endothelial cells, *Fed Proc. Fed. Am. Soc. Exp. Biol.*, 36, 2683, 1977.

16. Fishman, A. P. and Giuseppe, G. P., Handling of bioactive materials by the lung (Part II), *N. Engl. J. Med.*, 291, 953, 1974.

17. Alabaster, V. A. and Bakhle, Y. S., Removal of 5-hydroxytryptamine in the pulmonary circulation of rat isolated lungs, *Br. J. Pharmacol.*, 40, 468, 1970.

18. Junod, A. F., Uptake, metabolism and efflux of ¹⁴C-5-hydroxytryptamine in isolated perfused rat lungs, *J. Pharmacol. Exp. Ther.*, 183, 341, 1972.

19. Iwasawa, J. and Gillis, C. N., Pharmacological analysis of norepinephrine and 5-hydroxytryptamine removal from the pulmonary circulation: differentiation of uptake sites for each amine, *J. Pharmacol. Exp. Ther.*, 188, 386, 1974.

20. Pickett, R. D., Anderson, M. W., Orton, T. C., and Eling, T. E., The pharmacodynamics of 5-hydroxytryptamine uptake and metabolism by the isolated perfused rabbit lung, *J. Pharmacol. Exp. Ther.*, 194, 545, 1975.

21. Hughes, J., Gillis, C. N., and Bloom, F. E., The uptake and disposition of DL-noradrenaline in perfused rat lung, *J. Pharmacol. Exp. Ther.*, 169, 237, 1969.

22. Nicholas, T. E., Strum, J. M., Angelo, L. S., and Junod, A. F., Site and mechanism of uptake of ³H-1-norephinephrine by isolated perfused rat lungs, *Circ. Res.*, 35, 670, 1974.

23. Alabaster, V. A., Inactivation of endogenous amines in the lungs, in *Metabolic Functions of the Lung*, Vol. 4, Bakhle, Y. S. and Vane, J. R., Eds., Marcel Dekker, New York, 1977, 3.

24. Roth, J. A. and Gillis, C. N., Multiple forms of amine oxidase in perfused rabbit lung, *J. Pharmacol. Exp. Ther.*, 194, 537, 1975.

25. Bakhle, Y. S. and Youdim, M. B. H., Metabolism of phenylethylamine in rat isolated perfused lung: evidence for monoamine oxidase "type B" in lung, *Br. J. Pharmac.*, 56, 125, 1976.

26. Wiersma, D. A. and Roth, R. A., Clearance of 5-hydroxytryptamine by rat lung and liver: the importance of relative perfusion and intrinsic clearance, *J. Pharmacol. Exp. Ther.*, 212, 97, 1980.

27. Roth, R. A. and Wiersma, D. A., Role of the lung in total body clearance of circulating drugs, *Clin. Pharmacokinetics*, 4, 355, 1979.

28. Bakhle, Y. S. and Youdim, M. B. H., The metabolism of 5-hydroxytryptamine and β-phenylethylamine in perfused rat lung and in vitro, *Br. J. Pharmacol.*, 65, 147, 1979.

29. Kung, H. C. and Wilson, A. G. E., Characterization of rat pulmonary monoamine oxidase, *Life Sci.*, 24, 425, 1979.

30. Junod, A. F., Mechanism of uptake of biogenic amines in the pulmonary circulation, in *Lung Metabolism*, Junod, A. F and deHaller, R., Eds., Academic Press, New York, 1975, 387.

31. Rane, A., Wilkinson, G. R., and Shand, D. G., Prediction of hepatic extraction ratio from *in vitro* measurement of intrinsic clearance, *J. Pharmacol. Exp. Ther.*, 200, 420, 1977.

32. Rowland, M., Benet, L. Z., and Graham, G. G., Clearance concepts in pharmacokinetics, *J. Pharmacokinetics Biopharm.*, 1, 123, 1973.

33. Gillis, C. N. and Roth, J. A., The fate of biogenic monoamines in perfused rabbit lung, *Br. J. Pharmacol.*, 59, 585, 1977.

34. Piper, J. P., Vane, J. R., and Wyllie, J. H., Inactivation of prostaglandins by the lungs, *Nature*, 225, 600, 1970.

35. Samuelsson, B., Granstrom, E., Green, K., and Hamberg, M., Metabolism of prostaglandins, *Ann. N.Y. Acad. Sci.*, 180, 138, 1971.

36. Hansen, H. S., 15-Hydroxyprostaglandin dehydrogenase. A review, *Prostaglandins*, 12, 647, 1976.

37. Flower, R. J., Prostaglandin metabolism in the lung, in *Metabolic Functions of the Lung*, Vol. 4, Bakhle, Y. S. and Vane, J. R., Eds., Marcel Dekker, New York, 1977, 85.

38. Anderson, M. W. and Eling, T. E., Prostaglandin removal and metabolism by isolated perfused lung, *Prostaglandins*, 11, 645, 1976.

39. Bito, L. Z., Baroody, R. A., and Reitz, M. E., Dependence of pulmonary prostaglandin metabolism on carrier-mediated transport processes, *Am. J. Physiol.*, 232, E382, 1977.

40. Ferreira, S. H. and Vane, J. R., Prostaglandins: their disappearance from and release into the circulation, *Nature (London)*, 216, 868, 1967.

41. Hawkins, H. J., Wilson, A. G. E., Anderson, M. W., and Eling, T. E., Uptake and metabolism of prostaglandins by isolated perfused lung: species comparisons and the role of plasma protein binding, *Prostaglandins*, 14, 251, 1977.

42. Eling, T. E., Hawkins, H. J., and Anderson, M. W., Structural requirements for, and the effects of chemicals on, the rat pulmonary inactivation of prostaglandins, *Prostaglandins*, 14, 51, 1977.

43. Ryan, J. W. and Ryan, U. S., Is the lung a para-endocrine organ?, *Am. J. Med.*, 63, 595, 1977.

44. Piper, P. J., Anaphylaxis and the release of active substances in the lungs, *Pharmacol. Ther. B*, 3, 75, 1977.

45. Piper, P. J., Release induced by anaphylaxis, in *Metabolic Functions of the Lung*, Vol. 4, Bakhle, Y. S. and Vane, J. R., Eds., Marcel Dekker, New York, 1977, 261.

46. Said, S., Release induced by physical and chemical stimuli, in *Metabolic Functions of the Lung*, Vol. 4, Bakhle, Y. S. and Vane, J. R., Eds., Marcel Dekker, New York, 1977, 297.

47. Hamberg, M. and Samuelsson, B., Prostaglandin endoperoxides. Novel transformations of arachidonic acid in guinea pig lung, *Biochem. Biophys. Res. Commun.*, 61, 942, 1974.

48. Ng, K. K. F. and Vane, J. R., The conversion of angiotensin I to angiotensin II, *Nature*, 216, 762, 1967.

49. Longenecker, G. L. and Huggins, C. G., Biochemistry of the pulmonary angiotensin — converting enzyme, in *Metabolic Functions of the Lung*, Vol. 4, Bakhle, Y. S. and Vane, J. R., Eds., Marcel Dekker, New York, 1977, 55.

50. Ferreira, S. H. and Bakhle, Y. S., Inactivation of bradykinin and related peptides in the lung, in *Metabolic Functions of the Lung*, Vol. 4, Bakhle, Y. S. and Vane, J. R., Eds., Marcel Dekker, New York, 1977, 33.

51. Ryan, J. W. and Smith, U., Metabolism of adenosine 5′-monophosphate during circulation through the lungs, *Trans. Assoc. Am. Physicians*, 84, 297, 1971.

52. Dieterle, Y., Ody, C., Ehrensberger, A., Stadler, H., and Junod, A. F., Metabolism and uptake of adenosine triphosphate and adenosine by porcine aortic and pulmonary endothelial cells and fibroblasts in culture, *Circ. Res.*, 42, 869, 1978.

53. Binet, L. and Burstein, M., Poumon et action vasculaire de l'adenosine triphosphate (ATP), *Presse Med.*, 58, 1201, 1950.

54. Ryan, U. S. and Ryan, J. W., Correlations between the fine structure of the alveolar-capillary unit and its metabolic activities, in *Metabolic Functions of the Lung*, Vol. 4, Bakhle, Y. S. and Vane, J. R., Eds., Marcel Dekker, New York, 197, 1977.

55. Crutchley, D. S., Eling, T. E., and Anderson, M. W., ADPase activity of isolated perfused rat lung, *Life Sci.*, 22, 1413, 1978.

56. Gillis, C. N. and Iwasawa, Y., Technique for measurement of norepinephrine and 5-hydroxytryptamine uptake by rabbit lung, *J. Appl. Physiol.*, 33, 404, 1972.

57. Block, E. R. and Fisher, A. B., Prevention of hyperoxic-induced depression of pulmonary serotonin clearance by pretreatment with superoxide dismutase, *Am. Rev. Respir. Dis.*, 116, 441, 1977.

58. Gruby, L. A., Rowlands, C., Varley, B. Q., and Wyllie, J. H., The fate of 5-hydroxytryptamine in the lungs, *Br. J. Surg.*, 58, 526, 1971.

59. Steinberg, H., Bassett, D. J. P., and Fisher, A. B., Depression of pulmonary 5-hydroxytryptamine uptake by metabolic inhibitors, *Am. J. Physiol.*, 228, 1298, 1975.

60. Gillis, C. N., Huxtable, R. J., and Roth, R. A., Effects of monocrotaline pretreatment of rats on removal of 5-hydroxytryptamine and noradrenaline by perfused lung, *Br. J. Pharmacol.*, 63, 435, 1978.

61. Huxtable, R., Ciaramitaro, D., and Eisenstein, D., The effect of a pyrrolizidine alkaloid, monocrotaline, and a pyrrole dehydroretronecine, on the biochemical functions of the pulmonary endothelium, *Mol. Pharmacol.*, 14, 1189, 1978.

62. Hagedorn, B. and Kostenbauder, B., Studies on the effect of tobacco smoke on the biotransformation of vasoactive substances in the isolated perfused rabbit lung, II. Angiotensin-I conversion, *Res. Commun. Chem. Pathol. Pharmacol.*, 20, 195, 1978.

63. Klein, L. S., Fisher, A. B., Soltoff, S., and Coburn, R. F., Effect of O_2 exposure on pulmonary metabolism of prostaglandin E_2, *Am. Rev. Respir. Dis.*, 118, 622, 1978.

64. Leary, W. P., Asmal, A. C., and Botha, J., Pulmonary inactivation of prostaglandin by hypertensive rats, *Prostaglandins*, 13, 697, 1977.

65. Gillis, C. N. and Roth, J. A., Pulmonary disposition of circulating vasoactive hormones, commentary, *Biochem. Pharmacol.*, 25, 2547, 1976.

66. Gillis, C. N., Extraneuronal transport of noradrenaline in the lung, in *The Mechanism of Neuronal and Extraneuronal Transport of Catecholamines,* Paton, D. M., Ed., Raven Press, New York, 1976, 281.

67. Block, E. R. and Fisher, A. B., Depression of serotonin clearance by rat lungs during oxygen exposure, *J. Appl. Physiol.,* 42, 33, 1977.

68. Block, E. R. and Fisher, A. B., Effect of hyperbaric oxygen exposure on pulmonary clearance of 5-hydroxytryptamine, *J. Appl. Physiol.,* 43, 254, 1977.

69. Block, E. R., Recovery from hyperoxic depression of pulmonary 5-hydroxytryptamine clearance. Effect of inspired O_2 tension, *Lung,* 155, 131, 1978.

70. Block, E. R. and Cannon, J. K., Effect of oxygen exposure on lung clearance of amines, *Lung,* 155, 287, 1978.

71. Parkes, D. G. and Eling, T. E., The influence of environmental agents on prostaglandin biosynthesis and metabolism in the lung, *Biochem. J.,* 146, 549, 1975.

72. Klein, L. S., Fisher, A. B., Soltoff, S., and Coburn, R. F., Effect of O_2 exposure on pulmonary metabolism of prostaglandin E_2, *Am. Rev. Respir. Dis.,* 118, 622, 1978.

73. Chaudhari, A., Sivarajah, K., Warnock, R., Eling, T. E., and Anderson, M. W., Inhibition of pulmonary prostaglandin metabolism by exposure of animals to oxygen or nitrogen dioxide, *Biochem. J.,* 184, 51, 1979.

74. Smith, P. and Heath, D., Paraquat, *CRC Crit. Rev. Toxicol.,* 4, 411, 1976.

75. Pasi, A., *The Toxicology of Paraquat, Diquat and Morfumquat,* Hans Huber, Bern, 1978.

76. Autor, A. P., Ed., *Biochemical Mechanisms of Paraquat Toxicity,* Academic Press, New York, 1977.

77. Roth, R. A., Wallace, K. B., Alper, R. H., and Bailie, M. D., Effect of paraquat treatment of rats on disposition of 5-hydroxytryptamine and angiotensin I by perfused lung, *Biochem. Pharmacol.,* 28, 2349, 1979.

78. Smith, L. L., Lock, E. A., and Rose, M. S., The relationship between 5-hydroxytryptamine and paraquat accumulation into rat lung, *Biochem. Pharmacol.,* 25, 2485, 1976.

79. Schoental, R. and Head, M. A., Pathological changes in rats as a result of treatment with monocrotaline, *Br. J. Cancer,* 9, 229, 1955.

80. Hayashi, Y and Lalich, J. J., Renal and pulmonary alterations induced in rats by a single injection of monocrotaline, *Proc. Soc. Exp. Biol. Med.,* 124, 392, 1967.

81. Roth, J. A., Use of the isolated perfused lung in biochemical toxicology, in *Reviews in Biochemical Toxicology,* Vol. 1, Hodgson, E., Bend, J. R., and Philpot, R. M., Eds., Elsevier/North-Holland, New York, 1979, 287.

82. Post, C., Studies on the Pharmacokinetic Function of the Lung with Special Reference to Lidocaine, Linkoping University Medical Dissertation, No. 73, Linkoping, 1979.

83. Bend, J. R., Ben-Zvi, Z., Anda, J. V., Dansette, P. M., and Jerina, D. M., Hepatic and extraheptic glutathione S-transferase activity towards several arene oxides and epoxides in the rat, in *Polynuclear Aromatic Hydrocarbons: Chemistry, Metabolism and Carcinogenesis,* Vol. 1, Freudenthal, R. I. and Jones, P. W., Eds., Raven Press, New York, 1976, 63.

84. Oesch, F., Glatt, H., and Schmassmann, H., The apparent ubiquity of epoxide hydratase in rat organs, *Biochem. Pharmacol.,* 26, 603, 1977.

85. Mehendale, H. M. and El-Bassiouni, E. A., Uptake and disposition of aldrin and dieldrin by isolated perfused rabbit lung, *Drug Metab. Dispos.,* 3, 543, 1975.

86. Law, F. C. P., Eling, T. E., Bend, J. R., and Fouts, J. R., Metabolism of xenobiotics by the isolated perfused lung, *Drug Metab. Dispos.,* 2, 433, 1974.

87. McGovern, J. P., Lubawy, W. C., and Kostenbauder, H. B., Uptake and metabolism of nicotine by the isolated perfused rabbit lung, in press.

88. Blase, B. W. and Loomis, T. A., The uptake and metabolism of carbaryl by isolated perfused rabbit lung, *Toxicol. Appl. Pharmacol.,* 37, 481, 1976.

89. Wilson, A. G. E., Hirom, P. C., and Kung, H. C., Pharmacokinetics of uptake and metabolism of α-naphthol by the isolated perfused lung, *Toxicol. Appl. Pharmacol.,* 48, A161, 1979.

90. Wilson, A. G. E., Law, F. C. P., Eling, T. E., and Anderson, M. W., Uptake, metabolism and efflux of methadone in 'single pass' isolated perfused rabbit lungs, *J. Pharmacol. Exp. Ther.,* 199, 360, 1976.

91. Roth, R. A., Jr., Roth, J. A., and Gillis, C. N., Disposition of ^{14}C-mescaline by rabbit lung, *J. Pharmacol. Exp. Ther.,* 200, 394, 1977.

92. Law, F. C. P., Metabolism and disposition of Δ^9-tetrahydrocannabinol by the isolated perfused rabbit lung, *Drug Metab. Dispos.,* 6, 154, 1977.

93. Smith, B. R., Philpot, R. M., and Bend, J. R., Metabolism of benzo(a)pyrene by the isolated perfused rabbit lung, *Drug Metab. Dispos.,* 6, 425, 1978.

94. Ryrfeldt, A. and Nilsson, E., Uptake and biotransformation of ibuterol and terbutaline in isolated perfused rat and guinea pig lungs, *Biochem. Pharmacol.,* 27, 301, 1978.

95. Hartiala, J., Studies on Pulmonary Testosterone Metabolism, Ph.D. thesis, Department of Physiology, University of Turku, Finland, 1976.

96. **Vestal, R. E., Kornhauser, D. M., and Shand, D. G.**, Active uptake of ^{3}H-propranolol by isolated alveolar macrophages, *Clin. Res.*, 24, 259, 1976.

97. Biological Effects of Atmospheric Pollutants, Particulate Polycyclic Organic Matter, National Academy of Science, Washington, D.C., 1972.

98. **Wynder, E. L. and Hoffman, D.**, Experimental tobacco carcinogenesis, *Science*, 162, 862, 1968.

99. **Miller, J. A.**, Carcinogenesis by chemicals: an overview, *Cancer Res.*, 30, 559, 1970.

100. **Miller, J. A. and Miller, E. C.**, Ultimate chemical carcinogens as reactive mutagenic electrophiles, in *Origins of Human Cancer*, Book B, Hiatt, H. H., Watson, J. D., and Winsten, J. A., Eds., Cold Spring Harbor Laboratory, Cold Spring Harbor, N.Y., 1977, 605.

101. **Sims, P. and Grover, P. L.**, Epoxides in polycyclic aromatic hydrocarbon metabolism and carcinogenesis, *Adv. Cancer Res.*, 20, 165, 1974.

102. **Cohen, G. M., Moore, B. P., and Bridges, J. W.**, Organic solvent soluble sulphate ester conjugates of monohydroxybenzo(a)pyrenes, *Biochem. Pharmacol.*, 26, 551, 1977.

103. **Nemoto, N. and Gelboin, H. V.**, Enzymatic conjugation of benzo(a)pyrene oxides, phenols and dihydrodiols with UDP-glucuronic acid, *Biochem. Pharmacol.*, 25, 1221, 1976.

104. **Nemoto, N., Takayama, S., and Gelboin, H. V.**, Enzymatic conversion of benzo(a)pyrene phenols, dihydrodiols and quinones to sulfate conjugates, *Biochem. Pharmacol.*, 26, 1825, 1977.

105. **Lesko, S., Caspary, W., Lorentzen, R., and Ts'o, P. O. P.**, The autoxidation of 6-hydroxybenzo(a)pyrene and 6-oxobenzo(a)pyrene radical, reactive metabolites of benzo(a)pyrene, *Biochemistry*, 14, 3878, 1975.

106. **Maher, V. M. and McCormick, J. J.**, Mammalian cell mutagenesis by polycyclic aromatic hydrocarbons and their derivatives, in *Polycyclic Hydrocarbons and Cancer: Molecular and Cell Biology*, Vol. 2, Gelboin, H. V., and Ts'o, P. O. P., Eds., Academic Press, New York, 1978, 137.

107. **Lehr, R. E., Yagi, H., Thakker, D. R., Levin, W., Wood, A. W., Conney, A. H., and Jerina, D. M.**, The bay region theory of polycyclic aromatic hydrocarbon-induced carcinogenicity, in *Polynuclear Aromatic Hydrocarbons: Analysis, Chemistry, and Biology*, Vol. 3, Jones, P. W. and Freudenthal, R. I., Eds., Raven Press, New York, 1978, 231.

108. **Malaveille, C., Bartsch, H., Grover, P. L., and Sims, P.**, Mutagenicity of non-K-region diols and diol-epoxides of benz(a)anthracene and benzo(a)pyrene in *S. typhimurium* TA 100, *Biochem. Biophys. Res. Commun.*, 66, 693, 1975.

109. **Wood, A. W., Levin, W., Lu, A. Y. H., Yagi, H., Hernandez, O., Jerina, D. M., and Conney, A. H.**, Metabolism of benzo(a)pyrene and benzo(a)pyrene derivatives to mutagenic products by highly purified hepatic microsomal enzymes, *J. Biol. Chem.*, 251, 4882, 1976.

110. **Huberman, E., Sachs, L., Yang, S. K., and Gelboin, H. V.**, Identification of mutagenic metabolites of benzo(a)pyrene in mammalian cells, *Proc. Natl. Acad. Sci., U.S.A.*, 73, 607, 1976.

111. **Newbold, R. F. and Brookes, P.**, Exceptional mutagenicity of a benzo(a)pyrene diol epoxide in cultured mammalian cells, *Nature (London)*, 261, 52, 1976.

112. **Kapitulnik, J., Levin, W., Conney, A. H., Yagi, M., and Jerina, D. M.**, Benzo(a)pyrene 7,8-dihydrodiol is more carcinogenic than benzo(a)pyrene in newborn mice, *Nature (London)*, 266, 378, 1977.

113. **Buening, M. K., Wislocki, P. G., Levin, H., Yagi, H., Thakker, D. R., Akagi, H. Koreeda, M., Jerina, D. M., and Conney, A. H.**, Tumorigenicity of the optical enantio enantiomers of the diastereomeric benzo(a)pyrene 7,8-diol-9,10-epoxides in newborn mice: exceptional activity of (+)-7β,8α-dihydroxy-9α,10α-epoxy-7,8,9,10-tetrahydrobenzo(a)pyrene, *Proc. Natl. Acad. Sci. U.S.A.*, 75, 5358, 1978.

114. **Marquardt, H., Grover, P. L., and Sims, P.**, *In vitro* malignant transformation of mouse fibroblasts by non-K-region dihydrodiols derived from 7-methylbenz(a) 7-methylbenz(a)anthracene, 7,12-dimethyl 7,12-dimethylbenz(a) anthracene, and benzo(a)pyrene, *Cancer Res.*, 36, 2059, 1976.

115. **Huberman, E. and Sachs, L.**, DNA binding and its relationship to carcinogenesis by different polycyclic hydrocarbons, *Int. J. Cancer*, 19, 122, 1977.

116. **Grover, P. L. and Sims, P.**, Enzyme-catalyzed reactions of polycyclic hydrocarbons with deoxyribonucleic acid and protein, *Biochem. J.*, 110, 159, 1968.

117. **Thompson, M. H., King, M. W. S., Osborne, M. R., and Brookes, P.**, Rat liver microsome-mediated binding of benzo(a)pyrene metabolites to DNA, *Int. J. Cancer*, 17, 270, 1976.

118. **Pelkonen, O., Boobis, A. R., Yagi, H., Jerina, D. M., and Nebert, D. W.**, Tentative identification of benzo(a)pyrene metabolite-nucleoside complexes produced in vitro by mouse liver microsomes, *Mol. Pharmacol.*, 14, 306, 1978.

119. **Jeffrey, A. M., Weinstein, I. B., Jennette, K. W., Grzeskowiak, K., Nakanishi, K., Harvey, R. G., Autrup, H., and Harris, C.**, Structure of benzo(a)pyrene-nucleic acid adducts formed in human and bovine bronchial explants, *Nature (London)*, 269, 348, 1977.

120. **Phillips, D. M., Grover, P. L., and Sims, S. P.**, A quantitative determination of the covalent binding of a series of polycyclic hydrocarbons to DNA in mouse skin, *Int. J. Cancer*, 23, 201, 1979.

121. Weinstein, I. B., Jeffrey, A. M., Jennette, K. W., Blobstein, S. H., Harvey, R. G., Harris, C. C., Autrup, H., Kasai, H., and Nakanishi, K., Benzo(a)pyrene diol epoxides as intermediates in nucleic acid binding in vitro and in vivo, *Science*, 193, 592, 1976.

122. Eastman, A., Sweetenham, J., and Bresnick, E., Comparisons of *in vivo* and *in vitro* binding of polycyclic hydrocarbons to DNA, *Chem. Biol. Interact.*, 23, 345, 1978.

123. Kahl, G. F., Klaus, E., Legraverend, C., Nebert, D. W., and Pelkonen, O., Formation of benzo(a)pyrene metabolite-nucleoside adducts in isolated perfused rat and mouse liver and in mouse lung slices, *Biochem. Pharmacol.*, 28, 1051, 1979.

124. Vahakangas, K., Nebert, D. W., and Pelkonen, O., The DNA binding of benzo(a)pyrene metabolites catalyzed by rat lung microsomes in vitro and in isolated perfused rat lung, *Chem. Biol. Interact.*, 24, 167, 1979.

125. Deckers-Schmelzle, B., Klaus, E., Kahl, R., and Kahl, G. F., Binding of benzo(a)pyrene metabolites to cellular DNA in perfused rat lungs, *Naunyn-Schmiedeberg's Arch. Pharmacol.*, 303, 303, 1978.

126. Anderson, M. W., Hirom, P. C., Boroujerdi, M., Kung, H. C., and Wilson, A. G. E., Effect of pre-treatment of rats with butylated hydroxyanisole (BHA) on benzo(a)pyrene (BP) pharmacokinetics, *Fed. Proc. Fed. Am. Soc. Exp. Biol.*, 38, 1979.

127. Vahakangas, K., Nevasaari, K., Pelkonen, O., and Karki, N. T., The metabolism of benzo(a)pyrene in isolated perfused lungs from variously treated rats, *Acta Pharmacol. Toxicol.*, 41, 129, 1977.

128. Wattenberg, L. W., Dietary modification of intestinal and pulmonary aryl hydrocarbon hydroxylase activity, *Toxicol. Appl. Pharmacol.*, 23, 741, 1972.

129. Welch, R. M., Cavallito, J., and Loh, A., Effect of exposure to cigarette smoke on the metabolism of benzo(a)pyrene and acetophenetidin by lung and intestine of rats, *Toxicol. Appl. Pharmacol.*, 23, 749, 1972.

130. Cantrell, E., Busbee, D., Warr, G., and Martin, R., Induction of aryl hydrocarbon hydroxylase in human lymphocytes and pulmonary alveolar macrophages — a comparison, *Life Sci.*, 13, 1649, 1973.

131. Wattenberg, L. W. and Leong, J. L., Inhibition of the carcinogenic action of benzo(a)pyrenes by flavones, *Cancer Res.*, 30, 1922, 1970.

132. Wattenberg, L. W., Inhibition of chemical carcinogenesis by antioxidants, in *Carcinogenesis*, Vol. 5, Slaga, T. J., Ed, Raven Press, New York, 85, 1980.

133. Wilson, A. G. E., Kung, H. C., Boroujerdi, M., and Anderson, M. W., unpublished observation.

134. Benedict, W. F., Considine, N., and Nebert, D. W., Genetic differences in aryl hydrocarbon hydroxylase induction and benzo(a)pyrene-produced tumorigenesis in the mouse, *Mol. Pharmacol.*, 9, 266, 1973.

135. Fuller, R. W., Droddy, H. J., and Molloy, B. B., Effect of β,β-difluoro substitution on the disposition and pharmacological effects of 4-chloroamphetamine in rats, *J. Pharmacol. Exp. Ther.*, 184, 278, 1973.

136. Fuller, R. W., Molloy, B. B., and Parli, C. J., The effect of β,β-difluoro substitution on the metabolism and pharmacology of amphetamines, in *Psychopharmacology, Sexual Disorders and Drug Abuse*, Ban, T. A., Boissier, J. R., Gessa, G. J., Heimann, H., Hollister, L., Lehmann, H. E., Munkvad, I., Steinberg, H., Sulser, F., Sundwall, A., and Vinar, O., Eds., North-Holland, Amsterdam, 1973, 615.

137. Lüllman, H., Rossen, E., and Seiler, K. U., The pharmacokinetics of phentermine and chlorphentermine in chronically treated rats, *J. Pharm. Pharmacol.*, 25, 239, 1973.

138. Kuntzman, R., Klutch, A., Tsai, S., and Burns, J. J., Physiological distribution and metabolic inactivation of chlorcyclizine and cyclizine, *J. Pharmacol. Exp. Ther.*, 149, 29, 1965.

139. Glazko, A. J., McGirty, D. A., Dill, W. A., Wilson, M. L., and Ward, C. D., Biochemical studies on diphenhydramine (Benadryl), *J. Biol. Chem.*, 179, 409, 1949.

140. Way, E., Leong, J. L., and Daily, R. E., Absorption, distribution and excretion of tripelennamine (pyribenzamine), *Soc. Exp. Biol. Med.*, 73, 423, 1950.

141. Dreyfuss, J., Rose, J. J., and Schreiben, E. C., Biological disposition and metabolic fate of fluphenazine-^{14}C in the dog and Rhesus monkey, *J. Pharm. Sci.*, 60, 821, 1971.

142. Gardiner, T. H., Lewis, J. M., and Shore, P. A., Distribution of Clozapine in the rat. Localization in lung, *J. Pharmacol. Ther.*, 206, 151, 1978.

143. Wilson, A. G. E., Pickett, R. D., Eling, T. E., and Anderson, M. W., Studies on the persistence of basic amines in the rabbit lung, *Drug Metab. Dispos.*, 7, 420, 1979.

144. Bickel, M. H. and Weder, H. J., The total fate of a drug: kinetics of distribution, excretion, and formation of 14 metabolites in rats treated with imipramine, *Arch. Int. Pharmacodyn. Ther.*, 17, 433, 1968.

145. Richards, J. C., Boxer, G. E., and Smith, C. C., Studies on the distribution and metabolism of methadone in normal and tolerant rats by a new colorimetric method, *J. Pharmacol. Exp. Ther.*, 98, 380, 1950.

146. Hahn, E. F., Norton, B. I., and Fishman, J., Dose related changes in tissue morphine concentration, *Res. Commun. Chem. Pathol. Pharmacol.*, 13, 569, 1976.

147. Agurell, S., Nilson, I. M., Ohlsson, A., and Sandberg, F., On the metabolism of tritium-labelled Δ⁹-tetrahydrocannabinol in the rabbit, *Biochem. Pharmacol.,* 19, 1333, 1970.
148. Hayes, A. and Cooper, R. G., Studies on the absorption, distribution, and excretion of propranolol in rat, dog, and monkey, *J. Pharmacol. Exp. Ther.,* 176, 302, 1971.
149. Black, J. W., Duncan, W. A. M., and Shanks, R. G., Comparison of some properties of pronethalol and propranolol, *Br. J. Pharmacol. Chemother.,* 25, 577, 1965.
150. Stock, K. and Westermann, E., Quantitative estimation and tissue distritution of KO 592, 1-(3-methylphenoxy)-3 isopropyl aminopropanol-2-hydrochloride, a new sympathetic beta-receptor blocking agent, *Biochem. Pharmacol.,* 14, 227, 1965.
151. Sharp, W. C., Ottolenghi, A., and Posner, H. D., Correlation of paraquat toxicity with tissue concentrations and weight loss of the rat, *Toxicol. Appl. Pharmacol.,* 22, 241, 1972.
152. Turner, D. M., The metabolism of ¹⁴C-nicotine in the cat, *Biochem. J.,* 115, 889, 1969.
153. Drew, G., Uptake of amphetamine by guinea pig lung *in vitro, J. Pharm. Pharmacol.,* 30, 55p, 1978.
154. Gardiner, T. H. and McAnalley, B. H., Species comparison of phenol red transport and binding in the mammalian lung, *Gen. Pharmacol.,* 8, 235, 1977.
155. Eling, T. E., Pickett, R. D., Orton, T. C., and Anderson, M. W., A study of the dynamics of imipramine accumulation in the isolated perfused rabbit lung, *Drug Metab. Dispos.,* 3, 389, 1975.
156. Schwartz, S. L., Interaction of nicotine and other amines with the endocytic and exocytic functions of macrophages, *Fed. Proc. Fed. Am. Soc. Exp. Biol.,* 35, 85, 1976.
157. Wilson, A. G. E., Sar, M., and Stumpf, W. E., unpublished observation.
158. Lüllman, H., Lullman-Rauch, R., and Wasserman, O., Drug-Induced phospholipidoses, *CRC Crit. Rev. Toxicol.,* 4, 185, 1975.
159. Lüllmann, H., Rossen, E., and Seiler, K. U., The pharmacokinetics of phentermine and chlorphentermine in chronically treated rats, *J. Pharm. Pharmacol.,* 25, 239, 1973.
160. Seydel, J. K. and Wassermann, O., NMR studies on the molecular basis of drug-induced phospholipidosis, *Naunyn-Schmiedeberg's Arch. Pharmacol.,* 279, 207, 1973.
161. Lüllmann-Rauch, R. and Reil, G. H., Chlorphentermine-induced lipidosis-like ultrastructural alterations in lungs and adrenal glands of several species, *Toxicol. Appl. Pharmacol.,* 30, 408, 1974.
162. Schmien, R., Seiler, K. U., and Wasserman, O., I. Lipid composition and chlorphentermine content of rat lung tissue and alveolar macrophages after chronic treatment, *Naunyn-Schmiedeberg's Arch. Pharmacol.,* 283, 331, 1974.
163. Fishman, A. P., Dietary pulmonary hypertension, *Circ. Res.,* 35, 657, 1974.
164. Mielke, H., Seiler, K. U., Stumpf, U., and Wassermann, O., Uber eine Bejiehung zwischen dem serotoninstoffwechsel und der pulmonalen Hypertonie bei Ratten nach Gabe verschiedener Anorektika, *Z. Kardiol.,* 62, 1090, 1973.
165. Seiler, K. U., Tamm, G., and Wassermann, O., On the role of serotonin in the pathogenesis of pulmonary hypertension induced by anorectic drugs, an experimental study in the isolated perfused rat lung. I. Aminorex, Chlorphentermine and phenmetrazine, *Clin. Exp. Pharmacol. Physiol.,* 1, 463, 1974.
166. Brown, T. C. K. and Leversha, A., Comparison of the cardiovascular toxicity of three tricyclic antidepressant drugs; Imipramine, Amitryptyline and Doxepin, *Clin. Toxicol.,* 14, 253, 1979.
167. Smith, P. H. and Heath, D., Paraquat, *CRC Crit. Rev. Toxicol.,* 4, 411, 1976.
168. Pasi, A., *Toxicology of Paraquat, Diquat and Morfumquat,* Hans Huber, Bern, 1978.
169. Sharp, C. W. M., Ottolenghi, A., and Posner, H. S., Correlation of paraquat toxicity with tissue concentrations and weight loss of the rat, *Toxicol. Appl. Pharmacol.,* 22, 241, 1972.
170. Rose, M. S., Lock, E. A., Smith, L. L., and Wyatt, I., Paraquat accumulation. Tissue and species specificity, *Biochem. Pharmacol.,* 25, 419, 1976.
171. Rose, M. S., Smith, L. L., and Wyatt, I., Evidence for the energy dependent accumulation of parquat into the lung, *Nature (London),* 252, 314, 1974.
172. Rose, M. S. and Smith, L. L., The relevance of paraquat accumulation by tissues, in *Biochemical Mechanisms of Paraquat Toxicity,* Autor, A. P., Ed., Academic Press, New York, 71, 1977.
173. Rose, M. S. and Smith, L. L., Tissue uptake of paraquat and diquat, *Gen. Pharmacol.,* 8, 173, 1977.
174. Wilson, A. G. E., unpublished observation.
175. Lock, E. A., Smith, L. L., and Rose, M. S., Inhibition of paraquat accumulation in rat lung slices by a component of rat plasma and a variety of drugs and endogenous amines, *Biochem. Pharmacol.,* 25, 1769, 1976.
176. Maling, H. M., Saul, W., Williams, M. A., Brown, E. A. B., and Gillette, J. R., On the mechanism of the potentiation by beta adrenergic agonists of paraquat toxicity in rats and mice, in *Biochemical Mechanisms of Paraquat Toxicity,* Autor, A. P., Ed., Academic Press, New York, 137, 1977.
177. Shea, T. E., Jr., Acute and subacute toxicity of morpholine, *J. Ind. Hyg. Toxicol.,* 21, 236, 1939.

178. Kung, H. C., Tombropolous, E. G., and Wilson, A. G. E., Effect of pre-exposure of rabbits to morpholine on imipramine pharmacokinetics in the isolated perfused lung (IPL), Society of Toxicology, 18th Annual Meeting, New Orleans, 1979.

179. Mehendale, H. M., Modulation of pulmonary uptake by pre-exposure to xenobiotics, *Toxicol. Appl. Pharmacol.*, 45, 316, 1978.

180. Smith, B., personal communication.

Primary Responses of the Lung to Toxic Agents

Chapter 5

CELL DEATH AND CELL RENEWAL IN SMALL AIRWAYS AND ALVEOLI

Michael J. Evans

TABLE OF CONTENTS

I. INTRODUCTION

Many chemicals are known to injure the lung.[1] Injury may occur via the airways or the bloodstream. The cells most vulnerable to injury in distal airways are ciliated cells. In alveoli, Type I epithelial cells and endothelial cells of the vascular system are most frequently damaged. Clara cells, Type II cells, and alveolar macrophages appear to be relatively resistant to injury. Inhalation of oxidant gases such as NO_2 and O_3 causes damage in the terminal bronchioles and adjacent alveoli,[2,3] but peripheral alveoli are rarely affected. This is thought to be due to a concentration gradient for these gases that exists in the lung. Also, injury occurs mainly to the epithelium, with few effects reported for the endothelium. Effects similar to those seen with NO_2 and O_3 are reported following exposure to such chemicals as $FeCl_3$ and $CdCl_2$.[4-6] Oxygen, on the other hand, affects all regions of the alveoli;[7,8] damage occurs to both epithelial and endothelial cells. Agents that affect the lung by way of the bloodstream, such as butylated hydroxytoluene[9] or bleomycin,[10] induce diffuse damage to the alveoli similar to that reported for oxygen.

Under normal conditions, animals surviving the initial damage enter a phase of cellular proliferation in order to repair the injured tissue. The mechanism by which this type of reparative regeneration occurs has been shown to be an acceleration of the normal cell renewal processes of the tissue.[11,12] Cell renewal as a mechanism can be described as a homeostatic means for replacement of cells lost from a tissue.[13] It is most obvious in tissues that have a large loss of cells that must be constantly replaced, e.g., skin, intestine, and blood. In these tissues, replacement of the lost differentiated cells occurs through division of undifferentiated (progenitor) cells followed by migration and maturation of the sister cells. In slowly renewing cell populations, the mechanisms are not as clearly defined; however, they appear to follow the same basic pattern.

Mechanisms for cell renewal in the lung have been under investigation for many years.[14,15] The concept that the lung contained renewing populations of cells was first advanced by the observations that large numbers of pulmonary cells were extruded in the sputum. Most of these cells were macrophages, and early investigators directed their efforts toward understanding the origin of the extruded macrophages. In studies using colchicine to arrest dividing cells during metaphase, Bertalanffy[15] observed two populations of dividing cells in the alveoli. With light microscopy, he classified these cell populations as vacuolated and nonvacuolated alveolar cells. Using the incidence of mitotic figures observed, he calculated a turnover time of 27 days for vacuolated cells and 9 days for nonvacuolated cells. These results were interpreted to be a mechanism for replacement of the alveolar macrophage cell population lost from the lung. Using tritiated thymidine (^{3}H-TdR) to label cells synthesizing DNA in preparation for division and light microscopic autoradiography to visualize them, other investigators confirmed these results.[16,17]

Although these investigations had demonstrated a population of dividing cells in the lung, the identity of the dividing cells in the alveoli was not clear. To clarify the identity of these cells, Evans and Bils[18] used ^{3}H-TdR to label dividing cells and studied them with the electron microscope. In young mice, about 2% of the alveolar cells are labeled following an injection of ^{3}H-TdR. Of this population of labeled cells, the largest proportion (42.0%) consisted of mononuclear cells in the capillaries, followed by endothelial cells (30.8%), Type II cells (6.0%), and alveolar macrophages (5.2%). The remaining labeled cells could not be positively identified and were classified as "interstitial cells". How these various cell types participate in a mechanism for cell renewal and their relationship to reparative regeneration following injury have been studied extensively in recent years. Such studies have resulted in descriptions of the

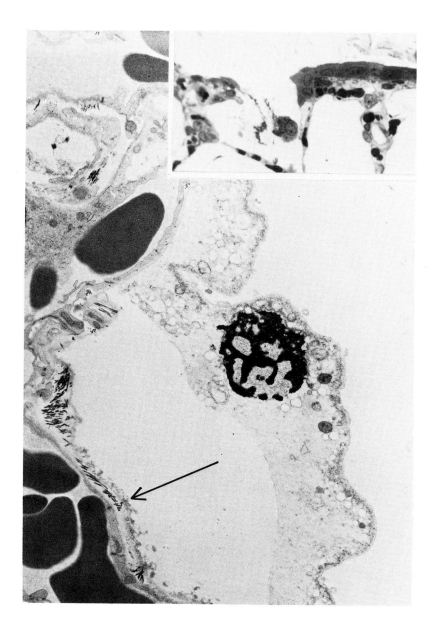

FIGURE 1.   Injured Type I alveolar cell after 24 hr of exposure to NO_2. Note the amount of basement membrane not covered by the Type I cell (arrow). (Magnification × 6384.) Insert — light micrograph of injured area. (Magnification × 527.)

mechanisms for renewal of the epithelial and macrophage cell populations of the lung. Studies on renewal of pulmonary endothelium have only recently begun.

II. PULMONARY EPITHELIUM

A. Alveoli

The epithelium lining the walls of the alveoli is composed primarily of large, squamous Type I cells and smaller, cuboidal Type II cells. Type I cells cover most of the alveolar surface, and Type II cells are dispersed throughout the alveoli between Type

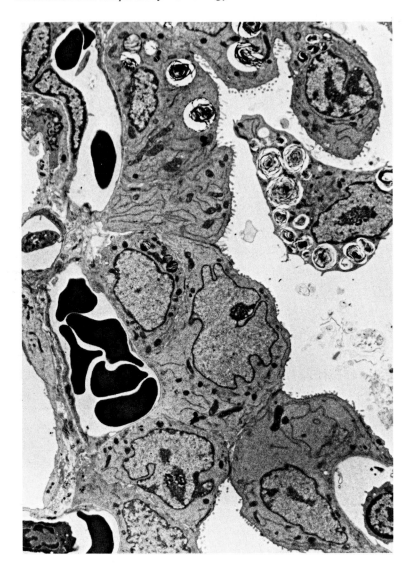

FIGURE 2.   Cuboidal epithelium covering a portion of the alveoli after 72-hr exposure to NO_2. (Magnification × 3230.)

I cells. Both cell types lie on a common basement membrane. Occasionally, a Type III cell is observed.[19]

A number of studies have described injury to Type I alveolar epithelium under a variety of conditions.[2-7,9,10,20] Generally, it involves swelling and disruption of Type I cells. The cells are then sloughed off the alveolar walls, leaving large areas of basement membrane uncovered (see Figure 1). Type II cells are relatively resistant to injury. Following injury to Type I epithelium, Type II cells appear to proliferate and cover the damaged areas of alveolar walls (see Figure 2).

The means by which the alveolar epithelium is renewed was recently described. Based on morphologic data, Kapanci et al.[7] suggested that Type II cells were the reserve cells for repair of the alveolar epithelium. In a study of rats exposed to NO_2, the proliferative response of Type II cells following injury to Type I epithelium was measured.[21] Proliferation reached a maximum in 2 days and then subsided (see Figure 3). Based

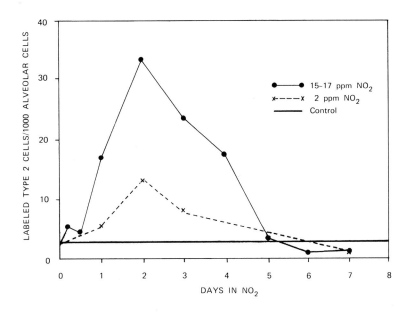

FIGURE 3. Mean labeling indexes of Type II alveolar cells from rats exposed to 2 and 17 ppm NO₂ for 7 days. The shaded area is the SD from the mean.

on these observations, studies were initiated to determine the fate of Type II cells after division.[22] A group of rats was exposed to NO_2 for 2 days and the dividing cells were labeled with ³H-TdR. The rats were sacrificed at various times after labeling; the lungs were removed and studied in light and electron microscopy, using autoradiographic techniques.

These studies showed that as Type II cells divided, they moved apart over the basement membrane, so that both sister cells remained on the alveolar wall after division. A curve of mitotic figures demonstrated that most of the labeled Type II cells had divided within 12 hr of injecting the ³H-TdR. Electron microscopic autoradiography revealed that at 1 hr after ³H-TdR, all labeled cells were Type II cells (see Figure 4). However, after 2 days, 64.2% of the labeled cells were Type II, and 35.8% were Type I (see Figure 5). Light microscopy revealed that the large increase in labeled Type I cells occurred between 1 and 2 days after ³H-TdR and persisted at 3 days. Because Type II cells were the only cells labeled initially, any other labeled cells that appeared would have been derived from them. From these data, it was interpreted that Type II cells acted as progenitor cells of the alveolar epithelium, forming new Type I and Type II cells after dividing.

In a later study, the morphologic and kinetic details of the process whereby Type II cells differentiate into Type I cells were described.[23] Rats exposed to NO_2 for 2 days were injected with ³H-TdR, placed in room air, and the lungs examined with electron microscopic autoradiography for 14 days after labeling. Labeled cells were classified as either Type II, undetermined, or Type I. Undetermined cells were epithelial cells not containing lamellar bodies or not having attenuated portions of cytoplasm covering the basement membrane (see Figure 6). The majority of these cells had a cuboidal shape. The results of this study are summarized in Figure 7. They demonstrate the progression of label from Type II cells through the undetermined cell population and ending in the Type I cell population. The time required for Type II cells to differentiate into Type I cells was about 2 days, after which the labeled cell populations were stable for up to 14 days. Not all labeled Type II cells transformed into Type I cells, and there was a slight overall increase of Type II cells in the tissue. The process of differentiation

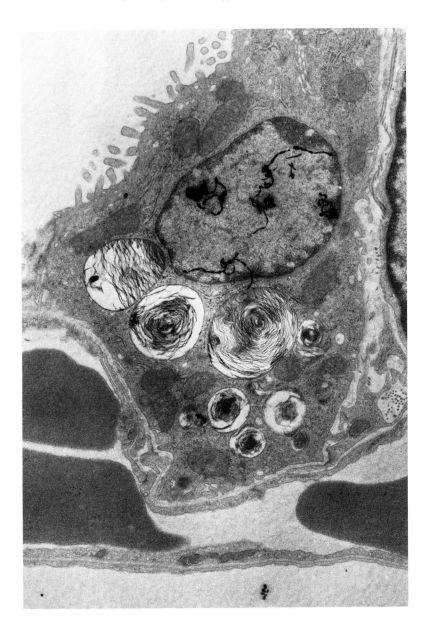

FIGURE 4.   Labeled Type II cell in the alveoli of a rat 1 hr after injection of ^{3}H-TdR.
(Magnification × 13,000.)

involved an intermediate step (undetermined cell type) that exists at 1 day after injection of ^{3}H-TdR. Presumably, this cell may either flatten out and become a Type I cell
or synthesize lamellar bodies and become a Type II cell.

In a study of mice exposed to 100% O_2 for 6 days, Adamson and Bowden[24] confirmed these observations and reached the same conclusion. They found that mice
surviving the exposure exhibited a large increase in Type II cell proliferation. Repeating
this study, they labeled Type II cells during the peak of cell division and followed them
for 4 days with light microscopic autoradiography. Initially, most of the labeled cells
were Type II, but on the 4th day a large increase in labeled Type I cells was observed.
Based on these data, they concluded that Type II cells are the progenitors of the alveolar epithelium.

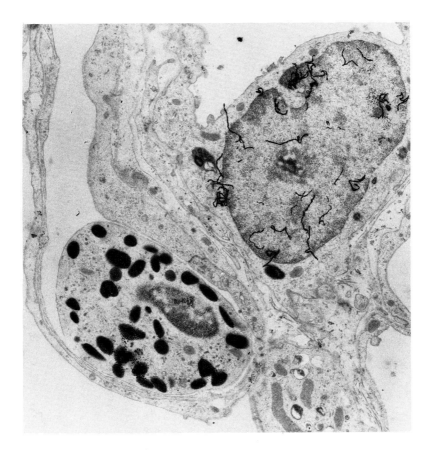

FIGURE 5.   Labeled Type I cell in the alveoli of a rat 2 days after an injection of ³H-TdR. (Magnification × 11,600.)

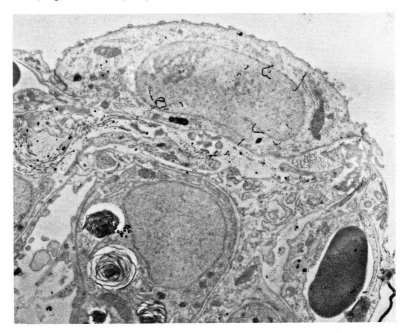

FIGURE 6.   Labeled undetermined cell in the alveoli of a rat 1 day following an injection of ³H-TdR. (Magnification × 9000.)

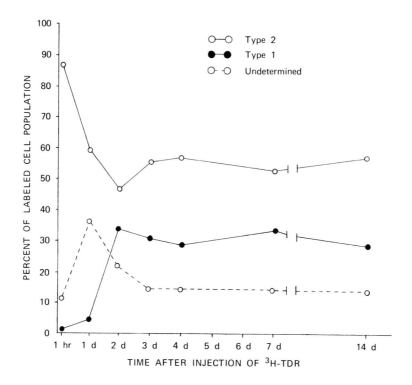

FIGURE 7.   Average percentage of each cell type in the labeled alveolar epithelium from 1 hr to 14 days following a single injection of ³H-TdR.

Using a different approach, Kauffman et al.[25] studied the postnatal growth of rat lung. They found a large increase in labeled Type II cells, but no labeled Type I cells. Following the increase in labeled Type II cells, there was a large increase in the total number of Type I cells, but not in the number of Type II cells. From these data, they concluded that Type II cells were the stem cells of the Type I epithelium. In a study of postnatal development in the lungs of rats, Adamson and Bowden[26] found similar results and reached similar conclusions.

B. Bronchiolar Epithelium

The bronchiolar epithelium is lined with cells that are continuous with those in the alveoli, but that differ morphologically from alveolar epithelial cells.[27-29] Bronchiolar cells may be divided into two groups: nonciliated cells and ciliated cells. The population of nonciliated cells has been further separated into as many as four cell types. The most numerous type is Clara cells which are characterized by the presence of secretory granules and smooth endoplasmic reticulum (SER). Intermediate cells are much less numerous and are characterized by their lack of secretory granules. "Serous" cells, which were only recently described, are not numerous and are characterized by the presence of secretory granules and the lack of SER. Brush cells contain stubby microvilli on their free surface and numerous cytoplasmic fibers; they are rarely encountered in normal animals. Both ciliated and nonciliated cells reside on a common basement membrane, and no basal cells are present.

A number of investigators have described injury to bronchiolar epithelial cells following various treatments.[2,3,20,30,31] Ciliated cells appear to be the most vulnerable to damage. Most commonly reported changes are loss of cilia, necrosis, and sloughing of cells into the airway lumen (see Figure 8). Changes in nonciliated cells are less commonly observed. Those reported are swelling, necrosis, and desquamation of cells.[32,33]

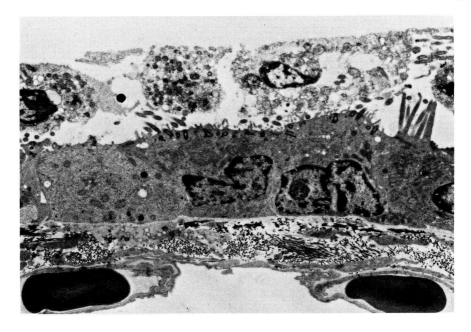

FIGURE 8. Damaged bronchiolar epithelium in a rat after 8 hr of exposure to NO_2. (Magnification × 5700.)

Occasionally, large sheets of bronchiolar epithelium containing both ciliated and nonciliated cells are sloughed off.[34]

A mechanism for renewal of the bronchiolar epithelium was recently described. Studies of control animals indicated that the rate of cell division in the bronchiolar epithelium is low.[35] However, following injury there is a large increase in the number of dividing cells.[21] The maximum amount of cell division is seen within 24 hr of injury (see Figure 9). Under the light microscope, most of the dividing cells in the bronchiolar epithelium appeared to be nonciliated.

To determine the fate of the dividing cells, Evans et al.[36] labeled them with ^{3}H-TdR and followed them over 15 days of recovery. Electron microscopy revealed that at 1 hr after ^{3}H-TdR, all of the labeled cells were nonciliated (see Figure 10). During the next few days, labeled ciliated cells appeared, and by the 4th day they made up 20 to 30% of the labeled cell population (see Figure 11). They remained at this level for the remaining 11 days of the study. Grain counts of nonciliated cells decreased from 9.0 at 1 hr to 5.2 at 4 days, indicating that the labeled cells had undergone division. Grain counts of ciliated cells after 4 days (5.3) were the same as that of nonciliated cells at 4 days. Because nonciliated cells were the only cells labeled at 1 hr after ^{3}H-TdR and labeled ciliated cells appeared later, it was concluded that ciliated cells are derived from nonciliated cells.

In a later study, the relationship between the various nonciliated cell types (Clara, serous, intermediate, and brush cells) and the dividing cell population was examined.[37] It was previously thought that intermediate cells were the nonciliated cell types that underwent division.[27] However, in the previous study, examples of dividing Clara cells were observed.[36] The main morphological difference between these cell types is the presence or absence of secretory granules. In animals exposed to NO_2, there appeared to be a loss of granules from the Clara cells. If this were the case, they would be classified as intermediate cells. In a study similar to the previous one, rats were exposed to NO_2 for 24 hr, labeled with ^{3}H-TdR, and allowed to recover for 14 days. At intervals, animals were sacrificed and studied with electron microscopic autoradiography.

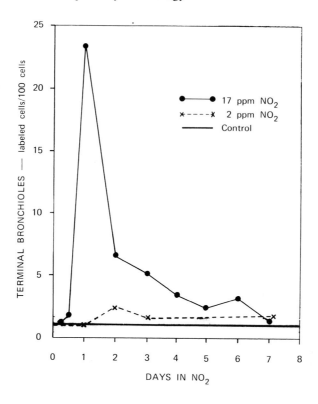

FIGURE 9.   Mean labeling indexes of nonciliated bronchiolar
cells from rats exposed to 2 and 17 ppm NO_2 for 7 days. The
shaded area is the SD from the mean.

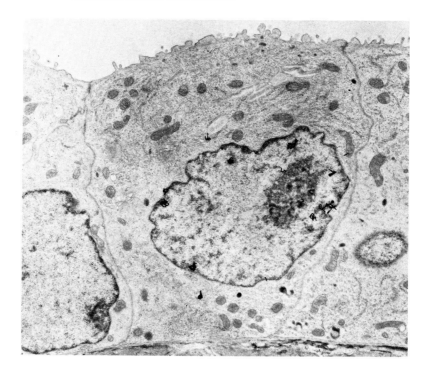

FIGURE 10.   Labeled nonciliated bronchiolar cell (Type A intermediate) 1 hr after
injection of ^{3}H-TdR. Note lack of oval granules. (Magnification × 7100.)

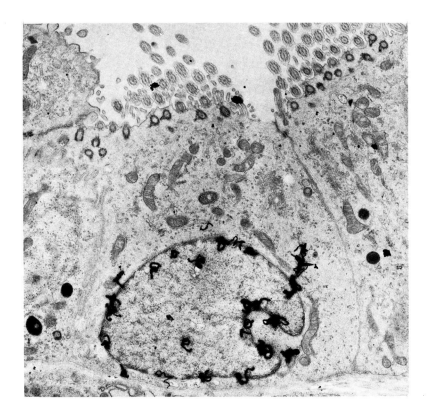

FIGURE 11. Labeled ciliated cell in bronchiolar epithelium 7 days after ³H-TdR. (Magnification × 9100.)

Criteria for identification of nonciliated cell types were established as follows. Clara cells were those containing both oval granules and SER (see Figure 12). The remaining nonciliated cells were separated into two groups, one lacking oval granules (Type A cells, Figure 10) and the other containing oval granules, but lacking SER (Type B cells, Figure 13). Brush cells were recognized by their characteristic microvilli (see Figure 14).

The frequencies of these cell types over the period studied are presented in Figure 15. In 1 hr after ³H-TdR, 90% of the labeled cells were Type A cells. During the next 6 days, they decreased in number to around 10% of the labeled population and remained at that level thereafter. Clara cells composed only 3% of the labeled cell population at 1 hr after ³H-TdR. They increased to approximately 60% of the labeled cell population by 7 days and remained at that level. Type B cells made up 6.5% of the labeled population at 1 hr after ³H-TdR. After 2 days, they had increased to 35%; by the 7th day, they decreased to 7%. Only a few labeled brush cells were observed. Labeled ciliated cells appeared in the manner described previously.[36] Based on these data, it was concluded that Clara cells were derived through differentiation of Type A cells, that Type B cells were a phase of this process, and that ciliated cells were also derived from Type A cells. There were not enough labeled brush cells seen to determine whether they could divide or were derived from other sources.

Because Type A cells are rarely seen in control animals, but are numerous after exposure to NO_2, their increase in number could have occurred through multiplication of Type A cells or by secretion of oval granules from Clara cells and their subsequent reclassification to Type A cells. To determine which event occurred, the above experi-

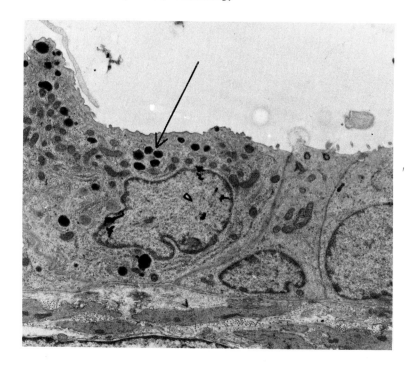

FIGURE 12.   Labeled Clara cell with numerous oval granules (arrow) and abundant SER 7 days after ³H-TdR. (Magnification × 6700.)

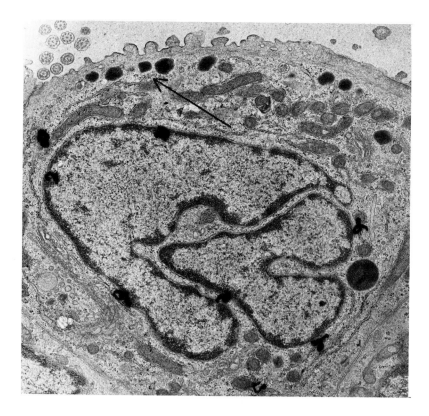

FIGURE 13.   Labeled Type B intermediate cell 3 days after ³H-TdR. Note oval granules (arrow) and lack of SER. (Magnification × 12,700.)

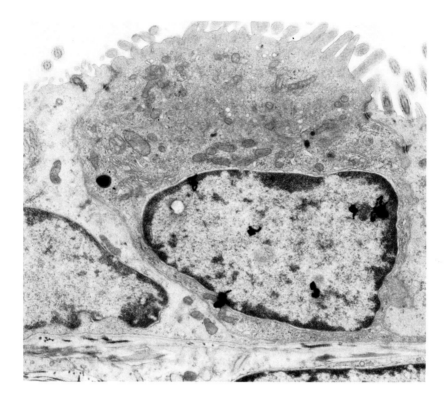

FIGURE 14. Labeled brush cell in bronchiolar epithelium 5 days after ³H-TdR. (Magnification × 10,750.)

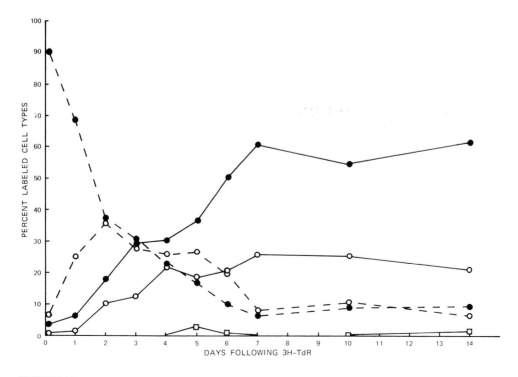

FIGURE 15. Average frequencies of bronchiolar cell types at various times after labeling with ³H-TdR: Type A cells (●---●); Type B cells (○---○); Clara cells (●—●); ciliated cells (○—○); brush cells (□—□).

Table 1
FREQUENCY OF LABELED CELL TYPES IN THE BRONCHIOLAR
EPITHELIUM AFTER REEXPOSURE TO NO₂

Duration of reexposure	Number of labeled cells	Percent of total population					Mean grain count[a]
		Type A cells	Type B cells	Clara cells	Brush cells	Ciliated cells	
None	43 ± 6	13.5 ± 5.0	8.2 ± 1.9	57.0 ± 8.6	0.6 ± 0.9	20.8 ± 5.9	10.0 ± 1.1
12 hr	33 ± 4	42.1 ± 7.5	7.4 ± 4.2	27.7 ± 9.0	0.7 ± 1.1	22.1 ± 10.5	9.9 ± 2.3
24 hr	47 ± 8	56.0 ± 7.8	5.9 ± 1.7	14.0 ± 5.4	0.5 ± 1.1	23.7 ± 4.5	10.9 ± 0.5

Note: Each value represents the mean ± SD from six rats.

[a]   Grain counts determined with the light microscope.

ment was repeated and the animals were allowed to recover for 14 days. At 14 days, there is a stable population of labeled cells in the epithelium (see Figure 15). Groups of animals were then reexposed to NO₂. At 0, 12, and 24 hr of exposure, rats were sacrificed and the proportion of labeled cells present was determined (see Table 1). In animals not reexposed, Type A cells made up 13.5% of the labeled population, and Clara cells made up 57%. After 12 hr of reexposure, Type A cells made up 42.1% and by 24 hr made up 56%. Clara cells decreased to 27.7% at 12 hr of reexposure and to 14.0% at 24 hr. Grain counts at 0, 12, and 24 hr were 10.0, 9.9, and 10.9, indicating that the labeled cells had not divided. These data were interpreted to mean that Clara cells had lost oval granules during exposure to NO₂ and were reclassified as Type A cells. Because cell division was not associated with these changes, it was concluded that the Type A cell is a functional phase of the Clara cells and that the Clara cell is the progenitor for the bronchiolar epithelium. In agreement with these results, Lum et al.[38] found, in rats exposed to O₃ and O₂, that most of the dividing nonciliated cells were Clara cells.

The process of cell renewal in the terminal bronchioles is basically the same as that reported for the tracheobronchial epithelium.[39-42] In this region of the airway, the epithelium is composed of ciliated, mucous, nonciliated, and basal cells. Cell kinetic studies indicate that basal cells are the progenitor cells for the tracheobronchial epithelium. Following division, the sister cells may become intermediate cells and divide again or may differentiate directly into mature epithelial cells (ciliated and mucous cells). It is thought that mucous cells may also differentiate into ciliated cells.[42,43]

C. Renewal of Pulmonary Epithelium

A scheme for renewal of the pulmonary epithelium is presented in Table 2. In the upper airways, basal cells are the progenitor cells. Following division, the sister cells become intermediate cells and may divide again or differentiate directly into mature epithelial cells (ciliated and mucous cells). In the bronchioles, there are no basal cells, and Clara cells act as progenitor cells. Following division, the sister cells may divide again or directly form new Clara and ciliated cells. It is not clear whether new brush cells are formed by this route. In the alveoli, Type II cells are the progenitor cells. Following division, the sister cells may divide again or directly form new Type II and Type I cells.

A common feature in this scheme for renewal of the pulmonary epithelium concerns the nature of the progenitor cells and the cells being replaced. In the region of the pulmonary epithelium without basal cells (bronchioles and alveoli), both Clara cells and Type II cells act as progenitor cells. These cells have a much smaller surface area

Table 2
MECHANISMS FOR RENEWAL OF THE PULMONARY
EPITHELIUM

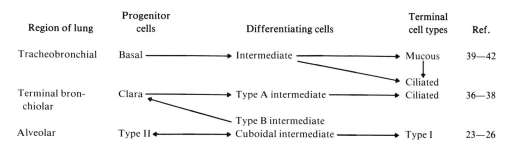

Region of lung	Progenitor cells	Differentiating cells	Terminal cell types	Ref.
Tracheobronchial	Basal ⟶	Intermediate ⟶	Mucous ↓ Ciliated	39—42
Terminal bron-chiolar	Clara	Type A intermediate ⟶ Type B intermediate	Ciliated	36—38
Alveolar	Type II ⟵	Cuboidal intermediate ⟶	Type I	23—26

than either ciliated or Type I cells and are not injured as easily. Also, both are thought to be secretory in nature. The intermediate cells formed following division of the progenitor cells are also similar. The cells being replaced (ciliated and Type I cells) present a large surface area to the environment and are sensitive to damage by injurious agents. There is no clear evidence that ciliated cells can divide, and there are only a few examples of dividing Type I cells. It is probable that ciliated and Type I cells do not divide because of their degree of differentiation. Ciliated cells have a complex surface anatomy (the cilia and associated structures) which could make cell division difficult.[27] In a different manner, Type I cells are also specialized. Weibel[44] described them as differentiated topographically. According to this theory, it would be physically difficult for them to divide because of the large surface area that each cell covers in the alveoli.

The process described here for renewal of the pulmonary epithelium was developed in part from studies in which the epithelium had been damaged experimentally. This raises the possibility that the same process may not occur in normal animals. However, in other tissues, this type of reparative regeneration occurs through acceleration of the normal mechanism for cell renewal.[12] In several studies, it was shown that removal of surface epithelial cells resulted in increased proliferation of the remaining progenitor cells.[11,45-47] This was followed by a buildup of intermediate cells which eventually differentiated into a normal surface epithelium. This sequence of events is essentially the same as that seen in the pulmonary epithelium following experimental injury, suggesting that cell renewal in the pulmonary epithelium of uninjured animals occurs by the same means.

D. Factors Affecting Epithelial Cell Renewal
1. Progenitor Cells

Many factors are involved in the process of epithelial cell renewal.[12,13] The event initiating cell proliferation appears to be cellular injury that results in a loss of cells from the tissue.[11,45-47] In the lung, most examples of progenitor cell division have occurred in animals exposed to agents that cause injury to the terminal cell types.[21,24,48-53] If no injury was observed following an insult, there was usually no cell division.[51] Cell proliferation not associated with tissue renewal mechanisms can also occur in the lung. Such proliferation is associated with growth of the lung or tumor formation.[25,26,54-62]

Under normal conditions, the amount of epithelial cell proliferation following loss of cells is controlled in part by a negative feedback mechanism.[11,13] According to this theory, a decrease in the number of differentiated cells is followed by increased proliferation of progenitor cells until the differentiated cells are replaced. To determine whether proliferation in the lung is under this type of control, a study was carried out to determine how closely the amount of Type I epithelial cell damage was related to the total proliferative response of the Type II cells.[63] In these experiments, rats of various ages were exposed to different concentrations of NO_2 for up to 14 days. At daily intervals for at least the first 5 days of exposure, the Type II labeling index (LI) had been determined. In each of these experiments, the Type II cell labeling increased by the 2nd or 3rd day and then decreased by the 5th day of exposure (see Figure 3). The sum of these LIs over the 5 days of exposure was considered a measure of the magnitude of the proliferative response. In the same experiments, animals exposed for only 1 day were studied with the electron microscope. At this time, Type II cell proliferation had not replaced the damaged Type I cells and injury was visible as areas of basement membrane not covered (BmNC) by Type I cells (see Figure 1). Using standard morphometric techniques, the proportion of alveolar BmNC was determined. There was a high degree of correlation ($r = 0.90$) between the amount of injury and the corresponding proliferative response (see Figure 16). The positive correlation obtained suggests that proliferation of Type II cells in the presence of Type I cell injury is in response to that injury and is under control of a negative feedback mechanism. Because of the high degree of correlation, the proliferative response of Type II cells can be used as an indirect means of quantitating the amount of Type I cell damage. These observations are supported by other studies[21,49-51] in which there was a dose-related correlation between the extent of proliferation and injury in the alveoli under a variety of experimental conditions.

Although no direct correlation between cellular injury and the proliferative response has been made in tracheobronchial and bronchiolar epithelium, a similar situation probably exists in those areas. Several studies have demonstrated a dose-related response in the airway epithelium,[21,38,41,64] suggesting that the magnitude of proliferation is related to the amount of injury in these tissues also.

The time at which cell division begins following injury is important to the process of repair in the lung. Under most conditions of injury, proliferation of cells in the lung occurs within the first day of injury.[21,48-51,64] Exceptions are found in aging animals and in those exposed to oxygen.[65-70] In a study of rats exposed to NO_2, the onset of cell proliferation took about a day longer in old rats than in young ones.[69] The older rats had a greater area of tissue damage (see Figure 17) and higher mortality due to edema than did young rats.[68] It was concluded that the higher mortality was due to a delay in repair combined with greater tissue damage, which resulted in a greater accumulation of edema. A similar situation seems to exist in lungs of animals exposed to O_2. It is known that O_2 inhibits cell division in the lung.[65,67] Also, O_2 causes injury to Type I epithelium similar to that seen with O_3 and NO_2, and death is due to pulmonary edema.[7,8] The major difference between the response of the lung to O_2 and to O_3 or NO_2 is that reparative regeneration is inhibited during exposure to O_2.

Additional studies on the effect of O_2 on the lung showed that deprivation of food caused an inhibition of cell division in unexposed mice that was the same as in animals exposed to O_2.[70] It was also noted that the latter group eat less and have about the same weight loss as those deprived of food. These findings raised a question concerning whether inhibition of cell division in rats exposed to O_2 was due to the O_2 or the lack of food. Therefore, animals were exposed to O_3 to injure the tissues and increase the number of dividing cells. The animals were allowed to recover in 100% O_2 or air, with or without food. These results demonstrated that recovery in 100% O_2 inhibits cell division, whereas recovery in air and deprivation of food does not.[71] This indicates that in vivo, O_2 acts on the cell to inhibit cell division.

In a similar study, Witschi and Côte[105] reported inhibition of total lung DNA synthesis in mice injured by butylated hydroxytoluene (BHT) and allowed to recover in 60, 80, and 100% oxygen. In mice recovering in 40% oxygen, DNA synthesis was not

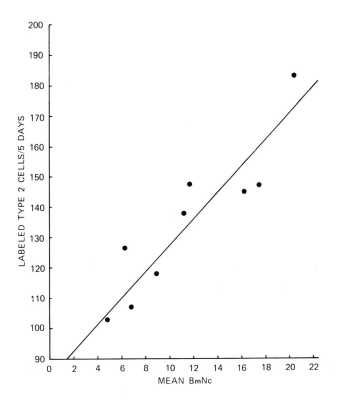

FIGURE 16. The relationship between the proliferative response of Type II cells and the proportion of alveolar epithelium damaged (BmNC) during continuous exposure to NO_2. Correlation coefficient, r = 0.90.

significantly inhibited. The results obtained by Witschi and Côte[105] and those of Hackney et al.[71] may be of practical importance. It is clear that concentrations of oxygen as low as 60% could inhibit the repair processes in the lung following acute lung injury. This could lead to lethal pulmonary edema such as that demonstrated in aging rats exposed to NO_2 in which the onset of Type II cell proliferation was delayed 1 day.[69] Also it has been suggested that inhibition of epithelial cell division associated with repair may lead to fibrosis.[106] A large number of toxic agents cause injury to Type I epithelium followed by Type II cell proliferation.[1] Understanding factors associated with control of reparative cell proliferation in the lung, particularly the identification of agents that inhibit this process, would be of importance in the treatment of injury to the alveolar epithelium such as that seen in acute respiratory failure.[72]

2. Cellular Differentiation

The proliferative phase of Type II cells is associated with replacement of damaged Type I epithelium. Under conditions of acute injury where the animals recover without further insult, this usually results in a cuboidal layer of cells in the alveoli which then differentiates into the normal squamous Type I epithelium (see Figure 7).[22-24] However, under conditions of chronic insult and with various types of injury, the cuboidal epithelium persists (see Figure 2).[68,73,74] Although no kinetic studies have been carried out on this process, it can be postulated that because of the treatment, the cuboidal intermediate cells do not differentiate into Type I cells. Under conditions of chronic insult by oxidant gases, this situation may be associated with the development of tolerance.[20,68,75] With certain types of chemical injury, it appears to be a failure in differ-

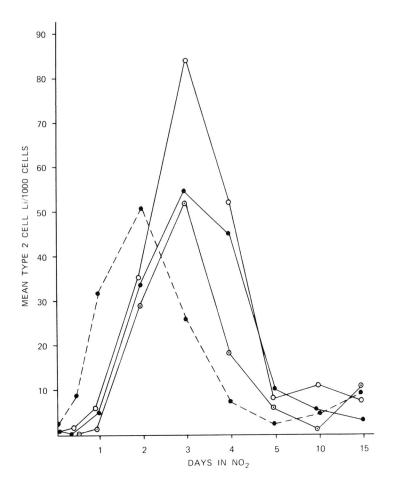

FIGURE 17.   Mean labeling indexes of Type II cells from rats of different ages exposed to NO_2: 1 month old (●---●); 11 months old (●—●); 19 months old (O—O); 25 months old (O--O).

entiation.[10,52] Another aspect of the persisting cuboidal epithelium is its relationship to tumor formation.[56,62]

The concept of tolerance is well documented in the literature on the lungs' response to injury.[75] Tolerance develops following injury. The tolerant cells are those resulting from division of progenitor cells in order to repair the damaged tissue. This was demonstrated in a study in which rats were exposed to O_3, labeled with ^{3}H-TdR, and allowed to recover in air.[76] After 3 days, a stable population of labeled Type I and Type II cells existed in the tissue. These animals were then reexposed to O_3 for 24 hr, and the proportion of labeled Type I cells was determined. There was no loss of labeled Type I cells such as would be expected if they were reinjured. The length of time that such cells remain tolerant following an acute exposure to O_3 was shown in a subsequent study. Animals were exposed to O_3 for 2 days and allowed to recover in air. At intervals of 3, 7, 15, and 30 days, they were reexposed to the same concentration of O_3, and Type II cell proliferation was measured. At 3 and 7 days, Type II cell proliferation was low, but at 15 and 30 days of recovery, it was elevated (see Figure 18). Because such proliferation is in response to injury, the data may be interpreted as showing that the tissue was tolerant for at least 7 days. Similar results were obtained in a study of hamsters exposed to NO_2.[77]

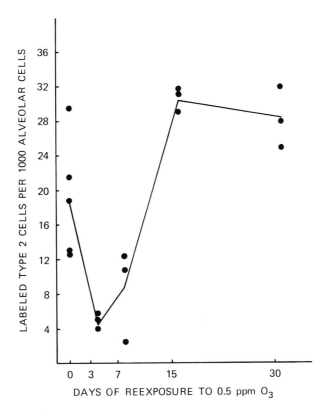

FIGURE 18. Labeling indexes of Type II cells from rats reexposed to 0.5 ppm O_3 at various days after an initial exposure to 0.5 ppm O_3.

Tolerance was also displayed during continuous exposure. In these experiments, rats were exposed to O_3 or NO_2 continuously for up to 15 days. Injury occurred early during exposure, followed by proliferation of progenitor cells. When repair was complete, the rate of proliferation returned to near control levels, and no further injury was seen despite continuous exposure to the gas.[21,49] If the concentration of the gas was elevated, injury was observed, but it was less than the amount of injury caused by that concentration of gas in previously unexposed animals (see Figure 19).[49]

The reason for the resistance of such cells to injury is not clear. The resistance may be due to biochemical changes within the cell or its membrane. Also, it is possible that injury is related to the surface area of the cell exposed to the gas. In alveolar tissue that has been injured and repaired, there are more cells in the injured area of tissue which results in a smaller surface area of each cell being exposed to the environment.[21-23] This is particularly obvious in chronic exposure where a cuboidal epithelium develops.[68,73,74] If animals exposed chronically to the gas are placed in air for a period of time, the tissue returns to a normal squamous appearance,[73] indicating that persistence of the cuboidal epithelium was associated with exposure to the gas. However, further research is needed to explain how the cuboidal epithelium is related to tolerance.

Certain chemicals, such as bleomycin[10,52] and $CaCrO_4$,[78] cause the cuboidal epithelium to persist in a manner similar to that seen with chronic exposure to oxidant gases.[10,52,78] Often the cuboidal cells lining the alveoli take on the characteristics of bronchiolar cells, namely, the formation of ciliated and Goblet cells. This condition has been called alveolar bronchiolization.[78] The source of the cells involved has been

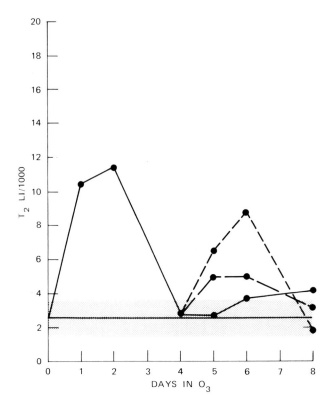

FIGURE 19.   Mean labeling indexes of Type II cells from rats exposed to O_3: 0.5 ppm (●—●); 0.5 ppm for 4 days followed by 0.75 ppm (● --- ●); 0.5 ppm for 4 days followed by 1.0 ppm (●---●); control (—). The shaded area is the SD from the control mean.

of interest for several years. Most investigators have considered the formation of this epithelium to be an outgrowth of the bronchiolar epithelium.[78] However, recently, Adamson and Bowden[52] showed that these cells were derived from proliferating Type II cells. In animals given bleomycin, a cuboidal epithelium formed in injured areas of the alveoli. Initial labeling studies showed increased division of Type II cells in the alveoli. In the bronchiole, the rate of division was near the control value. Because bronchiolar cells did not divide, but Type II cells did, the authors concluded that (1) bronchiolar cells did not contribute to formation of the cuboidal epithelium and (2) ciliated cells that differentiated in this epithelium were derived from Type II cells.

The relationship between the formation of a cuboidal epithelium and tumor formation is not clearly understood. Studies by Kauffman[56] have demonstrated Type II cell hyperplasia and the formation of tumors in animals exposed to urethane. However, they could not relate the two forms of proliferation and suggested that Type II cell hyperplasia was in response to injury caused by the urethane.

In the bronchioles, a situation similar to that in the alveoli probably exists. The cells most vulnerable to injury are ciliated cells. Proliferation of Clara cells occurs to replace damaged ciliated cells. When the insulting agent is removed, the epithelium returns to normal. If the insulting agent persists, hyperplasia of nonciliated cells is seen.[73]

III. PULMONARY ENDOTHELIUM

The most numerous cells in the lung are the endothelial cells lining the blood vessels.[19] Injury to these cells may occur via the airways or the bloodstream.[1] Damage usually involves subendothelial swelling, cellular swelling, and occasionally necrosis.

Renewal of the endothelium lining the blood vessels appears to be less complicated morphologically than renewal of the epithelium. Basically, the endothelium is different from the epithelium in that there are no specific progenitor cells in the former. Endothelial cells lost or damaged are replaced through division of other endothelial cells. Most studies on endothelial cell renewal have been carried out on large vessels outside of the lung.[79-83] These studies show that the endothelium has a slow rate of turnover in the normal animal. Of interest is the observation that dividing endothelial cells are localized in certain areas of the aorta. Several hypotheses have been given to explain this phenomenon. First, regional distribution of dividing cells may be due to a shortening of the life span of cells because of local disturbances in hemodynamic flow. Second, it is possible that these cells represent growth centers comparable to the intestinal crypts. Third, they may be areas of aorta that are still growing and developing. If the endothelium has been injured, the rate of cell division is elevated until the damaged area is repaired, thus supporting the first theory. Dividing cells are adjacent to endothelial cells for the most part, indicating a form of reparative regeneration. However, patches of endothelium also form in the middle of denuded areas, suggesting that circulating cells or underlying interstitial cells may participate in forming new endothelium. There is no evidence that circulating monocytes can perform this function. Possibly, the division of endothelial cells at other sites, with subsequent sloughing of the sister cell, may be the source of circulating cells. However, to date no clear-cut evidence is available on the source of these cells.

The mechanism for renewal of the pulmonary endothelium has not been studied in detail. The vast majority of the endothelium in the lungs is associated with capillaries. It was shown that about 30% of the ^{3}H-TdR-labeled cells in the pulmonary alveoli of young control animals were endothelial cells (see Figure 20).[18] Based on the assumption that the labeled cells would divide, it was concluded that endothelial cells in the lung were a renewing cell population. In agreement with these findings, Engerman et al.[84] demonstrated that capillary endothelial cells of several other organs were also renewing cell populations. Subsequent studies by several investigators have shown that after injury to vascular endothelium in the lung, the number of dividing endothelial cells increases greatly.[53,85,86] In mice exposed to O_2 and allowed to recover in air, a large increase in endothelial cell labeling was observed on the 3rd day of recovery.[86] Similarly, in mice injected with butylated hydroxytoluene, injury was observed in the endothelium on the 5th day, followed by a large increase in endothelial cell labeling.[53] These studies indicate the potential for endothelial cell renewal in the lung. To date, however, no studies have been performed to determine the process of division or the fate of the sister cells after division.

Associated with endothelial cell renewal are increases in the thickness of the connective tissue framework of the vessel.[79,80,87,88] This is particularly obvious in large vessels, but has also been reported in capillaries. In the lung, changes in the thickness of the connective tissue are of great importance. Considering the relationship of the pulmonary capillary endothelium to the environment and the potential for injury, future research in this area may help explain the pathogenesis of various lung disorders related to increase in thickness of lung connective tissue.

IV. PULMONARY MACROPHAGES

Macrophages in the lung may be separated into two functional groups.[89] The first group, alveolar macrophages, lie in the surface-active film covering epithelial cells lining the alveoli. They move through this film over the alveolar surface and phagocytize inhaled particles and other extraneous material. When they reach the regions of the terminal bronchioles, the majority either are carried upward in the airways in a mucous

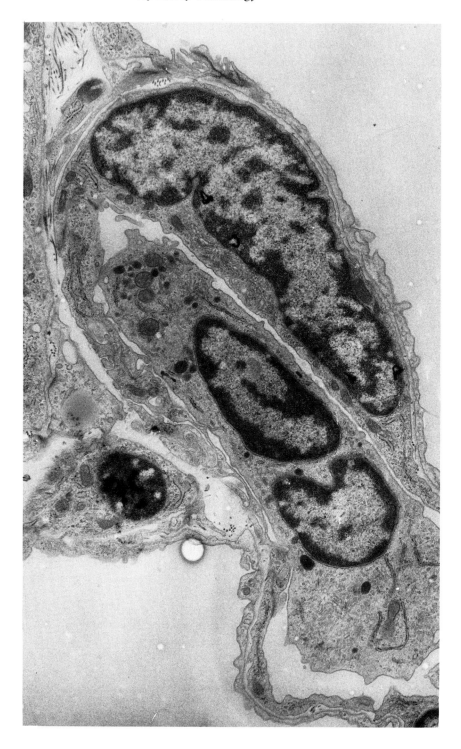

FIGURE 20.   Labeled endothelial cell 1 hr following an injection of ³H-TdR. (Magnification
× 10,750.)

layer or enter the lymphatic system. In both cases, they are lost from the lung. Large numbers of alveolar macrophages are extruded from the lung by this means each day. Because they are replaced in the alveoli, they are classified as a renewing cell population.[14,15] The second group of macrophages reside in the connective tissue. They are equivalent to the fixed macrophages or histiocytes of other connective tissues in the body.[89] Most are found in the connective tissues surrounding airways and in blood vessels. Very few are found in the interstitial regions of the alveoli.

The mechanism by which the alveolar macrophage population maintains and increases its numbers has been of interest for many years.[14,15] Control of macrophage renewal is different from control of epithelial and endothelial tissue renewal in that a demand for more macrophages does not appear to be dictated by the loss of macrophages. Instead, it appears to be associated with an increased need for a specific macrophage function. Research to date has demonstrated two distinct means for supplying alveolar macrophages to the lung. The first is through migration of marrow-derived cells through the vascular system into the alveoli; the second is division of alveolar macrophages *in situ*. Pinkett et al.[90] used mouse irradiation chimeras in which donor hematopoietic cells were marked by the T_6 chromosome; they concluded that all dividing free cells were of hematopoietic origin. Virolainen[91] also used the T_6 method and reached a similar conclusion. Using an esterase marker and reciprocal chimeras, Brunstetter et al.[92] concluded that alveolar macrophages were primarily of bone marrow origin. In a quantitative study using an antigenic marker to identify cells of hematopoietic origin, Godleski and Brain[93] concluded that alveolar macrophages in mouse chimeras were entirely of hematopoietic origin.

In the studies by both Pinkett et al.[90] and Virolainen,[91] the chromosome marker is only visible during mitosis, indicating that alveolar macrophages may divide. In specific studies of alveolar macrophage division, several investigators have shown that macrophages do divide. Evans et al.[94] observed that during continuous exposure to NO_2, there was a large increase in dividing alveolar macrophages (see Figures 21 and 22). The kinetics of their division was determined from a curve of labeled mitotic figures and was found to be similar to that of other dividing cell populations. In cultures of alveolar macrophages obtained from mice, Soderland and Naum[95] demonstrated that macrophages were capable of cell division. Macrophages obtained from humans by pulmonary lavage were also shown to be capable of cell division.[96,97] These results indicate that in addition to migrating from the vascular system, alveolar macrophages may also divide in order to maintain or increase their numbers.

An additional step in the process whereby mononuclear cells migrate into the lung to become macrophages was recently postulated by Bowden and Adamson.[98,99] From studies conducted on lung explants, they suggested that a pulmonary interstitial cell acted as the immediate precursor of the alveolar macrophage. This cell is thought to be derived from circulating monocytes which enter the interstitium and reside there until needed. When needed, they may divide and act as an immediate source of macrophages. This theory is based on two observations. First, in studies of radiation injury, whole-body exposure decreased the number of macrophages present; however, if a chest shield was in place, normal numbers were maintained.[100] Second, in a cultured explant of lung tissue, alveolar macrophages do not divide, cells classified as "interstitial" do divide, and associated with division of interstitial cells is an increase in alveolar macrophages near the periphery of the explant.[98,99] Indirect evidence supporting the concept of an intrapulmonary compartment for macrophage precursors has been presented by several other investigators in studies utilizing radiation to inhibit cell division.[101,102]

Although the evidence indicates that there is an intrapulmonary source of macrophages, the identity of the "interstitial cells" acting as the source is not clear. The

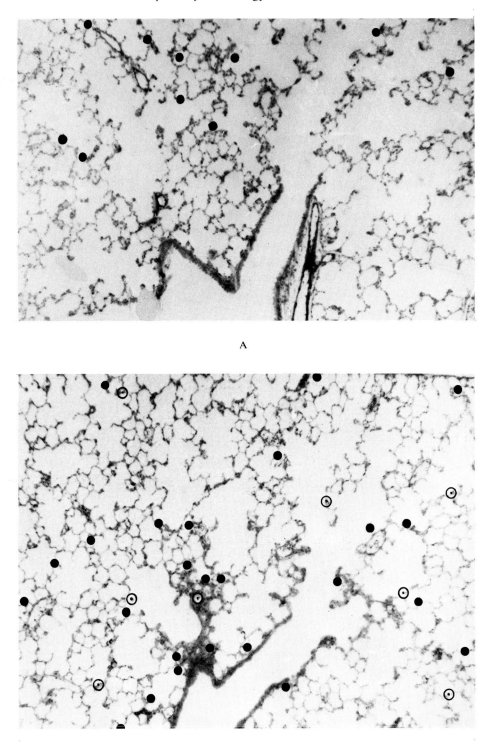

A

B

FIGURE 21.   (A) Pulmonary alveolar tissue in a control rat. Each point represents the site where an alveolar macrophage was observed. No alveolar macrophages were labeled in this section. (Magnification × 88.) (B) Pulmonary alveolar tissue in a rat exposed to 15 to 17 ppm NO_2 for 48 hr. Each point represents the site where an alveolar macrophage was found. Circled points represent alveolar macrophages that were labeled. (Magnification × 88.)

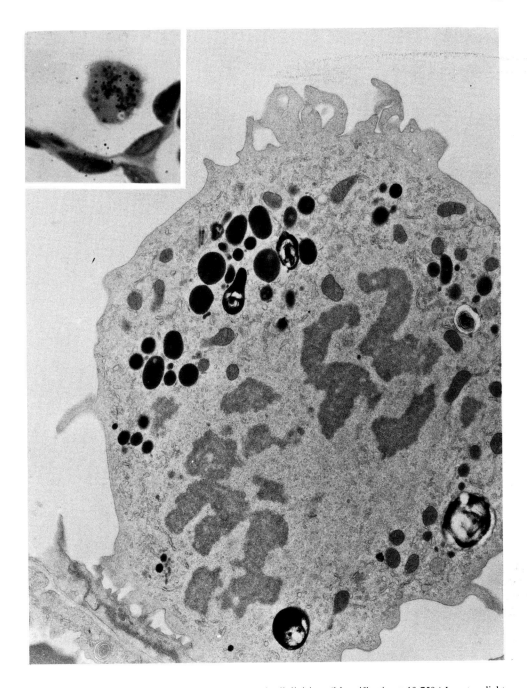

FIGURE 22.   Alveolar macrophage in the process of cell division. (Magnification × 10,750.) Insert — light micrograph of a labeled alveolar macrophage during metaphase. (Magnification × 1250.)

studies by Bowden and Adamson did not demonstrate the site of dividing cells in the lung explant with the electron microscope at a time when the structure of the tissue was clearly defined. According to the morphometric studies of Weibel,[19] most interstitial cells in the alveoli are either fibroblasts associated with the connective tissue or pericytes associated with capillaries. Other cell types are only rarely seen in the alveolar interstitium of normal animals. However, in the interstitium around large blood vessels and airways, fixed histiocytes and monocytes are occasionally observed. These would be the most likely interstitial cells to divide in the lung explant.

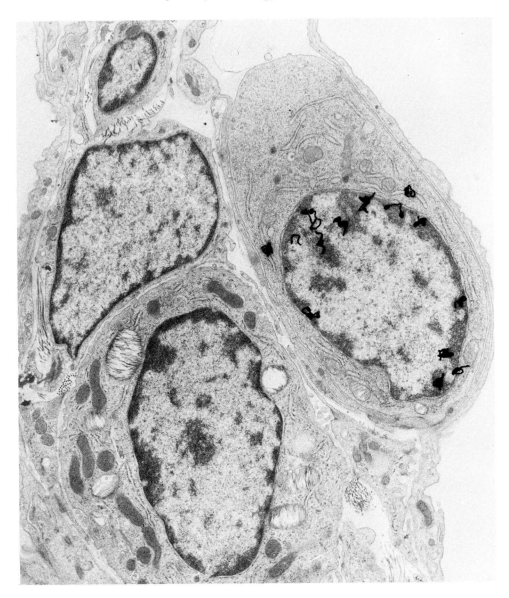

FIGURE 23.   Labeled mononuclear cell in a capillary lumen 1 hr after injection of ³H-TdR. (Magnification × 10,750.)

Another possible source of alveolar macrophages is the circulating monocytes within the capillary lumen. They occur in large numbers in the lung[103,104,107] and are capable of DNA synthesis and cell division (see Figure 23).[18] Based on studies on rats, Fritsch et al.[104] and Masse et al.[107] suggested that lung capillaries acted as a reserve for monocytes. Whether such cells represent the intrapulmonary precursor compartment for alveolar macrophages is not known. However, since circulating monocytes are a source of alveolar macrophages, the large numbers found in capillaries of the lung need to be considered in any theory of intrapulmonary alveolar macrophage precursors. Future research in this area should clarify the nature of the intrapulmonary compartment and the conditions under which the various sources for macrophages prevail.

REFERENCES

1. Witschi, H., Proliferation of Type II alveolar cells: a review of common responses in toxic lung injury, *Toxicology,* 5, 267, 1976.
2. Stephens, R. J., Freeman, G., and Evans, M. J., Early response of lungs to low levels of nitrogen dioxide, *Arch. Environ. Health,* 24, 160, 1972.
3. Plopper, C. G., Dungworth, D. L., and Tyler, W. S., Pulmonary lesions in rats exposed to ozone, *Am. J. Pathol.,* 71, 375, 1973.
4. Penha, P. D. and Werthamer, S., The role of pneumocyte II in alveolar injury and repair, *Am. Rev. Respir. Dis.,* 107, 1109, 1973.
5. Stelzner, M. F., Baron, D. A., and Esterly, J. R., Cadmium induced lung injury, *Lab. Invest.,* 32, 457, 1975.
6. Strauss, R. H., Palmer, K. C., and Hayes, J. A., Acute lung injury induced by cadmium aerosol. I. Evaluation of alveolar cell damage, *Am. J. Pathol.,* 84, 561, 1976.
7. Kapanci, Y., Weibel, E. R., Kaplan, H. P., and Robinson, F. R., Pathogenesis and reversibility of the pulmonary lesions of oxygen toxicity in monkeys. II. Ultrastructural and morphometric studies, *Lab. Invest.,* 20, 101, 1969.
8. Kaplan, H. P., Robinson, F. R., Kapanci, Y., and Weibel, E. R., Pathogenesis and reversibility of the pulmonary lesions of oxygen toxicity in monkeys. I. Clinical and light microscopic studies, *Lab. Invest.,* 20, 94, 1969.
9. Hirai, K., Witschi, H., and Côte, M. G., Electron microscopy of butylated hydroxytoluene-induced lung damage in mice, *Exp. Mol. Pathol.,* 27, 295, 1977.
10. Aso, Y., Yoneda, K., and Kikkawa, Y., Morphologic and biochemical study of pulmonary changes induced by bleomycin in mice, *Lab. Invest.,* 35, 558, 1976.
11. Hennings, H. and Elgjo, K., Epidermal regeneration after cellophane tape stripping of hairless mouse skin, *Cell Tissue Kinet.,* 3, 243, 1970.
12. Oehlert, W., Cell proliferation in carcinogenesis, *Cell Tissue Kinet.,* 6, 325, 1973.
13. Bullough, W. S. and Laurence, E. B., Mitotic and functional homeostasis: a speculative review, *Cancer Res.,* 25, 1683, 1965.
14. Bertalanffy, F. D., Respiratory tissue: structure, histophysiology, cytodynamics. I. Review and basic cytomorphology, *Int. Rev. Cytol.,* 16, 233, 1964.
15. Bertalanffy, F. D., Respiratory tissue: structure, histophysiology, cytodynamics. II. New approaches and interpretations, *Int. Rev. Cytol.,* 17, 213, 1964.
16. Shorter, R. G., Titus, J. L., and Divertie, M. B., Cell turnover in the respiratory tract, *Dis. Chest,* 46, 138, 1964.
17. Shorter, R. G., Titus, J. L., and Divertie, M., Cytodynamics in the respiratory tract of the rat, *Thorax,* 21, 32, 1966.
18. Evans, M. J. and Bils, R. F., Identification of tritiated thymidine labeled cells in the pulmonary alveolar walls of the mouse, *Am. Rev. Respir. Dis.,* 100, 372, 1969.
19. Weibel, E. R., Gehr, P., Haies, D., Gil, J., and Bachofen, M., The cell populations of the normal lung, in *Lung Cells in Disease,* Bouhuys, A., Ed., Elsevier/North-Holland, Amsterdam, 1976, chap. 1.
20. Stephens, R. J., Sloan, M. F., Evans, M. J., and Freeman, G., Early response of lung to low levels of ozone, *Am. J. Pathol.,* 74, 31, 1974.
21. Evans, M. J., Stephens, R. J., Cabral, L. J., and Freeman, G., Cell renewal in the lungs of rats exposed to low levels of NO_2, *Arch. Environ. Health,* 24, 180, 1972.
22. Evans, M. J., Cabral, L. J., Stephens, R. J., and Freeman, G., Renewal of alveolar epithelium in the rat following exposure to NO_2, *Am. J. Pathol.,* 70, 175, 1973.
23. Evans, M. J., Cabral, L. J., Stephens, R. J., and Freeman, G., Transformation of alveolar Type 2 cells to Type 1 cells following exposure to NO_2, *Exp. Mol. Pathol.,* 22, 142, 1975.
24. Adamson, I. Y. R. and Bowden, D., The Type 2 cell as progenitor of alveolar epithelial regeneration. A cytodynamic study in mice after exposure to oxygen, *Lab. Invest.,* 30, 35, 1974.
25. Kauffman, S. L., Burri, P. H., and Weibel, E. R., The postnatal growth of the rat lung. II. Autoradiography, *Anat. Rec.,* 180, 63, 1974.
26. Adamson, I. Y. R. and Bowden, D., Derivation of Type 1 epithelium from Type 2 cells in developing rat lung, *Lab. Invest.,* 32, 736, 1975.
27. Breeze, R. C. and Wheeldon, E. B., The cells of the pulmonary airways, *Am. Rev. Respir. Dis.,* 116, 705, 1977.
28. Jeffery, P. K. and Reid, L., New observations of rat airway epithelium: a quantitative and electron microscopic study, *J. Anat.,* 120, 295, 1975.
29. Lauweryns, J. J., Cokelaere, M., and Boussauw, L., L'Ultrastructure de l'epithelium bronchique et bronchiolaire de la souris, *Bull. Assoc. Anat.,* 146, 548, 1969.

30. **Parkinson, D. R. and Stephens, R. J.,** Morphological surface changes in the terminal bronchiolar region of NO₂-exposed rat lung, *Environ. Res.,* 6, 37, 1973.

31. **Freeman, G., Juhos, L. T., Furiosi, N. J., Mussenden, R., Stephens, R. J., and Evans, M. J.,** Pathology of pulmonary disease from exposure to interdependent ambient gases (nitrogen dioxide and ozone), *Arch. Environ. Health,* 29, 203, 1974.

32. **Ludwin, S. K., Northway, W. H., and Bensch, K. G.,** Oxygen toxicity in the newborn. Necrotizing bronchiolitis in mice exposed to 100 percent oxygen, *Lab. Invest.,* 31, 425, 1974.

33. **Mahvi, D., Bark, H., and Harley, R.,** Morphology of napthalene-induced bronchiolar lesion, *Am. J. Pathol.,* 86, 559, 1977.

34. **Boatman, E. S., Sato, S., and Frank, R.,** Acute effects of ozone on cat lungs, *Am. Rev. Respir. Dis.,* 110, 157, 1974.

35. **Bolduc, P. and Reid, L.,** Mitotic index of the bronchial and alveolar lining of the normal rat lung, *Am. Rev. Respir. Dis.,* 114, 1121, 1976.

36. **Evans, M. J., Johnson, L. V., Stephens, R. J., and Freeman, G.,** Renewal of the terminal bronchiolar epithelium in the rat following exposure to NO₂ or O₃, *Lab. Invest.,* 35, 246, 1976.

37. **Evans, M. J., Cabral-Anderson, L. J., and Freeman, G.,** Role of the Clara cell in renewal of the bronchiolar epithelium, *Lab. Invest.,* 38, 648, 1978.

38. **Lum, H., Schwartz, L. W., Dungworth, D. L., and Tyler, W. S.,** A comparative study of cell renewal after exposure to ozone or oxygen, *Am. Rev. Respir. Dis.,* 118, 335, 1978.

39. **Blenkinsopp, W. K.,** Proliferation of respiratory tract epithelium in the rat, *Exp. Cell Res.,* 46, 144, 1967.

40. **Bindreiter, M., Schuppler, J., and Stokinger, L.,** Zellproliferation und Differenzierung im Tracheal-epithel der Ratte, *Exp. Cell Res.,* 50, 377, 1968.

41. **Wells, A. B.,** The kinetics of cell proliferation in the tracheobronchial epithelia of rats with and without chronic respiratory disease, *Cell Tissue Kinet.,* 3, 185, 1970.

42. **Harris, C., Frank, A., Barrett, L., McDowell, E., Trump, B., Paradise, L., and Boren, H.,** Cytokinetics in the respiratory epithelium of the hamster, cow and man, *J. Cell Biol.,* 67(2, Part 2), Abstracts, 158a, 1975.

43. **Matulionis, D. H.,** Light and electron microscopic study of the effects of ZnSO₄ on mouse nasal respiratory epithelium and subsequent responses, *Anat. Rec.,* 183, 63, 1975.

44. **Weibel, E. R.,** A note on differentiation and divisibility of alveolar epithelial cells, *Chest,* 65, 19S, 1974.

45. **Lane, B. P. and Gordon, R.,** Regeneration of rat tracheal epithelium after mechanical injury. I. The relationship between mitotic activity and cellular differentiation, *Proc. Soc. Exp. Biol. Med.,* 145, 1139, 1974.

46. **Kurman, M. and Argyris, T. S.,** The proliferative response of epidermis of hairless mice to full thickness wound, *Am. J. Pathol.,* 79, 301, 1975.

47. **Rothberg, S., Nancarrow, G. E., Meydrech, E. F., and Iwanik, M. J.,** Extracellular stimulation of epidermal DNA synthesis, *Cell Tissue Kinet.,* 9, 439, 1976.

48. **Palmer, R. C., Snider, G. L., and Hayes, J. A.,** Cellular proliferation induced in the lung by cadmium aerosol, *Am. Rev. Respir. Dis.,* 112, 173, 1975.

49. **Evans, M. J., Johnson, L. V., Stephens, R. J., and Freeman, G.,** Cell renewal in the lungs of rats exposed to low levels of ozone, *Exp. Mol. Pathol.,* 24, 70, 1976.

50. **Aronson, J. F., Johns, L. W., and Pietra, G. G.,** Initiation of lung cell proliferation by trypsin, *Lab. Invest.,* 34, 529, 1976.

51. **Aronson, J. F. and Johns, L. W.,** Injury of lung alveolar cells by lysolecithin, *Exp. Mol. Pathol.,* 27, 35, 1977.

52. **Adamson, I. Y. R. and Bowden, D. H.,** Origin of ciliated alveolar epithelial cells in bleomycin-induced lung injury, *Am. J. Pathol.,* 87, 569, 1977.

53. **Adamson, I. Y. R., Bowden, D. H., Cote, M. G., and Witschi, H.,** Lung injury induced by butylated hydroxytoluene. Cytodynamic and biochemical studies in mice, *Lab. Invest.,* 36, 26, 1977.

54. **Kauffman, S. L.,** Alteration in cell proliferation in mouse lung following urethane exposure. II. Effects of chronic exposure on terminal bronchiolar epithelium, *Am. J. Pathol.,* 64, 531, 1971.

55. **Kauffman, S. L.,** Kinetics of alveolar epithelial hyperplasia in lungs of mice exposed to urethane. I. Quantitative analysis of cell populations, *Lab. Invest.,* 30, 170, 1974.

56. **Kauffman, S. L.,** Autoradiographic study of Type II cell hyperplasia in lungs of mice chronically exposed to urethane, *Cell Tissue Kinet.,* 9, 489, 1976.

57. **Kauffman, S. L.,** Proliferation, growth, and differentiation of pulmonary epithelium in fetal mouse lung exposed transplacentally to dexamethasone, *Lab. Invest.,* 37, 497, 1977.

58. **Brody, J. S. and Buhain, W. J.,** Hormone-induced growth of the adult lung, *Am. J. Physiol.,* 223, 1444, 1972.

59. **Cunningham, E. L., Brody, J. S., and Jain, B. P.,** Lung growth induced by hypoxia, *J. Appl. Physiol.,* 37, 362, 1974.

60. Fisher, J. M. and Simnett, J. D., Morphogenetic and proliferative changes in the regenerating lung of the rat, *Anat. Rec.*, 176, 389, 1973.
61. Simnett, J. D., Stimulation of cell division following unilateral collapse of the lung, *Anat. Rec.*, 180, 681, 1974.
62. Dyson, P. and Heppleston, A. G., Cell kinetics of urethane-induced murine pulmonary adenomata. I. The growth rate, *Br. J. Cancer*, 31, 405, 1975.
63. Evans, M. J., Dekker, N. P., Cabral-Anderson, L. J., and Freeman, G., Quantitation of damage to the alveolar epithelium by means of Type 2 cell proliferation, *Am. Rev. Respir. Dis.*, 118, 787, 1978.
64. Wells, A. B. and Lamerton, L. F., Regenerative response of the rat tracheal epithelium after acute exposure to tobacco smoke: a quantitative study, *J. Natl. Cancer Inst.*, 55, 887, 1975.
65. Evans, M. J., Hackney, J. D., and Bils, R. F., Effects of a high concentration of oxygen on cell renewal in the pulmonary alveoli, *Aerosp. Med.*, 40, 1365, 1969.
66. Evans, M. J., Mayr, W., Bils, R. F., and Loosli, C. G., Effects of ozone on cell renewal in pulmonary alveoli of aging mice, *Arch. Environ. Health*, 22, 405, 1971.
67. Evans, M. J. and Hackney, J. D., Cell proliferation in lungs of mice exposed to elevated concentrations of oxygen, *Aerosp. Med.*, 43, 620, 1972.
68. Cabral-Anderson, L. J., Evans M. J., and Freeman, G., Effects of NO_2 on the lungs of aging rats. I. Morphology, *Exp. Mol. Pathol.*, 27, 353, 1977.
69. Evans, M. J., Cabral-Anderson, L. J., and Freeman, G., Effects of NO_2 on the lungs of aging rats. II. Cell proliferation, *Exp. Mol. Pathol.*, 27, 366, 1977.
70. Hackney, J. D., Evans, M. J., Bils, R. F., Spies, C. E., and Jones, M. P., Effects of oxygen at high concentrations and food deprivation on cell division in lung alveoli of mice, *Exp. Mol. Pathol.*, 26, 350, 1977.
71. Hackney, J. D., Evans, M. J., Spier, C. E., Clark, K. W., and Anzar, U. T., Effect of high concentrations of oxygen on reparative regeneration of damaged alveolar epithelium, *J. Undersea Biomed. Res.*, 6, 38, 1979.
72. Bachofen, M. and Weibel, E. R., Alterations of the gas exchange apparatus in adult respiratory insufficiency associated with septicemia, *Am. Rev. Respir. Dis.*, 116, 589, 1977.
73. Freeman, G., Crane, S. C., Stephens, R. J., and Furiosi, N. J., Pathogenesis of the nitrogen-induced lesion in the rat lung: a review and presentation of new observations, *Am. Rev. Respir. Dis.*, 98, 429, 1968.
74. Frasca, J. M., Auerbach, O., Parks, V. R., and Jamieson, J. D., Alveolar cell hyperplasia in the lungs of smoking dogs, *Exp. Mol. Pathol.*, 21, 300, 1974.
75. Morrow, P. E., Adaptations of the respiratory tract to air pollutants, *Arch. Environ. Health*, 14, 127, 1967.
76. Evans, M. J. and Freeman, G., Injury and cell renewal in rat lungs exposed to ozone, in *Biochemical Effects of Environmental Pollutants*, Lee, S. D., Ed., Ann Arbor Sciences, Ann Arbor, 1977, Chap. 3.
77. Creasia, D. A., Nettesheim, P., and Kim, J. S. C., Stimulation of DNA synthesis in the lungs of hamsters exposed intermittently to nitrogen dioxide, *J. Toxicol. Environ. Health*, 2, 1173, 1977.
78. Nettesheim, P. and Szakal, A. K., Morphogenesis of alveolar bronchiolization, *Lab. Invest.*, 26, 210, 1972.
79. Fishman, J. A., Ryan, G. B., and Karnovsky, M. J., Endothelial regeneration in the rat carotid artery and the significance of endothelial denudation in the pathogenesis of myointimal thickening, *Lab. Invest.*, 32, 339, 1975.
80. Friedman, R. J., Moore, S., and Singal, D. P., Repeated endothelial injury and induction of atherosclerosis in normolipemic rabbits by human serum, *Lab. Invest.*, 30, 404, 1975.
81. Gimbrone, M. A., Cotran, R. S., and Falkman, J., Human vascular endothelial cells in culture. Growth and DNA synthesis, *J. Cell Biol.*, 60, 637, 1974.
82. Schwartz, S. M. and Benditt, E. P., Cell replication in the aortic endothelium. A new method for study of the problem, *Lab. Invest.*, 28, 699, 1973.
83. Spaet, T. H., Stemerman, M. B., Veith, F. J., and Lejnicks, I., Intimal injury and regrowth in the rabbit aorta, *Circ. Res.*, 36, 58, 1975.
84. Engerman, R. L., Pfaffenbach, D., and Davis, M. D., Cell turnover of capillaries, *Lab. Invest.* 17, 738, 1967.
85. Gaynor, E., Increased mitotic activity in rabbit endothelium after endotoxin, *Lab. Invest.*, 24, 318, 1971.
86. Bowden, D. H. and Adamson, I. Y. R., Endothelial regeneration as a marker of the differential vascular responses in oxygen-induced pulmonary edema, *Lab. Invest.*, 30, 350, 1974.
87. Vracko, R. and Benditt, E. P., Capillary basal lamina thickening. Its relationship to endothelial cell death and replacement, *J. Cell Biol.*, 47, 281, 1970.
88. McKinney, R. V. and Panner, B. J., Regenerating capillary basement membrane in skeletal muscle wounds, *Lab. Invest.*, 26, 100, 1972.

89. Sorokin, S. and Brain, J. D., Pathways of clearance in mouse lungs exposed to iron oxide aerosols, *Anat. Rec.*, 181, 581, 1975.
90. Pinkett, M. D., Cowdrey, C. R., and Nowell, P. C., Mixed hematopoietic and pulmonary origin of "alveolar macrophages" as demonstrated by a chromosomal marker, *Am. J. Pathol.*, 48, 859, 1966.
91. Virolainen, M., Hematopoietic origin of macrophages as studied by chromosomal markers in mice, *J. Exp. Med.*, 127, 943, 1968.
92. Brunstetter, M. A., Hardie, J. A., Schiff, R., Lewis, J. P., and Cross, C. E., The origin of pulmonary alveolar macrophages, *Arch. Intern. Med. Symp.*, 9, 130, 1971.
93. Godleski, J. J. and Brain, J. D., The oxygen of alveolar macrophages in mouse radiation chimeras, *J. Exp. Med.*, 136, 630, 1972.
94. Evans, M. J., Cabral, L. J., Stephens, R. J., and Freeman, G., Cell division of alveolar macrophages in the rat lung following exposure to NO_2, *Am. J. Pathol.*, 70, 195, 1973.
95. Soderland, S. C. and Naum, Y., Growth of pulmonary alveolar macrophages *in vitro*, *Nature (London)*, 245, 150, 1973.
96. Golde, D. W., Byers, L. A., and Finley, T. N., Proliferative capacity of human alveolar macrophages, *Nature (London)*, 247, 373, 1974.
97. Golde, D. W., Finley, T. N., and Cline, M. J., The pulmonary macrophage in acute leukemia, *N. Engl. J. Med.*, 290, 875, 1974.
98. Bowden, D. H. and Adamson, I. Y. R., The pulmonary interstitial cell as immediate precursor of the alveolar macrophage, *Am. J. Anat.*, 68, 521, 1972.
99. Bowden, D. H. and Adamson, I. Y. R., The macrophage delivery system: kinetic studies in cultured explants of murine lung, *Am. J. Pathol.*, 83, 123, 1976.
100. Bowden, D. H., Adamson, I. Y. R., Grantham, W. G., and Wyatt, J. P., Origin of lung macrophages. Evidence derived from radiation injury, *Arch. Pathol.*, 88, 540, 1969.
101. Goldstein, E. and Lewis, J. P., Patterns of pulmonary alveolar macrophage function following radiation injury, *J. Lab. Clin. Med.*, 82, 276, 1973.
102. Kim, M., Goldstein, E., Lewis, J. P., Lippert, W., and Warshauer, D., Murine pulmonary alveolar macrophages. Rates of bacterial ingestion, inactivation, and destruction *J. Infect. Dis.*, 133, 310, 1976.
103. Whitelaw, D. M. and Batho, H. F., The distribution of monocytes in the rat, *Cell Tissue Kinet.*, 5, 215, 1972.
104. Fritsch, P., Masse, R., Levistre, J. P., LaFuma, J., and Chretien, J., Lung capillaries as a reserve for monocytes, *J. Microsc. Biol. Cell*, 25, 289, 1976.
105. Witschi, H. and Côte, M. G., Inhibition of butylated hydroxytoluene-induced mouse lung cell division by oxygen: time-effect and dose-effect relationships, *Chem. -Biol. Interact.*, 19, 279, 1977.
106. Haschek, W. M. and Witschi, H., Pulmonary fibrosis — a possible mechanism, *Toxicol. Appl. Pharmacol.*, 51, 475, 1979.
107. Masse, R., Fritsch, P., Nolibe, D., Lafuma, J., and Chretien, J., Cytokinetic study of alveolar macrophage renewal in rats, in *Pulmonary Macrophages and Epithelial Cells*, Proc. 16th Annu. Hanford Biology Symp., Richland, Wash., September 27 to 29, 1976, 106.

Chapter 6

PULMONARY EDEMA: EMPHASIS ON PHYSIOLOGIC AND TOXICOLOGICAL CONSIDERATIONS

Carroll E. Cross, Gibbe H. Parsons, Arnold B. Gorin, and Jerold A. Last

TABLE OF CONTENTS

I. INTRODUCTION

Toxic pulmonary edema represents an acute, exudative phase of lung injury and generally reflects a "permeability" * alteration in the alveolar-capillary barrier. It is biologically important because it interferes with the respiratory gas-exchanging function of the lung. Edema fluid, when present, will alter ventilation-perfusion relationships and limit diffusive transfer of O_2 and CO_2, even in structurally normal alveoli. While sophisticated morphologic or biochemical methods may be necessary to demonstrate the site and mechanism of a toxic injury, the presence of alveolar edema is usually obvious and is easily quantified. Measurement of edema is an excellent index of acute lung injury, and is particularly useful when the site or mechanism of action of a toxin is still unknown.

The present review provides the toxicologist with a conceptual approach to the study of pulmonary edema. It focuses on compartmental distribution of lung liquid, and the role of physical forces and cellular and structural lung constituents in regulating lung water and solute flux; considers attempts to explain some mechanisms of toxic edema formation; and mentions consequences of the process. Specific discussions of cellular changes subsequent to toxic lung injury, an inseparable aspect of toxic pulmonary edema, are available.[4] More comprehensive discussions of clinical and pathophysiologic aspects of pulmonary edema are published elsewhere.[5-9]

II. WATER DISTRIBUTION IN THE LUNG

A. Lung Water Compartments

There are four liquid compartments in the lung: (1) vascular bed, (2) intracellular space, (3) interstitium and its lymphatics, and (4) luminal liquid lining layer in alveoli and airways.

The normal pulmonary blood volume (PBV) is approximately 10 to 15% of the total intravascular volume. In life, approximately one half of lung weight is attributable to contained blood.[1,10] PBV varies directly with lung volume.[11] Thus, thoracotomy, with loss of the negative intrapleural pressure and resultant fall in lung volume below functional residual capacity, will cause an immediate fall in PBV.

Lung capillaries contain approximately 30% of PBV. Under normal circumstances, this capillary bed is highly compliant; cardiac output must increase by a factor of 2 to 3 before pulmonary artery pressure will rise. The compliance of the lung circulation is approximately 7 mm/torr in normal anesthetized dogs.[12] Based upon analysis of vascular and interstitial volumes in lung within the framework of a sheet-flow model of the alveolar septa, pulmonary capillary blood volume was suggested to be simply correlated with pulmonary arteriolar pressure.[13] However, others have found that independent changes in pulmonary arterial or venous pressure (transpulmonary pressure held constant) produced changes in capillary blood volume over an extremely wide range.[14]

Increases in PBV may occur in the presence of a variety of extrapulmonary injuries. Renal failure (e.g., $HgCl_2$, ethylene glycol toxicity) may result in generalized expansion

---

* More rigorous physiological considerations of "permeability" are available.[1-3] From a toxicological standpoint, alterations in diffusional, convectional and osmotic resistance and/or frank anatomical rupture or destruction of vascular endothelium, interstitium or alveolar epithelium can be operationally lumped together as "altered permeability".

of plasma volume, with a proportional increase in PBV. Cardiotoxicity (e.g., cobalt, adriamycin), and the resulting left-sided heart failure, will manifest itself as a rising pulmonary vascular pressure, causing an increased PBV. Neurogenic pulmonary edema may involve increases in pulmonary vascular pressures and PBV as well as increases in pulmonary vascular permeability.[15,16] Cerebral anoxia, and perhaps other central nervous system injuries, results in marked increase in pulmonary vascular resistance secondary to venular constriction,[17,18] and thus increases PBV. Other agents, such as pyrolizidine alkaloids, directly affect the pulmonary vasculature, causing pulmonary hypertension and expansion of the PBV.[19,20]

After toxic injury, simple measurement of lung weight does not provide a rigorous index of pulmonary edema, because vascular engorgement alone might increase organ weight by 20 to 50%. In older studies, it was assumed that blood could be cleared from the lung by passive drainage.[21] It is now evident that substantial quantities of blood remain after this procedure.[1,22] Even saline perfusion of the pulmonary circulation leaves significant residual blood, presumably in unperfused capillaries or as extravasated blood.[23] Thus, blood content of lung must be determined before changes in extravascular lung water (pulmonary edema) can be assessed.

The volume of the vascular compartment can be assessed from histologic sections by morphometry.[14,24] It is more common to estimate the distribution volume in a lung homogenate of some tracer molecule assumed to be restricted to the vascular space. Usually, hemoglobin content of the homogenate is assayed after hemoglobin conversion to acid hematin or cyanmethemoglobin.[25,26] These are quantitated by spectrophotometric methods best suited for large amounts of blood contamination. In saline-perfused preparations, with lesser amounts of blood contamination, accurate measurement of hemoglobin absorbance may be impaired by turbidity in the lung homogenates, even after centrifugation. A method for quantitating residual hemoglobin in saline-perfused lungs which utilizes the decrease in oxyhemoglobin absorbance at 415 nm following reduction of oxyhemoglobin to deoxyhemoglobin by dithionite has been recently described.[23]

When hemoglobin is used as marker for blood contamination, two assumptions are made: (1) the concentration of hemoglobin in lung blood is similar to that measured in large veins or cardiac ventricles, and (2) the measured hemoglobin is restricted to the intravascular space. The assumption that normal lung hematocrit is approximately the same as large-vein hematocrit appears valid.[27] In toxic pulmonary edema, hemorrhagic diathesis is common and the second assumption must be tested. This is usually done by light microscopy.

If extravasation of blood is expected, it is safest to infuse a tracer that is believed to be restricted to the vascular space immediately prior to killing the animal. At least 8 min must be allowed for uniform dispersion of the tracer in the circulating blood volume.[27] ^{51}Cr- or ^{99}Tc-labeled erythrocytes are excellent vascular markers. In the absence of active airway hemorrhage, it is unlikely that labeled erythrocytes will leak into the lung in sufficient quantity to invalidate assessment of lung vascular volume in this short time. Labeled macromolecules, such as [^{125}I] albumin, are frequently used to measure plasma volume. However, these molecules rapidly equilibrate between plasma and lung interstitium.[28,29] In the presence of a toxic lung injury, equilibration may occur in 10 min, thus causing an overestimation of the volume of the vascular compartment.

The nonblood tissue volume of the mammalian lung approximates 0.5 to 1.5% of body weight. This tissue volume is divided into interstitial, intracellular, and luminal compartments. The interstitium contains 30 to 60% of the total tissue volume.[1] Constituents of this compartment include cellular elements (e.g., fibroblasts, mesenchymal cells, macrophages, and other cells), structural proteins (e.g., collagen, elastin), and proteoglycan ground substance. Interlacing of fibrillar proteins and coiled proteoglycans creates an area in the interstitial space from which macromolecules are excluded on the basis of molecular size.[30] In the lung, this "excluded volume" is quite large, the albumin distribution space being only 25% of the total interstitial compartment in normal sheep.[31] By infusion of a crystalloid solution (Ringer's lactate) equal to 15% of total body weight, the distribution volume of albumin increased from 62% of the extravascular, extracellular space to 90% in dogs.[32] This decrease in the "excluded volume" is presumed to be related to hydration of the proteoglycan gel matrix.

The presence of an "excluded volume" indicates that care must be taken in choosing a molecular indicator for the interstitial space. Measurement of the albumin distribution volume in the interstitium depends upon knowledge of the albumin concentration in interstitial liquid. This is usually taken to be the same as the concentration of albumin in lung lymph (Section III). In the past, controversy has existed as to whether interstitial fluid was concentrated in lymphatics.[33] Recent evidence appears to have answered this controversy: the free interstitial fluid aspirated from the peribronchial tissue has the same protein concentration as post-nodal lymph in sheep;[34] no concentration of [^{125}I] albumin occurs in afferent lymphatics in the mouse lung;[35] and the composition of lymph is identical in pre- and postnodal lymphatics in dog lung.[36]

Interstitial volume is more accurately assessed by using some small molecule (<5000 daltons). It can be assumed that the concentration in interstitial liquid approximates that in plasma. Even for small tracers, differences in lung distribution volume have been reported. For example, the ratio of $^{36}Cl^-$/[^{14}C] sucrose volumes in blood-free sheep lung equals 1.57,[31] and the distribution volume of $^{22}Na^+$ significantly exceeds that of ^{99m}Tc-diethylenetriamine pentaacetic acid (DTPA).[34] Explanations for these discrepancies include: (1) limited intracellular penetration of $^{22}Na^+$ and $^{36}Cl^-$; (2) active transport of $^{22}Na^+$ and $^{36}Cl^-$ across the alveolar epithelium into the luminal compartment (given adequate time, all tracers should equilibrate in the luminal compartment, (3) exclusion of the larger sucrose and DTPA molecules from some portion of the distribution volume on the basis of molecular size, charge, or shape.

When edema formation results from increased hydrostatic filtration pressure, from decrease or reversal in the transcapillary oncotic pressure gradient, or from endothelial injury, the first site of extravascular fluid accumulation is the loose interstitial tissue surrounding bronchioles, vasculature, and the subpleural interstitium. The peribronchiolar and perivascular "cuffing" is easily seen in rapidly frozen edematous lung.[38] Fluid then accumulates in the interstitium of the alveolar septum, sparing the "minimal space" where the basal laminae and endothelial membranes appear to merge.[39]

The interstitium in lung has a relatively low compliance and limited capacitance,[40] the latter being no more than two times its normal water content. Liquid accumulation beyond this level is followed by decompression into the luminal compartment (alveolar flooding). There is some evidence that interstitial compliance surrounding intra-alveolar septal vessels and that surrounding the extra-alveolar arteries, arterioles, venules, and veins may not be identical. It has been suggested that this two compartment model of lung interstitial space, separated by a high resistance gel matrix, would allow for more gradual dissipation of liquid accumulated around the permeable extra-alveolar vessels into a potentially larger and more compliant second compartment in continuity with lymphatic channels.[40a] The interstitial compliance may decrease with lung inflation. In experimental toxic pulmonary edema in rodents, pleural effusions may arise via passage of interstitial liquid from the subpleural interstitium through stomata in their very thin pleural mesothelium. This phenomenon develops dramatically in rodents exposed to high concentrations (over 95%) of O_2 at normobaric pressures.

The intracellular fluid compartment in lung is usually determined by subtraction (intracellular volume = total extravascular lung water − interstitial volume) or by morphometry. The frequency of occurrence of five major cell types (endothelial "interstitial", Type I pneumocytes, Type II pneumocytes, and alveolar macrophages), and the estimated average cell volumes for each, has recently been reported.[41]

When pulmonary edema results from imbalance of the hemodynamic Starling forces (Section II), it is unlikely that significant changes occur in intracellular volume.[37] In a study of the effect of isotonic volume loading on lung weight in dogs, a proportional relationship between increase in total lung weight and increase in interstitial water was found.[32,42] Intracellular dehydration occurs when lungs are perfused with hyperosmolar solutions.[37]

Swelling of cells and cellular organelles occurs in the presence of toxic injuries, severe hypoxemia, and/or ischemia and exposure to hypotonic environments.[43,45] It is unlikely, however, that cellular edema contributes significantly to the measured lung weight gain after exposure to pneumotoxins.

The luminal liquid layer in small airways and alveoli is difficult to quantitiate in the normal lung, but may represent approximately 6 mℓ/100 g tissue.[33] Micropuncture techniques have been used to aspirate liquid from the alveolar lining layer in rat lung.[46] Freeze-etch fixation methods have allowed its visualization by electron microscopy.[47] It is extremely variable in its thickness, tending to fill in intracellular clefts thus smoothing out the alveolar surface. More recently, the liquid in the small airways of rats has been morphologically studied.[48,49]

The gas volume of the lung is extremely large when compared to the tissue volume. Thus, what is normally the alveolar gas volume has the largest capacitance of the four lung liquid storage compartments. Any major change in the quantity of lung extravascular water usually includes some alveolar flooding.

The relative dimensions of these compartments are not constant over the lung. There is a normal gradient of vascular perfusion in lung, increasing from apex to base in bipeds. Likewise, lung blood volume in uppermost portions of the lung may be considerably less than blood volume in dependent portions of the lung.[14] This reflects the fact that vascular luminal distending pressures are greater below than above the hilus of the lung. Surprisingly, recent studies have demonstrated that fractional water content (extravascular lung water/dry weight) of lung tissue is uniform throughout the organ in normal lung,[50,51] despite obvious differences in hydrostatic filtration pressures between apex and base. A corollary of these observations is that the ratio of vascular space to tissue volume is greater at the base that at the apex of the lung. In most pathological circumstances, edema formation is also more prominent at the base or dependent portions of the lung than at the apex or superior portion. This is due both to the increased hydrostatic filtration pressures and to the greater vascular surface area per unit lung volume available for liquid and solute exchange in the dependent lung tissue.

When assessing edema formation in large animals, including man, it is most precise to quantify changes in the entire organ. This is not always possible, particularly when concomitant morphological and/or biochemical studies are intended. These considerations are more important in large animals than in small species such as rodents, as presumably the effects of gravitational forces on distribution of pleural-interstitial pressures and on perfusion and blood volume per unit lung are more homogeneous in small species.

The best method of data expression when measuring pulmonary edema is the ratio of wet weight to dry weight of blood-free lung (Section IIB). The lung is homogenized; an aliquot is taken for hemoglobin analysis; and another aliquot is dried to constant weight in an oven at 90 to 105°C. Residual blood content should be determined by methods previously discussed. The coefficient of variation of this parameter in normal animals is approximately 10%, less than that for other means of normalizing data (e.g., wet weight/body weight, wet weight/body surface area).[1]

Routine histologic methods yield limited information regarding edema formation, since fixation is designed to remove water from tissue and fixatives themselves are hyperosmolar and may cause translocations of liquid. Histology is more successful in quantitating inflammation and exudation (including "hyaline membrane" formation). Rapid-freezing of lung (by immersion in liquid nitrogen-cooled liquid propane) preserves the normal distribution of lung water. The tissue may then be processed by freeze-drying or freeze-etching, which yield data on the distribution of edema liquid.[35,46]

Techniques exist for "in vivo" assessment of extravascular lung water. These are reviewed extensively elsewhere.[1,52-54c] In general, these approaches are more useful in large animals than in small ones.

B. Relevance to Experimental Toxicology

Pulmonary edema is customarily quantitated in experimental animals by some form of gravimetric measurement of lung water content.[1] There is at present no universal agreement as to a standard method for quantitating the severity of this condition. Very commonly, the wet (undesiccated) weight of the whole lung is determined.[55] This value is often normalized to the weight of the animal from which the lung was taken.[56] Alternatively, some investigators determine the lung water content by weighing whole lungs or lung slices before and after completely drying in an oven or a desiccator. Commonly used methods of expression of such data include: (1) percentage water content: [100 × (wet weight-dry weight)/(wet weight)],[57-59] (2) percentage dry weight: [100 × (dry weight)/(wet weight)],[56,60,61] and (3) water content ≈[(mℓ of water)/(dry weight)].[62] It has been argued on theoretical grounds[1,63] that such data are more precisely expressed as the fraction (wet weight)/(dry weight) so as to avoid the errors introduced by subtraction of a dry weight that is about 15 to 20% of the wet weight when the fraction (or percentage) [(wet weight − dry weight)/(wet weight)] is used.

The conventional method for this determination, as described above, requires an aliquot of homogenate from the entire lung. One acceptable alternative method useful in rodents is to use (wet weight)/(dry weight) ratios determined with the right cranial lobe to quantitate the pulmonary edema provoked by administration of pneumotoxins. This technique has several advantages. It is extremely precise with low coefficients of variance. It requires only a small percentage of the total lung mass (about 10%) and the right cranial lobe can be readily clamped or tied off in such a way as to allow perfusion of the remainder of the lung via either the pulmonary vasculature or the airways. In this way, each animal can be independently evaluated in several ways, even in situations where both vascular and airway perfusion protocols are necessary to investigate the parameters of interest. As a result, fewer animals must be killed to acquire correlative biochemical, morphological, and/or tissue culture data for comparison with the extent of pulmonary edema.

The wet/dry weight ratio of the right cranial lobes from normal rats is 4.63 ± 0.29 (mean ± SD), as determined from the pooled data of 156 rats (25 separate experiments) over a period of almost 2 years.[215] This value corresponds to a percentage water content [100 × (wet weight − dry weight)/(wet weight)] of 78.6%,* or a percentage dry weight

---

* Percent water content = (wet weight − dry weight)/(wet weight) × 100 = 1− (dry weight)/(wet weight) × 100.

TABLE 1
WET WEIGHT/DRY WEIGHT
RATIOS OF RAT LUNG LOBES

Lung lobe sampled	Normal lung wet- to dry-weight ratio
Right cranial	4.71 ± 0.08 (3)
Right middle	4.66 ± 0.19 (3)
Right caudal	4.54 ± 0.07 (3)
Right accessory	4.74 ± 0.03 (3)
Left lobe	4.58 ± 0.11 (3)
Cumulative lung	4.64 ± 0.12 (15)

Note: Each lobe was separately excised, patted dry with gauze, weighed, dried at 110° for 12 to 24 hr and reweighed. Data are tabulated as mean ± SD, with values for n, the number of individual lobes sampled, in parenthesis.

[100 × (dry weight) / (wet weight)] of 21.4%. In Table 1 the (wet weight)/(dry weight) ratios of individual lung lobes from healthy rats are compared. There is no statistically significant difference between the (wet weight)/(dry weight) ratios of any of the lobes within a given group. In particular, it is clear that sampling the right cranial lobe does not introduce any systematic bias into the ratio, as compared with any other lung lobe or with the entire lung per se. This is true even in cases of more severe edema induced by paraquat,[64] where the (wet weight)/(dry weight) ratio observed with the right cranial lobe may be as high as 6.54 ± 0.60 (n = 6).

The use of (wet weight) / (dry weight) ratios for expression of data quantitating lung water content, first introduced in 1950[63] and more recently strongly advocated,[1] unfortunately is not yet customary in toxicology. In normal dogs, the normal (wet weight)/(dry weight) ratio is about 4.5 to 5.0 at capillary pressures below 20 to 25 mm of Hg.[63] Above this critical region of capillary pressures, ratios of 5 to 10 were observed.[63] In dogs, pulmonary edema induced by alloxan caused the (wet weight)/(dry weight) ratio to increase from 3.7 (control value) to 7.4.[65] Presumably, the variation in normal may reflect variations in the state of hydration of the dogs or variability in, or failure to correct for, blood content in the lung. It has been reported that (extravascular lung water)/(dry weight) ratios for lungs of normal sheep are comparable to those of dogs, with increases of 3 to 30% during mild edema induced by intravenous infusion of *Pseudomonas* bacteria, and of 13 to 55% during mild to moderate cardiogenic pulmonary edema.[34]

From the standpoint of small-animal toxicology, this form of data expression also has several practical advantages. Since the (wet weight)/(dry weight) ratio of whole blood is similar to that of lung,[1,63] minor variations in handling and surgical technique, in retention of whole blood within the lobe vasculature or in time the lobe is in contact with mildly absorbent surfaces does not significantly affect the (wet weight)/(dry weight) ratios obtained. Changes in the amount of blood inadvertantly retained in the lung vessels would, however, profoundly influence the ratio of lung weight to body weight. The (wet weight)/(dry weight) ratio may be more precisely obtained as the slope of plots of wet weight versus dry weight from a least-squares fitted straight line when multiple replicate animals are studied (Figure 1). Values of (wet weight)/(dry weight) ratio obtained with the right cranial lobe from rats agrees with the ratios observed in sheep and dogs, as well as those obtained with whole rat lungs.

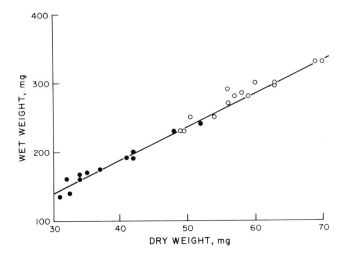

FIGURE 1.   Plot of wet weight vs. dry weight for individual right cranial lobes from lungs of control (●-●) or O_3-exposed (O-O) rats. Ozone exposure was 1 to 2 ppm daily for 7 to 14 days. Stability of wet weight/dry weight ratio in O_3-exposed rats is not readily explicable. Among the possible explanations for this result are: (i) increased blood in lungs derived from O_3-exposed rats; (ii) inflammatory edema with contained macromolecules (plasma proteins, fibrin, etc.) and phagocytes; (iii) reparative-proliferative responses in injured lung parenchyma.

The appearance of the dry weight term in the denominator, however, has an inherent disadvantage in that the dry weight of an edematous lung can be markedly increased. Normalization to lung dry weight will cause an under-estimation of the amount of edema fluid for any lung in which the edema liquid has a substantial protein and inflammatory cell content. This effect can be seen in the case of rats exposed to high concentrations of O_3 (Figure 1)[216] in which the wet weight of the lung lobe is high, indicating edema, yet the (wet weight)/(dry weight) ratio is indistinguishable from controls due to the concomitant elevation of the lobe dry weight. It has been suggested that this problem can be alleviated by estimating the excess lung dry weight by determining the (wet weight)/(dry weight) of the edema liquid itself.[1] Alternatively, a simpler method of correction could be to compare the wet weight of the lung lobes with lobes from matched controls. Clearly, in any situation where the other liquid is not plasma ultrafiltrate but is liquid-containing protein, connective tissue components and substantially increased inflammatory and/or proliferative cell constituents (the usual case in pneumotoxin-induced pulmonary edema), the dry weight term may increase concomitantly with the wet weight. Measurements of increased levels of protein and DNA in the lung homogenate can alert the investigator to this potential problem. One should also take care to determine blood levels in the lungs,[23] as there could also be ultrafiltration and hemoconcentration occurring in the lungs of pneumotoxin-intoxicated animals. A low (wet weight)/(dry weight) ratio in retained hemoconcentrated blood would then offset a high (wet weight)/(dry weight) ratio in edematous lungs, artifactually "normalizing" the values. Although dry weight corrections are necessary to allow for variability between rats and sampling errors, it is important to note that such corrections can mask significant lung changes unless one of these other criteria are also used.

In summary, expression of pulmonary edema as (wet weight)/(dry weight) ratios should be the toxicological standard. This method can be criticized as not allowing distinction of change in the numerator or denominator (or both) term(s). Thus, the ratio may be insensitive to the severity of the lesion when vascular permeability is increased or inflammatory edema is present. However, other methods of data expression have their own inherent shortcomings. Measurements of changes in lung weight per weight of rat are less precise and subject to the same uncertainty as to whether change is in wet weight or dry weight. Wet weight or dry weight without use of some normalizing denominator is very imprecise. As the composition of edema liquid becomes more proteinaceous, and/or more cellular, the investigator must rigorously determine both the wet- and dry-components of edema liquids, or serious errors may be introduced in determination of other parameters measured. For example, expression of enzyme activities per mg protein in lung homogenates is subject to large errors caused by the denominator term in edematous lungs, where protein may be a major component of contaminating blood, inflammatory edema liquid (and fibrin) or recruited (phagocytes), and/or proliferating cells.[23]

III. SYNOPSIS OF PATHOPHYSIOLOGIC BASIS

Discussions of the pathogenic mechanisms of pulmonary edema have generally focused on factors governing the exchange of water and macromolecules across the lung microcirculation.[1] The Starling equation* summarizes the physical forces governing liquid transport in the pulmonary microcirculation: $Q_f = K_f [(P_{mv} - P_{pmv}) - \sigma(\pi_{mv} - \pi_{pmv})]$ where Q_f is the net flux of liquid across the capillary, K_f is the liquid filtration coefficient (a term describing the hydraulic conductance of the capillary wall); P_{mv} and P_{pmv} represent the hydrostatic pressures in the microvascular lumen and perimicrovascular interstitial liquid, respectively; σ is the macromolecular (plasma protein) reflection coefficient (a constant, which may take any value from 0 to 1, that indicates the probability that osmotically active macromolecules approaching the capillary wall will be "reflected" back and not cross the membrane); and π_{mv} and π_{pmv} represent the protein oncotic pressure in the plasma and perimicrovascular compartments, respectively.

The variables P_{mv}, P_{pmv}, π_{mv}, and π_{pmv}, express physical forces ("Starling forces"). They are grouped as the differential hydrostatic (ΔP) and oncotic ($\Delta \pi$) pressures acting across the liquid-exchanging vessel wall. The two constants (K_f, σ), characterize the functional anatomy of the liquid-exchanging vessels. They are determined by the aggregate surface area available for transendothelial liquid exchange and the physical and biological characteristics of the pathways (including "pores") through which liquid and macromolecules flux.[1,2] The value of σ describes the extent to which the endothelium is semipermeable. When $\sigma = 0$ (membrane freely permeable to macromolecules) there can be no oncotic pressure differential.

Pulmonary edema is frequently physiologically classified as being one of two types. When edema results from an imbalance of the Starling forces (ΔP and $\Delta \pi$), it is said to be "high pressure", "hydrostatic" or "cardiogenic" pulmonary edema. When edema formation follows some change in the permeability or sieving properties of the vascular wall (either an increase in K_f or a decrease in σ), it is said to be "nonhydros-

---

* The Starling equation applies to the flow of liquid from a homogeneous microcirculatory bed to the interstitium at any given instant. Methodological problems exist in that there is heterogeneity in the pulmonary microcirculation (arteriolar vs. venular end of capillary; pulmonary vs. bronchial capillary bed) and a broader anatomical unit than the endothelial wall has to be considered (e.g., basement membrane). Protein fluxes, reviewed elsewhere,[2] are governed by the equation of Kedem and Katchalsky and are dependent upon bulk liquid flow (solvent drag), diffusional fluxes (surface area and permeability) and active transport (e.g., vesicular transport).

tatic'' or ''permeability'' pulmonary edema. This classification emphasizes the movement of liquid and solute across the endothelium. Starling forces also operate across the less permeable alveolar epithelium, but is has been more difficult to determine values for the interstitial and alveolar forces involved.

The magnitude of the Starling forces across lung capillaries may be estimated. There is no accurate direct method of measuring pulmonary capillary pressure. Indirect estimates suggest that mean capillary hydrostatic pressure is approximately 10 torr.[40] Frequently, capillary hydrostatic pressure (P_{mv}) is calculated from pressures measured in the pulmonary artery (P_{pa}) and left atrium (P_{la}), assuming that 40% of total pulmonary vascular resistance is postcapillary:[64] $P_{mv} = P_{la} + 0.4 (P_{pa} - P_{la})$. Experimental evidence suggests that relative resistances in the pulmonary circulation may change during perturbations such as cerebral anoxia and hemorrhagic shock.[17,18] Thus, this calculation may become unreliable when the gradient of pressure from pulmonary artery to left atrium is increased. Measurements of this parameter in rodents is technically difficult.

No reliable measurements of interstitial hydrostatic pressure in lung are available.[1] Chronically implanted capsules have been used to measure it,[67] but the development of scar tissue around the capsule may result in formation of a ''semipermeable membrane''. Thus, negative ''hydrostatic'' pressure measured may represent an oncotic pressure differential.[68] It is generally believed that normal lung P_{pmv} is slightly subatmospheric because of the existence of negative intrapleural hydrostatic pressures.[1] Under certain experimental conditions an equality of pleural pressure and interstitial liquid pressure may exist.[69]

The oncotic pressure of plasma, (π_{mv}), is easily measured. The oncotic pressure of lung lymph may be assumed to equal that of interstitial fluid in the perimicrovascular space (π_{pmv}, Section II). Thus, the oncotic pressure differential may be experimentally determined.

Those terms in the Starling equation which characterize the permeability characteristics of the vessel wall are more difficult to approach. Practically, the degree to which the microvascular membrane restricts passage of macromolecules of widely varying dimensions is determined. It must first be recognized that even the largest particles can pass from the vascular to the interstitial space (even occasional red blood cells, 7 μm in diameter, are found in prenodal lymph). The smaller the molecule, the more rapid its passage from intravascular to extravascular space. Typically, a tracer molecule is administered intravenously, and at some fixed time interval, the degree to which it has penetrated the extravascular space is measured.

If a correction is made for residual blood, or the vascular bed is thoroughly perfused with saline, the extravascular content of a radiotracer at a given time after intravenous injection in a lung homogenate can be determined. ^{125}I-albumin is readily available, and is a suitable tracer molecule. However, because albumin equilibration in the lung interstitium is normally rapid in rodents,[28,29] animals must be killed shortly after tracer injection (within 5 min). If a larger interval is allowed for equilibration, increased tracer content in the lung homogenate may reflect simple increase in extravascular, extracellular liquid volume rather than increase in vascular permeability. This method is easily applied in small animals and is very suitable for toxicologic studies of lung endothelial injury.[8,70]

Tracer molecules may be visualized by light, fluorescence, and electron microscopy.[29,70,71] These techniques are semiquantitative. Using ^{125}I-labeled molecules, it is possible to do quantitative autoradiography.[35] When a lymphatic has been cannulated, the rate of transvascular tracer flux can be measured.[26]

It is usually assumed that edema formation is preceded by some increase in Q_f. This is necessarily so when Q_f is determined from rate of weight gain in isolated perfused lungs, or continuously weighed isolated lung lobes[73] in which the lymphatic system of the lung has been ligated. Under baseline in vivo conditions, lung water is constant and Q_f must be exactly offset by some water clearance mechanism. This is presumed to be lymphatic drainage (although some portion of Q_f may be cleared via the airways). Thus, changes in Q_f in vivo can be approximated via measurements of lung lymph flow. Lung lymph can be obtained by cannulation of the caudal mediastinal lymph node efferent duct (in ruminants), the right lymphatic duct, or the efferent duct of any single mediastinal lymph node.[16,18,26,31,36,74,75] In the presence of an imbalance in the Starling forces that favors marked increase in transvascular water flux or an increase in vascular permeability, augmentation of lymphatic clearance may prevent edema accumulation in lung.[26] It is immediately apparent from this that we cannot simply tether a discussion of pulmonary edema to the Starling equation. It is also apparent that these techniques are directly applicable to studies of toxicological pulmonary edema in animals in which lymph flow rates may be measured.

Factors other than lymphatic clearance which may influence lung liquid accumulation (as opposed to flux) include interstitial compliance, alveolar epithelial permeability, surface tension forces in the alveolar luminal compartment, and, depending on the experimental preparation utilized, the pleural and alveolar luminal pressures.[69]

As discussed in Section II, the pulmonary interstitium has relatively limited elasticity.[40] Presumably, changes in the structural proteins of the interstitium might result in changes in the compliance of the interstitial space, and in the amount of extravascular lung water, even when the Starling forces are within the normal range. This may contribute to edemagenesis in inflammation or after intratracheal instillation or i.v. injection of leukocyte homogenates, elastase, or collagenase.[76-78] Selective injury to the alveolar epithelium, increasing its permeability, will probably result in pulmonary edema even when the Starling forces across the microcirculation are normal. This may occur after administration of certain pneumotoxins (e.g., butylated hydroxytoluene[79]) and in some clinical states (e.g., influenza[80]).

Finally, surface tension forces in the alveolus may contribute significantly to hydrostatic forces tending to draw liquid into the alveolar lining layer. Minimization of surface tension by the secreted alveolar surfactant is thus a factor in keeping the luminal compartment from flooding.[81] Loss of surfactant may contribute to edemagenesis in hyaline membrane disease of the newborn or after pneumotoxin-induced injury to type II pneumocytes (e.g., paraquat[56]).

IV. THE ENDOTHELIAL BARRIER

The role of the pulmonary endothelium in lung injury and repair and its related function in preventing excessive loss of intravascular liquid is of importance in toxic pulmonary edema. Presumably, increases in capillary permeability observed during injury and/or related inflammatory processes can be ascribed to: (1) the injury itself or (2) liberation of cellular or humoral "mediators" which reach the microenvironment of the pulmonary capillaries. Although numerous inhaled or circulating toxic substances, bacterial products, and drugs are believed to cause pulmonary edema by exerting their effects directly or indirectly on endothelial cells,[1,5,6,82-88] definitive mechanisms remain elusive.

The relative permeability of the capillary-interstitium barrier to liquid and solutes is dependent upon the structure and function of the continuous nonfenestrated endothelium of the pulmonary microcirculation. Although recent studies using freeze fracture and molecular probe techniques have provided much information, the ultrastructural determinant(s) of endothelial permeability remain(s) controversial. Whether transport of liquid and/or solutes across the microvasculature is predominantly via plasmalemmal pinocytotic vesicles (including transendothelial channels) or via interendothelial junctions* seems a perennial question,[92,93] as is the quantatative contribution to pulmonary edema of leaky bronchial microvessels.[93]**

Hydrostatic and osmotic force imbalances, toxic agents and/or "mediators" could increase lung transmicrovascular liquid flow by "opening" interendothelial spaces[91,96] (such as via contraction of intracytoplasmic microfilaments found in endothelial cells, by alterations of junction apparatus or both), by stimulating endocytosis (such as by causing membrane perturbation),[97-99] by causing endothelial cell desquamation and/or death, or by exerting effects on contiguous structures (e.g., pericytes, platelets, endocapillary material, basement membrane) which affect endothelial cell structure or metabolism. Clearly, more studies of junction apparatus and endocytosis are needed to elucidate cellular mechanisms of toxic "permeability" pulmonary edema.

Intracellular junctions between endothelial cells of the pulmonary microcirculatory network vary in complexity. As with the systemic microcirculation, the junctions at the venular end of the pulmonary capillary bed appear less "tight" and are therefore considered more permeable than junctions at the arteriolar end.[91] The leakiness and lability of the junctions may be of particular importance in the pathophysiology of inflammatory pulmonary edemas. The role of endocapillary material (glycocalyx) occupying the plasma endothelium interface, the role of membrane factors (such as overall degree of membrane fluidity, which in other systems affects pinocytosis), and the role of the endothelial basement membrane in determining overall permeability of the endothelial barrier, have yet to be assessed. One of the characteristics of normal endothelium is that it does not promote platelet or phagocyte adherence nor activate coagulation or immune systems, perhaps related to properties of the glycocalyx or to the ability of the endothelium to produce prostacyclin.[100]

Physiologists have, with the aid of several simplifying assumptions, determined various (hypothetical) "pore sizes" (generally based on measurement of the molecular size of substances leaving the pulmonary microvasculature or appearing in lung lymph) under a variety of circumstances and have formulated useful concepts involving "large pores" and "small pores" to describe "permeability".[101,102] In spite of the plethora of experimental approaches and the postulated pore theory of capillary permeability, understanding of the molecular events involved remains rather speculative; structural determinants of "pores" are controversial. Thus far, most lung "permeability" studies have been based on molecular size. Unlike studies of permeability in the glomerulus[103,104] or the peripheral circulatory bed,[92,93] no rigorous studies of effects of charge (anionic, neutral, cationic) and shape on pulmonary microvascular permeability have been published. Possibly because the pulmonary endothelium is normally far more permeable to liquid and solute than is the alveolar epithelium, more importance has been ascribed to pneumotoxin-induced increases in endothelial permeability than to increases in epithelial permability.[82-88]

Little attention has yet been focused on surface interactions occurring between blood and endothelium and interactions of the endothelial surface and the cytoplasmic contractile and/or structural filamentous systems. Endothelial interfaces with both the

---

* Many morphologic and physiologic studies have suggested that tight junctions (zonula occludentes) near the apex of endothelial cells, which form a belt-like region of interlinked rows of integral proteins appearing to obliterate intercellular space between adjacent endothelial cells, constitute a major important "permeability" barrier to passage of water and solutes.[89-91]

** That the bronchial circulation may be involved in the production of both hemodynamic[94] and "permeability"[93a] pulmonary edema warrants further investigation. To what extent events occurring in the bronchial circulation effect interstitial liquid kinetics has not been determined. Recent data implies that the bronchial circulation is strongly influenced by both hemodynamic events in the pulmonary circulation[95] and by agents in circulating blood which influence capillary "permeability".[71,93a]

interstitial space and with blood represent a complex milieu. Observations emphasizing the interdependence of endothelium and the homeostatic mechanisms of blood and tissue[105] and the role of several blood constituents such as platelets[106,110] in endothelial cell functions emphasize the importance of this complex interrelationship.

Although phagocyte adherence to endothelium characterizes the lung microcirculation in many clinical disorders associated with apparent "permeability" pulmonary edema,[111] only recently has an understanding of mechanisms whereby phagocyte-endothelium interactions could result in endothelial injury emerged.[105,112,113] Attachment of "activated" phagocytes to lung endothelium may contribute to endothelial derangements by release and/or secretion of proteases, lipases, or activated oxygen species.[113,114] Recently protective inhibitor proteases located at the interface between blood and endothelium have been described[115] and may modulate proteolytic reactions occurring at the vascular surface between platelets, phagocytes, and endothelium. That toxic short-lived oxygen radicals injure endothelium is buttressed by the finding that cytotoxicity in endothelial cell cultures can be induced by "activated" phagocytes.[116] In vitro studies[117] thus may potentially shed light on the mechanism of proposed endothelial injury in "permeability" pulmonary edema, such as that associated with sepsis[118] and other clinical forms of noncardiac pulmonary edema.[119]

More specific toxicologic studies of endothelium will be greatly facilitated via further utilization of endothelial cell cytokinetic techniques[83,85] by use of isolated perfused lung systems[98] as a model for studying toxic injury to lung endothelium and by the use of "markers" to assess endothelial cellular integrity (as might be reflected by prolonged platelet or phagocyte transit times across the lung or by changes in perfusate content of endothelial cell secretions or metabolites). Further studies utilizing isolation, culture, and characterization of endothelial cells[116,117,120,121] will undoubtedly contribute to further understanding of endothelial cell toxicology. Although success in maintaining and propagating endothelial cells in culture[121] and in isolating and characterizing endothelial cells from various organs[122,123] has begun to revolutionize understanding of the metabolic activities of the microvasculature, few studies are available concerning pulmonary vessels,[124] specifically pulmonary capillaries.[125]

V. INTERSTITIAL SPACE

The pulmonary interstitial matrix is a complex mixture of insoluble structural proteins (such as collagen, elastin, and proteoglycans), soluble proteins, and diffusible cellular metabolites.[126,127] Matrix metabolism, turnover, and constituent injury and reparative processes are expected to be of fundamental importance to normal and to pathological liquid movement in the lung.

The connective tissue-basement membrane constituents of the subendothelium and subepithelium probably function not only as key supportive and attachment structures for capillaries and alveolar lining epithelium,[127a] but may also function as physical barriers for liquid and solute exchange, in interactions with blood and alveolar components, and in certain inflammatory and immunological reactions. Few rigorous studies of lung basement membrane exist. There is contradictory evidence as to whether the basement membrane of the alveolar-capillary membrane represents a fused basement membrane of both endothelium and epithelium[99] or a composite structure, possibly with cross-links between constituent macromolecules of the two respective basal laminas.[128] There is no information pertaining to the potential role that fixed basement membrane anionic sites[103,104] might play in intravascular retention of anionic plasma proteins or facilitation of cationic macromolecular transport across the pulmonary microcirculation. Many workers in the field believe that the respective basement membrane scaffolds are especially important in preserving alveolar capillary architecture in

response to injury. In addition, endothelial noncollagenous and collagenous components of basement membrane and the subbasement membrane fibrous elements may
play an important role not only in arrest of bleeding following lung endothelial injury
but in modulating cellular traffic from blood to lung. As mentioned earlier, there is
evidence that the interstitial macromolecules (collagen, proteoglycans, etc.) may significantly influence liquid and solute movement, i.e., some of the transport resistance
(permeability) ascribed to the endothelium may be actually created by the interstitial
matrix, basement membrane, and endocapillary network of fibrous glycoproteins.

Other constituents of the lung interstitium that may play a role in pulmonary edema
include the pulmonary lymphatics, the residing and/or recruited interstitial cells including fibroblasts, phagocytes and contractile cells, and the extracellular connective
tissue elements.

The contractile cells of the lung interstitium[129,130] may acutely modulate interstitial
compliance, possibly by behaving as a functional coordinated syncytium of coupled
pulmonary myofibroblasts.[131] It is possible that acute expansion of the interstitial space
alters its compliance secondary to changes in states of activation of interstitial contractile cells. Likewise, the lung pericytes may have a complex functional interrelationship
with lung endothelial cells and may conceivably have a contractile function that could
modulate either permeability of the endothelium or compliance of the interstitial or
intravascular compartments of the lung. The role of interstitial hydrophilic proteoglycans in "binding" water has also been hypothesized to play a role in interstitial liquid
transport.[93]

Other than studies of the lung lymphatics,[132] few experimental techniques have been
directed towards specific assessment of the role of interstitial structures in modifying
the course of toxicological pulmonary edema. It can be predicted that many elements
present in lung interstitium would be capable of modifying interstitial liquid and solute
movement and their accumulation.[93,133]

VI. THE EPITHELIAL BARRIER

The interstitium is bounded by the alveolar epithelium, composed mostly of Type I
and Type II pneumocytes. Although in the human 9% of lung parenchymal cells are
Type I and 15% are Type II,[41] the extremely flattened Type I cells comprise twice as
much volume, line most of the alveolar surface, and represent the major barrier to
transport from interstium to alveoli (and vice versa).

As with most epithelial barriers, alveolar epithelium appears to have a much lower
permeability to liquid and solutes than does pulmonary endothelium. Ultrastructural
studies reveal a more continuous, complex network of junctional fibrils ("tight" junctions) between alveolar epithelial cells than is seen between the endothelial cells.[91] Physiological measurements of macromolecular transport confirm the anatomical observations and are consistent with an "equivalent pore" radius of 8 to 10 Å in lung
epithelium, as compared to 20 to 200 Å in lung endothelium.[134,135] Hydraulic liquid
conductance of the endothelium appears to be approximately fivefold greater than that
of the epithelium and solute conductance 10-fold greater.[136] Thus pneumotoxins that
appear to preferentially "hit" the endothelium (e.g., oxidants) may act at both surfaces, but the 10-fold larger "pores" in the endothelium may cause epithelial events
to be totally overshadowed experimentally by events at the endothelium.

Although most forms of toxic alveolar edema are thought to be an "all or nothing"
phenomenon,[1] transepithelial pinocytotic transport may play a significant role in the
alveolar edema.[98,137] At present, even considering recent publications concerned with
alveolar epithelial permeability,[137-139] the mechanisms of liquid and solute transport
from interstitium to alveolus and the site of this transport are little understood. That

bronchoalveolar epithelium actively transports ions, somewhat analogous to gastric and intestinal epithelium, has recently been documented.[140]

The presence of macromolecules in even the normal alveolar liquid lining layer has been clearly demonstrated.[141] These are too large to pass through a 10 Å "pore". It is not yet known whether these pass from lung interstitium to alveolus through a few, large, nonselective leaks ("pores", perhaps at bronchoalveolar junctions) or by pinocytosis and subsequent transcellular transport.[141,142] Under experimental conditions, both alveolar and bronchial epithelium have been shown to be permeable to macromolecules.[143,144]

At present there is a paucity of techniques available for differentiating whether or not endothelial or epithelial barriers are specifically responsible for toxic pulmonary edema.[145-147] Certain toxic agents, such as butylated hydroxytoluene,[79] N-nitroso-N-methylurethane,[148] and paraquat[149] may cause toxic pulmonary edema primarily via effects on the alveolar epithelium. However, it seems probable that in most types of toxic lung injury components of endothelium, interstitium, and epithelium are all compromised, to varying degrees. Where pneumotoxins injure alveolar epithelium, it is the Type I cell that appears to be most vulnerable to injury.[4]

Methods have been described for the isolation of Type I[150,151] and Type II[152] pneumocytes. The metabolism of Type II cells, and their responses to toxic agents such as paraquat and O_2, are being characterized.[153,154] However, these cells cover only 5% of the surface area of the alveolus.[41] They are relatively more resistant to most injuries than are the Type I pneumocytes.[4] Clearly, further studies of the response of type II, and especially of Type I pneumocytes to various toxins will be critical to an understanding of the mechanisms by which the alveolar epithelial barrier is compromised in toxic pulmonary edema.

VII. TOXICOLOGICAL CONSIDERATIONS

A. General Considerations

Pulmonary edema occurring after administration of various pneumotoxins has been described. It is beyond the scope of this review to detail primary and secondary multifactorial mechanisms which may play a role in formation of toxic "permeability" pulmonary edemas (Figure 2). The hallmark in this type of edema is an alteration in structure-function of the microvascular or epithelial membrane that permits easier passage of liquid and solutes between vascular, interstitial, and/or alveolar compartments and in which hemodynamic disturbances including hypervolemia and/or decreased plasma oncotic pressures are relatively noncontributory (concomitant effects of the Starling forces may be difficult to exclude in many clinical and toxic types of "permeability" pulmonary edema). The physiological correlates are increased liquid and solute fluxes at a given Starling force. In contrast to hemodynamic pulmonary edema the alveolar liquids contain high concentrations of plasma proteins (see Section II), including fibrinogen.[1,5] The increased "permeability" can be conveniently documented by comparing "clearance" rates of labeled serum proteins from the vascular to the interstitial or alveolar compartments of the lung[118] or by measurements of protein levels in pulmonary edema liquid.[119]

As emphasized in Figure 2, defects may occur as an immediate response to severe chemical or physical injury (which may cause destruction of a small or large area of endothelial or epithelial cytoplasm) or as a consequence of secondary inflammatory processes.[6,112,113] Of central importance is that toxic or "permeability" forms of pulmonary edema run the whole spectrum from almost no (or minor and reversible) ultrastructural changes in pulmonary vascular endothelium (and/or epithelium) to widespread cytoplasmic swelling, bleb formation, degeneration, necrosis, and disruption

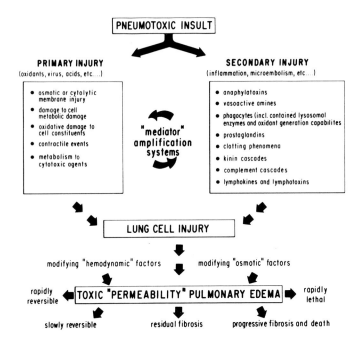

FIGURE 2. Theoretical diagram depicting potential modes of pneumotoxin-induced lung cell injury emphasizing the role of inflammatory-
immunological amplification systems that could potentially initiate, amplify, or propagate lung edemagenic mechanisms. The possible outcome
of pneumotoxin-induced ''permeability'' pulmonary edema is indicated.

of the entire cell layer (which is rapidly fatal). Two aspects that would appear to play
a role in many forms of pneumotoxin-induced pulmonary edema and which have received recent emphasis are examined in more detail below.

B. Oxidative and Phagocytic Mechanisms

The toxicity of oxygen and oxygen radicals at the cell level is being increasingly well-
understood.[155,156] Although much descriptive information characterizing oxidant lung
injury has accumulated,[157-162] specific biochemical mechanisms by which oxidants
damage lung cells remain inferential. Recently, it has become apparent that all forms
of toxic pulmonary edema may be accompanied by oxidant stresses.

Theories of lung oxidant toxicity relate to tissue formation of reactive and unstable
free radicals, with subsequent chain reactions leading to uncontrolled destructive oxidation. Recent work has emphasized the pivotal roles of superoxide and hydroxyl radicals and of singlet oxygen in mediating O_2-induced tissue damage.[155,156] Although
there is indirect evidence that lipid peroxides play a role in O_3-induced lung injury,[160]
that fatty acid hydroperoxides are highly toxic to lung tissue,[163] and that superoxide
anion may play a role in O_2-induced lung injury,[159] little information is available regarding which lung cell types and subcellular elements are responsible for generating
these species.

Reduction of O_2 to active O_2 metabolites occurs as a byproduct of cellular metabolism during both microsomal and mitochondrial electron transfer reactions;[164] considerable amounts of superoxide anion are generated by NADPH-cytochrome P-450 reductase reactions.[165] Because these oxidant species are potentially cytotoxic, they may
mediate or promote actions of various pneumotoxins. Such mechanisms have been
proposed for paraquat-[166] and nitrofurantoin-induced[167] lung injury. When cellular

injury of any type occurs, the release of contained microsomes and flavoproteins into the extracellular space may lead to extracellular generation of deleterious O_2 radicals. It remains to be conclusively demonstrated that these hypothesized peroxidative mechanisms are the critical lethal reactions occurring in oxidant-related lung injuries. These mechanisms do appear critical in so far as antibacterial activities of phagocytes are concerned.[168]

Among mammalian cells, neutrophils, monocytes, and macrophages seem particularly adept at converting molecular O_2 to reactive O_2 metabolites, probably related to both their phagocytosis and antimicrobial activities.[169] As a byproduct of this capability, toxic O_2 species are released (possibly by the plasmalemma itself) into surrounding tissues.[170] As most forms of toxic pulmonary edema are accompanied by phagocyte accumulation in the lung microcirculation (pulmonary leukostasis) and lung parenchyma,[111] oxidative damage may represent a significant component of all types of pneumotoxic lung injury accompanied by a phagocyte-mediated inflammatory component.[171,172]

Chemotactic and phagocytic "activation" processes result in a substantial increase in release of potent oxidants by the stimulated phagocytes,[168,169,173-177] these radicals causing oxidative damage to surrounding tissues. The key role of hydrogen peroxide as the mediator of the extracellular cytotoxic mechanism of "activated" phagocytes has been emphasized in a recent elegant study.[176,177] Phenomena occurring at the phagocyte surface, such as might occur in endogenous lung phagocytes following exposure to numerous inhalants such as dusts and toxic gases, or in circulating phagocytes prior to their accumulation in the lung, or subsequent to their attachment to normal or damaged lung endothelium, seem important in determining their degree of enhanced oxidative activity (which is dormant in the unstimulated cell).[170] For example, exposure of blood to dialyzer cellophane activates complement components, resulting in phagocytic hyperadherence, aggregation, and enhanced endothelial attachments and in their subsequent margination and sequestration in the lung.[178] Accumulation of "activated" phagocytes in the lung may be related to the lung edema seen occasionally following hemodialysis, cardiopulmonary bypass procedures, and in patients with leukoagglutinins. Although it has been long appreciated that phagocytes may cause lysosomal enzyme release and tissue damage,[113,179,180] assessment of the significance of phagocytic-related lysosomal enzyme and oxidant-induced processes in initiating or amplifying lung injury and edema have not been adequately characterized.

"Activated" phagocytes may not produce cytotoxic amounts of superoxide anion.[176,177,181] Although steroids appear to inhibit the generation of toxic oxygen metabolites by "activated" phagocytes,[182] there is little convincing evidence that steroids limit pneumotoxin-induced pulmonary edema. That oxidative processes are even more complex is suggested by the finding that phagocytic production of active oxygen species causes inactivation of proteinase inhibitors[183,184] and degranulation of mast cells.[185] The phagocyte capabilities for producing oxygen radicals are enhanced not only by interactions of cell surface membranes with various appropriate stimuli, but also by hyperoxia.[186] Platelets (and platelet microthrombi) also have capabilities for the generation of activated O_2 species.[187]

It can be concluded that the evidence linking the toxic and edemagenic effects of oxidants with increased generation of activated oxygen free radicals is extensive, but by no means unequivocal. Inflammation with phagocyte "activation" and the recruitment of these cells to the lung by the various chemotactic factors may mimic or amplify environmental oxidant-induced lung edema including that caused by oxygen itself.

The clinical literature has recently emphasized that the autopsy lesions of patients dying with acute lung injury may result as much from oxidant-related damage as from the proximate cause of injury.[188] Oxidants probably play a role in all pneumotoxic forms of pulmonary edema!

C. Microembolism

Pulmonary microemboli are believed to be a significant factor in the development of pulmonary edema in various forms of diffuse parenchymal injury, most notably those types associated with shock, trauma, and septicemia.[6,8,189,190] In these conditions the lung microcirculation contains products of intravascular coagulation (such as platelet-fibrin microaggregates) and varying amounts of sequestered phagocytes. Multifactorial interrelated mechanical, reflex, and vasoactive mechanisms are thought to contribute to the pulmonary edema.[191-193] The trapped microaggregated materials may indirectly potentiate edema formation by causing high linear blood flow velocities through the unobstructed but markedly restricted lung microvascular bed, with physical damage to the endothelium in unobstructed capillaries (over perfusions injury).[193] Platelets and phagocytes adhering to endothelium may initiate, sustain, and/or enhance inflammatory responses related to increased endothelial permeability. Recent attention has focused on release of substances from aggregated platelets, sequestered phagocytes, or the endothelial cells themselves. Fibrin may be necessary for the development of the increased "permeability",[192,192a] although the role of platelets[8,192b] and phagocytes,[194,195,195a] and vessel releases of such substances as prostaglandins and prostacyclin[100,109,110] to the pulmonary edemagenesis is not yet well understood. It can be concluded that blood-endothelial interactions are complex processes, with each cell type (including platelets and leukocytes) responding to the other or to the factors produced by it, so that data derived solely from studies of one cell system may not always reflect interactions occurring in vivo.

D. Enigmas

Understanding toxicological pulmonary edema involves both minor and major dilemmas. Minor problems relate to adequate quantitative measurements of lung extravascular liquid, establishment of time-dose dependencies, assessment of multiple and variable host factors (age, sex, species, strain, etc.), and determination of pathophysiologic parameters involved in the edema formation.

Major methodological dilemmas remain. Toxicological assessment are not complete until the proximate molecular and biochemical mechanisms are known. Ways of dissecting primary pneumotoxin-related events from secondary lung tissue damage occurring as a result of ensuing inflammatory and immunologic reactions, including those due to inadvertent extracellular releases of various hydrolytic enzymes[113,179,180] and oxidants from phagocytes[168,173,177] or oxygen administered during treatment remain elusive. The role of coagulation factors including platelets, phagocytes, and immunoreactants such as complement[195a] in all forms of toxic pulmonary injuries needs to be better defined,[113] as does the most susceptible site of primary and secondary injury (alveolar, interstitial, or endothelial). It is likely that complex, as yet unrecognized, interrelationships among the mediators of inflammation may prove to be a "final common pathway" in the pathogenesis of many of the toxicologic pulmonary edemas. The heterogeneity of lung cell components and lack of information about lung functional cells has limited interpretations of studies of the effects of toxic substances on the whole lung. The fact that lung interstitial and alveolar spaces represent a relatively larger volume reservoir for influx of more inflammation-related components than exists in other organs makes it especially difficult to assess biochemical parameters measured in lung homogenate from a standpoint of specific injury mechanisms in the lung. An added dilemma is that the demarcation between acute and chronic injury and/or inflammation in the lung is rarely sharply defined. Often pulmonary edema and exudation, hallmarks for acute injury, exist simultaneously with tissue proliferation and repair processes. The potential usefulness of cell separation and culture systems for the study of lung toxicity is readily apparent. Ultimate definitions of mechanisms of toxic pulmonary edema will undoubtedly be based on these techniques.

Relatively little is known concerning lung cell metabolism of pneumotoxins, such as the importance of activation or inhibition of mixed function microsomal enzyme systems that are responsible for drug biotransformation,[196] the modifying role of noninflammatory humoral mediators,[197] or the effects of edema formation itself on pneumotoxin pharmacodynamics.[198,199] Controversies exist as to both the operative pathophysiologic and the proximate molecular mechanisms in such well-defined experimental models as cerebrogenic,[17,200,201] hemorrhagic shock,[18,75,202] and paraquat pulmonary edema.[203-205]

Future progress in understanding of basic mechanisms of toxic lung damage is not likely to occur without a more clear understanding of some of these dilemmas.

VIII. CONSEQUENCES OF PULMONARY EDEMA

Biological consequences of toxic pulmonary edema depend not only on acute compromise of lung structure and function, but may also depend on abnormalities remaining after resolution of the edematous process. Toxic edema caused by alterations in endothelial or epithelial permeability due to modified, impaired, or lost cell function is often extreme. Following exposure to some toxic agents in which the alveolar-capillary surface is denuded (such as alloxan), recovery is unlikely, whereas in situations with a more modest injury (such as following histamine administration) full recovery is readily achieveable. Between these two extremes are forms of severe lung injury accompanied by amplified inflammatory damage and/or overzealous restorative-reparative processes (e.g., paraquat ingestion). In these severe forms, the extensive interstitial and intraalveolar inflammatory exudates resolve via fibrogenesis, an outcome that may be beneficial or damaging to the lung. That a degree of lung fibrosis accompanies many diverse forms of clinical severe pulmonary injury has been recently emphasized.[188,190,206-208] It seems certain that, depending on the magnitude and type of toxic lung injury, early pulmonary fibrosis during resolution of pulmonary edema can be either reversible, self-limited, slowly progressive, or rapidly progressive (Figure 2).

Accumulation and turnover of inflammatory cells and related immune responses in the edematous lung likely play a role in eliciting both mitogenic activity and fibrogenic responses.[209-211] Important unknowns are the molecular connections that link cell injury, inflammation, and increased fibrogenesis. Studies based upon determination of humoral and cellular constituents in broncho-alveolar lavage fluid sampled serially after lung insult point toward a close relationship between inflammation and fibrosis in noncardiogenic pulmonary edema.[212-214] Relatively little is known concerning interactions of fibroblasts and other collagen-synthesizing cells with components of these inflammatory humoral and cellular systems. The report that interstitial fluid (lung lymph) collected from animal models of experimental shock lung contains factors that cause proliferation of fibroblasts[190] may be important in this regard. Mechanisms whereby factors derived from injured tissue and from activated lymphocytes, monocytes, or macrophages, from activation of complement and/or from specific degradation products of collagen contribute to chemotactic migration, proliferation, and/or synthetic activations of fibroblasts are still speculative. Factors that control inflammatory fibrogenic responses remain an enigma. More toxicologic model systems, such as the paraquat model,[64] are necessary for studying induced fibrogenesis in the lung at the molecular level. It is unlikely that these model systems will provide the ultimate explanations of the influence of one cell upon proliferation and differentiation of its neighboring fibroblasts. Again, isolated cells in tissue culture seem to be required to answer these questions. Techniques designed to examine these interactions may produce an understanding of the mechanisms and consequences of toxicologic pulmonary edema, and will also provide approaches for treatment.

IX. CONCLUSIONS

During the past decade there has been an exponential increase in our awareness of lung metabolism and effects of toxic agents on this metabolism. The recent publication of the series *Lung Biology in Health and Disease* [217] bears eloquent witness to the present vigorous state of this awareness. The tools for expanding the scientific basis for understanding toxicologic pulmonary edema from mere delineation of the temporal sequences of the edema itself to actual awareness of cellular mechanisms responsible for the edema formation are now present. One can predict that sometime in the near future, the ultrastructure, biochemistry, and physiology of toxic pulmonary edema will be well defined, allowing for more clear-cut classifications into disorders of cell membrane, energy metabolism, biotransformation, antioxidant, or other specific metabolism; and into disorders dependent on inflammatory, coagulation, humoral, vasoactive, or immunologic amplifications. Many toxins and clinical circumstances are responsible for causing pulmonary edema, yet little is known concerning the nature of the chemical insult at the responsible cellular and subcellular level. Despite the impressive advances in fundamental understandings of lung cell biology, we are only at the threshold of a more rigorous and mechanistic approach in understanding toxicological pulmonary edemas and in devising appropriate pharmacological strategies.

REFERENCES

1. Staub, N. C., Pulmonary edema, *Physiol. Rev.*, 54, 678, 1974.
2. Crone, C. and Christensen, O., Transcapillary transport of small solutes and water, in *Cardiovascular Physiology*, Vol. 3, Guyton, A. C. and Young, D. B., Eds., University Park Press, Baltimore, 1979, 149.
3. Parker, J. C., Guyton, A. C., and Taylor, A. E., Pulmonary transcapillary exchange and pulmonary edema, in *Cardiovascular Physiology*, Vol. 3, Guyton, A. C. and Young, D. B., Eds., University Park Press, Baltimore, 1979, 261.
4. Witschi, H. and Côte, M. G., Pulmonary responses to toxic agents, *Crit. Rev. Toxicol.*, 5, 23, 1977.
5. Robin, E. D., Cross, C. E., and Zelis, R., Medical progress: pulmonary edema, *N. Engl. J. Med.*, 288, 239, 1973.
6. Blaisdell, F. W. and Lewis, F. R., *Respiratory Distress Syndrome of Shock and Trauma*, W. B. Saunders, Philadelphia, 1977, 237.
7. Staub, N. C., Ed., *Lung Water and Solute Exchange*, Marcel Dekker, New York, 1978, 568.
8. Hurley, J. V., Current views on the mechanisms of pulmonary edema, *J. Pathol.*, 125, 59, 1978.
9. Fishman, A. P. and Renkin, E. M., Eds., *Pulmonary Edema*, American Physiological Society, Bethesda, 1979, 269.
11. Hughes, J. M. B., Glazier, J. B., Maloney, J. E., and West, J. B., Effect of lung volume on the distribution of pulmonary blood flow in man, *Respir. Physiol.*, 4, 58, 1968.
12. Sarnoff, S. J. and Berglund, E., Pressure-volume characteristics and stress relaxation in the pulmonary vascular bed of the dog, *Am. J. Physiol.*, 171, 238, 1952.
13. Fung, Y. C., Fluid in the interstitial space of the pulmonary alveolar sheet, *Microvasc. Res.*, 7, 89, 1974.
14. Vreim, C. E. and Staub, N. C., Pulmonary vascular pressures and capillary blood volume changes in anesthetized cats, *J. Appl. Physiol.*, 36, 275, 1974.
15. Ducker, T. B., Increased intracranial pressure and pulmonary edema. I. Clinical study of 11 cases, *J. Neurosurg.*, 28, 112, 1968.
16. Bowers, R. E., McKeen, C. R., Park, B. E., and Brigham, K. L., Increased pulmonary vascular permeability follows intracranial hypertension in sheep, *Am. Rev. Respir. Dis.*, 119, 637, 1979.
17. Moss, G., Staunton, C., and Stein, A., Cerebral etiology of the "shock lung syndrome", *J. Trauma*, 12, 885, 1972.
18. Demling, R. H., Niahaus, G., and Will, J. A., Pulmonary microvascular response to hemorrhagic shock, resuscitation and recovery, *J. Appl. Physiol.*, 46, 498, 1979.

19. Meyrick, B. and Reid, L., Pulmonary hypertension and arterial changes in rats fed *Crotalaria spectabilis* seeds, *Fed. Proc. Fed. Am. Soc. Exp. Biol.*, 38, 1155, 1979.

20. Gardiner, M. R., Royce, R., and Bokor, A., Studies on *Crotalaria crispata*, a newly recognized cause of Kimberley Horse Disease, *J. Pathol. Bactiol.*, 89, 43, 1965.

21. Levine, O. R., Mellins, R. B., and Fishman, A. P., Quantitative assessment of pulmonary edema, *Circ. Res.*, 17, 414, 1965.

22. Peterson, B. T., Petrini, M. F., Hyde, R. W., and Schreiner, B. F., Pulmonary tissue volume in dogs during pulmonary edema, *J. Appl. Physiol.*, 44, 782, 1978.

23. Cross, C. E., Watanabe, T. T., Hasegawa, G. K., Goralnik, G. N., Kaizu, T., Reiser, K. M., Gorin, A. B., and Last, J. A., Biochemical assays in lung homogenates: artifacts caused by trapped blood after perfusion, *Toxicol. Appl. Pharmacol.*, 48, 99, 1979.

24. Weibel, E. R., Morphological basis of alveolar capillary gas exchange, *Physiol. Rev.*, 53, 419, 1973.

25. Marshall, B. E., Determination of the blood content of the lungs *in vitro*, *J. Appl. Physiol.*, 31, 643, 1971.

26. Brigham, K. L., Woolverton, W. C., Blake, L., and Staub, N. C., Increased sheep lung vascular permeability caused by pseudomonas bacteremia, *J. Clin. Invest.*, 54, 792, 1974.

27. Swan, H. and Nelson, A. W., Blood volume I: critique: spun vs. isotope hematocrit; ^{125}RIESA vs. ^{51}CrRBC, *Ann. Surg.*, 173, 481, 1971.

28. Studer, R. and Potchen, J., The radioisotopic assessment of regional microvascular permeability to macromolecules, *Microvasc. Res.*, 3, 35, 1971.

29. Nicolaysen, G. and Staub, N. C., Time course of albumin equilibration in interstitium and lymph of normal mouse lungs, *Microvasc. Res.*, 9, 29, 1975.

30. Laurent, T. C., The interaction between polysaccharides and other macromolecules. IX. The exclusion of molecules from hyaluronic acid gels and solutions, *Biochem. J.*, 93, 106, 1964.

31. Selinger, S. L., Bland, R. D., Demling, R. H., and Staub, N. C., Distribution volumes of [^{131}I] albumin, [^{14}C] sucrose, and ^{36}Cl in sheep lung, *J. Appl. Physiol.*, 39, 773, 1975.

32. Parker, J. C., Falgout, H. J., Parker, R. E., Granger, D. N., and Taylor, A. E., The effect of fluid volume loading on exclusion of interstitial albumin and lymph flow in the dog lung, *Circ. Res.*, 45, 440, 1979.

33. Guyton, A. C., Taylor, A. E., Drake, R. E., and Parker, J. C., Dynamics of subatmospheric pressure in the pulmonary interstitial fluid, in *Lung Liquids,* Porter, R. and O'Connor, M., Eds., Ciba Found. Symp. No. 38 (New Ser.), Elsevier, Amsterdam, 1976, 77.

34. Vreim, C. E., Snashall, P. D., Demling, R. H., and Staub, N. C., Lung lymph and free interstitial fluid protein composition in sheep with edema, *Am. J. Physiol.*, 230, 1650, 1976.

35. Nicolaysen, G., Nicolaysen, A., and Staub, N. C., A quantitative radioautographic comparison of albumin concentration in different sized lymph vessels of normal mouse lung, *Microvasc. Res.*, 10, 138, 1975.

36. Taylor, A. E., Parker, J. C., Parker, R. E., and Granger, D. N., Permselectivity of pulmonary capillaries to endogenous macromolecules, *Fed. Proc. Fed. Am. Soc. Exp. Biol.*, 38, 1327, 1979.

37. Effros, R. and Chang, R., Distribution of water and protein in the lungs in pulmonary edema, in *Pulmonary Edema,* Fishman, A. P. and Renkin, E. M., Eds., American Physiological Society, Bethesda, 1979, 137.

38. Staub, N. C., Nagano, H., and Pearce, M. L., Pulmonary edema in dogs, especially the sequence of fluid accumulation in the lungs, *J. Appl. Physiol.*, 22, 227, 1967.

39. Weibel, E. R. and Bachofen, H., Structural design of the alveolar septum and fluid exchange, in *Pulmonary Edema,* Fishman, A. P. and Renkin, E. M., Eds., American Physiological Society, Bethesda, 1979, 1.

40. Parker, J. C., Guyton, A. C., and Taylor, A. E., Pulmonary interstitial and capillary pressures estimated from intra-alveolar fluid pressures, *J. Appl. Physiol.*, 44, 267, 1978.

40a. Mitzner, W. and Robotham, J. L., Distribution of interstitial compliance and filtration coefficient in canine lung, *Lymphology*, 12, 140, 1979.

41. Barry, B. E., Crapo, J. D., Gehr, P., Bachofen, M., and Weibel, E. R., Population characteristics of the cells in normal human lung, *Am. Rev. Respir. Dis.*, 119(Abstr.), 287, 1979.

42. Snashall, P. D., Weidner, W. J., and Staub, N. C., Extravascular lung water after extracellular fluid volume expansion in dogs, *J. Appl. Physiol.*, 42, 624, 1977.

43. Robin, E. D. and Theodore, J., Intracellular and subcellular oedema and dehydration, in *Lung Liquids,* Porter, R. and O'Conner, M., Eds., Ciba Found. Symp. No. 38 (New Ser.), Elsevier, Amsterdam, 1976, 273.

44. Amthor, M., The temporary ischemia as experimental model for human shock lung, *Pathol. Res. Pract.*, 162, 88, 1978.

45. Modry, D. L. and Chiu, R. C-J., Pulmonary reperfusion syndrome, *Ann. Thorac. Surg.*, 27, 206, 1979.

46. Reifenrath, R. and Zimmermann, I., Blood plasma contamination of the lung alveolar surfactant obtained by various sampling techniques, *Respir. Physiol.*, 18, 238, 1973.

47. Untersee, P., Gil, J., and Weibel, E. R., Visualization of extracellular lining layer of lung alveoli by freeze-etching, *Respir. Physiol.*, 13, 171, 1971.

48. Yoneda, K., Mucus blanket of rat bronchus: an ultrastructural study, *Am. Rev. Respir. Dis.*, 114, 837, 1976.

49. Van As, A., Pulmonary airway clearance mechanisms: a reappraisal, *Am. Rev. Respir. Dis.*, 115, 721, 1977.

50. Baile, E. M., Paré, P. D., Dahlby, R. W., and Hogg, J. C., Regional distribution of extravascular water and hematocrit in the lung, *J. Appl. Physiol. Respir. Environ. Exercise Physiol.*, 46, 937, 1979.

51. Flick, M. R., Perel, A., Kageler, W., and Staub, N. C., Regional extravascular lung water in normal sheep, *J. Appl. Physiol. Respir. Environ. Exercise Physiol.*, 46, 932, 1979.

52. Chinard, F. P., Estimation of extravascular lung water by indicator dilution techniques, *Circ. Res.*, 37, 137, 1975.

53. Casaburi, R., Wasserman, K., and Effros, R., Detection and measurement of pulmonary edema, in *Lung Water and Solute Exchange*, Staub, N. C., Ed., Marcel Dekker, New York, 1978.

54. Petrini, M. F., Peterson, B. T., and Hyde, R. W., Lung tissue volume and blood flow by rebreathing: theory, *J. Appl. Physiol. Respir. Environ. Exercise Physiol.*, 4, 795, 1978.

54a. MacArthur, C. G. C., Rhodes, C. G., Swinburne, A. J., Heather, J. D., and Hughes, J. M. B., Measurement of regional lung water using gamma-emitting tracers, *Bull. Eur. Physiopathol. Respir.*, 16, 321, 1980.

54b. Gamsu, G., Kaufman, L., Swann, S. J., and Brito, A. C., Absolute lung density in experimental canine pulmonary edema, *Invest. Radiat.*, 14, 261, 1979.

54c. Simon, D. S., Murray, J. F., and Staub, N. C., Measurement of pulmonary edema in intact dogs by transthoracic x-ray attenuation, *J. Appl. Physiol. Respir. Environ. Exercise Physiol.*, 47, 1228, 1979.

55. Cross, C. E., Hasegawa, G., and Reddy, K. A., Enhanced lung toxicity of O_2 in selenium-deficient rats, *Res. Comm. Chem. Pathol. Pharmacol.*, 16, 695, 1977.

56. Fisher, H. K., Clements, J. A., and Wright, R. R., Pulmonary effects of the herbicide paraquat studied three days after injection in rats, *J. Appl. Physiol.*, 35, 268, 1973.

57. Kirk, B., Effect of alterations in pulmonary blood flow on lung-exchangeable water in the dog, *J. Appl. Physiol.*, 27, 607, 1969.

58. Thet, L. A., Delaney, M. D., Gregorio, C. A., and Massaro, D., Protein metabolism by rat lung: influence of fasting, glucose, and insulin, *J. Appl. Physiol. Respir. Environ. Exercise Physiol.*, 43, 463, 1977.

59. Hollinger, M. A. and Chvapil, M., Effect of paraquat on rat lung prolyl hydroxylase, *Res. Commun. Chem. Pathol. Pharmacol.*, 16, 159, 1977.

60. Massaro, D., Weiss, H., and White, G., Protein synthesis by lung following pulmonary artery ligation, *J. Appl. Physiol.*, 31, 8, 1971.

61. Gacad, G., Dickie, K., and Massaro, D., Protein synthesis in lung: influence of starvation on amino acid incorporation into protein, *J. Appl. Physiol.*, 33, 381, 1972.

62. Smith, L. L. and Rose, M. S., A comparison of the effects of paraquat and diquat on the water content of rat lung and the incorporation of thymidine into lung DNA, *Toxicology*, 8, 223, 1977.

63. Guyton, A. C. and Lindsey, A. W., Effect of elevated left atrial pressure and decreased plasma protein concentration on the development of pulmonary edema, *Circ. Res.*, 7, 649, 1959.

64. Greenberg, D. B., Lyons, S. A., and Last, J. A., Paraquat-induced changes in the rate of collagen biosynthesis by rat lung explants, *J. Lab. Clin. Med.*, 92, 1033, 1978.

65. Vreim, C. E. and Staub, N. C., Protein composition of lung fluids in acute alloxan edema in dogs, *Am. J. Physiol.*, 230, 376, 1976.

66 Gaar, K. A., Jr., Taylor, A. E., Owens, L. J., and Guyton, A. C., Pulmonary capillary pressure and filtration coefficient in the isolated perfused lung, *Am. J. Physiol.*, 213, 910, 1967.

67. Guyton, A. C., Granger, H. J., and Taylor, A. E., Interstitial fluid pressure, *Physiol. Rev.*, 51, 527, 1971.

68. Snashall, P. D., Mucopolysaccharide osmotic pressure in the measurement of interstitial pressure, *Am. J. Physiol.*, 232, H608, 1977.

69. Lee, J. S. and Lee, L. P., Effect of vascular, pleural, and alveolar pressures on filtration in isolated, perfused lobes of dogs, *Microvasc. Res.*, 14, 265, 1977.

70. Scherzer, H. and Ward, P. A., Lung and dermal vascular injury produced by preformed immune complexes, *Am. Rev. Respir. Dis.*, 117, 551, 1978.

71. Pietra, G. G., Szidon, J. P., and Fishman, A. P., Leaky pulmonary vessels, *Trans. Am. Assoc. Physicians*, 85, 369, 1972.

72. Michel, R. P., Inoue, S., and Hogg, J. C., Pulmonary capillary permeability to HRP in dogs: a physiological and morphological study, *J. Appl. Physiol.*, 42, 13, 1977.

73. **Albert, R. K., Lakshminavayan, S., Huang, T. W., and Butter, J.,** Fluid-leaks from extra-alveolar vessels in living dog lungs, *J. Appl. Physiol.*, 44, 759, 1978.

74. **Brigham, K. L. and Snell, J. D.,** In vivo assessment of pulmonary vascular integrity in experimental pulmonary edema, *J. Clin. Invest.*, 52, 2041, 1973.

75. **Todd, T. R. J., Baile, E., and Hogg, J. C.,** Pulmonary capillary permeability during hemorrhagic shock, *J. Appl. Physiol. Respir. Environ. Exercise Physiol.*, 45, 298, 1978.

76. **Polzin, J. K., Napier, J. S., Taylor, J. C., and Rodarte, J. R.,** Effect of elastase and ventilation on elastic recoil of excised dog lungs, *Am. Rev. Respir. Dis.*, 119, 377, 1979.

77. **Karlinsky, J. B., Snider, G. L., Franzblau, C., Stone, P. J., and Hoppin, F. G., Jr.,** In vitro effects of elastase and collagenase on mechanical properties of hamster lungs, *Am. Rev. Respir. Dis.*, 113, 769, 1976.

78. **Weinbaum, G., Marco, V., Ikeda, T., Mass, B., Meranze, D. R., and Kimbel, P.,** Enzymatic production of experimental emphysema in the dog. Route of exposure, *Am. Rev. Respir. Dis.*, 109. 351, 1974.

79. **Adamson, I. Y. R., Bowden, D., Côte, M., and Witschi, H.,** Lung injury induced by butylated hydroxytoluene, *Lab. Invest.*, 36, 26, 1977.

80. **Stinson, S. F., Ryan, D. P., Hertweck, M. S., Hardy, J. D., Hwang-Kow, S., and Loosli, C.,** Epithelial and surfactant changes in influenzal pulmonary lesions, *Arch. Pathol. Lab. Med.*, 100, 147, 1976.

81. **Alpert, R. K., Lakshminarayan, S., Hillebrandt, J., Kink, W., and Butler, J.,** Increased surface tension favors pulmonary edema formation in anesthetized dogs' lungs, *J. Clin. Invest.*, 63, 1015, 1979.

82. **Brigham, K. L.,** Factors affecting lung vascular permeability, *Am. Rev. Respir. Dis.*, 115, 165, 1977.

83. **Miller, W. C., Rice, D. L., Kreusel, R. G., and Bedrossian, C. W. M.,** Monocrotaline model of noncardiogenic pulmonary edema in dogs, *J. Appl. Physiol. Respir. Environ. Exercise Physiol.*, 45, 962, 1978.

84. **Malik, A. B. and van der Zee, H.,** Mechanism of pulmonary edema induced by microembolization in dogs, *Cir. Res.*, 42, 72, 1978.

85. **Freudenberg, N.,** Endothelium and shock, *Pathol. Res. Pract.*, 162, 105, 1978.

86. **Staub, N. C.,** Pulmonary edema due to increased microvascular permeability to fluid and protein, *Cir. Res.*, 43, 143, 1978.

87. **Sandritter, W., Mittermayer, C., Riede, U. N., Freudenberg, N., and Grimm, H.,** Shock lung syndrome (a general review), *Pathol. Res. Pract.*, 162, 7, 1978.

88. **Robin, E. D.,** Permeability pulmonary edema, in *Pulmonary Edema*, Fishman, A. P. and Renkin, E. M., Eds., American Physiological Society, Bethesda, Md., 1979, 217.

89. **Staehelin, L. A.,** Structure and function of intracellular junctions, *Int. Rev. Cytol.*, 39, 191, 1974.

90. **Simionescu, M., Simionescu, N., and Palade, G. E.,** Segmented differentiations of cell junctions in the vascular endothelium: the microvasculature, *J. Cell Biol.*, 67, 863, 1975.

91. **Schneeberger, E. E.,** Structural basis for some permeability properties of the air-blood barrier, *Fed. Proc. Fed. Am. Soc. Exp. Biol.*, 37, 2471, 1978.

92. **Renkin, E. M.,** Multiple pathways of capillary permeability, *Cir. Res.*, 41, 735, 1977.

93. **Renkin, E. M.,** The microcirculatory society Eugene D. Landis Award lecture, *Microvasc. Res.*, 15, 123, 1978.

93a. **Pietra, G. G.,** The basis of pulmonary edema, with emphasis on ultrastructure, in *The Lung: Structure, Function and Disease*, Thurlbeck, W. M. and Abell, M. R., Eds., Williams & Wilkins, Baltimore, 1978, 215.

94. **Conway, D. and Johnson, R.,** The nature and significance of peribronchial cuffing in pulmonary edema, *Radiology*, 125, 577, 1977.

95. **Magno, M.,** Effect of pulmonary blood flow on the post-occlusion response of the bronchial circulation in anesthetized sheep, *Fed. Proc. Fed. Am. Soc. Exp. Biol.*, 38, 1378, 1979.

96. **Barrios, R., Inove, S., and Hogg, J. C.,** Intercellular junctions in "shock lung", *Lab. Invest.*, 36, 628, 1977.

97. **Silverstein, S. C., Steinman, R. M., and Cohn, Z. A.,** Endocytosis, *Ann. Rev. Biochem.*, 46, 669, 1977.

98. **DeFouw, D. O. and Berendsen, P. B.,** Morphological changes in isolated perfused dog lungs after acute hydrostatic edema, *Circ. Res.*, 43, 72, 1978.

99. **DeFouw, D. O. and Berendsen, P. B.,** A morphometric analysis of isolated perfused dog lungs after acute oncotic edema, *Microvasc. Res.*, 17, 90, 1979.

100. **Moncada, S. and Vane, J. R.,** The role of prostacyclin in vascular tissue, *Fed. Proc. Fed. Am. Soc. Exp. Biol.*, 66, 1979.

101. **Blake, L. H.,** Mathematical modeling of steady state fluid and protein exchange in the lung, in *Lung Water and Solute Exchange*, Staub, N. S., Ed., Marcel Dekker, New York, 1978, 99.

102. Taylor, A. E. and Drake, R. E., Fluid and protein movement across the pulmonary microcirculation, in *Lung Water and Solute Exchange*, Staub, N. S., Ed., Marcel Dekker, New York, 1978, 99.

103. Brenner, B. M., Hostetter, T. H., and Humes, H. D., Molecular basis of proteinuria of glomerular origin, *N. Engl. J. Med.*, 298, 826, 1978.

104. Kanwar, Y. S. and Farquar, M. G., Anionic sites in the glomerular basement membrane, *J. Cell Biol.*, 81, 137, 1979.

105. Thorgeirsson, G. and Robertson, A. L., The vascular endothelium: pathobiologic significance, *Am. J. Pathol.*, 93, 803, 1978.

106. White, M. K., Shepro, D., and Hechtman, H. B., Pulmonary function and platelet-lung interaction, *J. Appl. Physiol.*, 34, 697, 1973.

107. D'Amore, P., Platelet-endothelial interaction and the maintenance of the microvasculature, *Microvasc. Res.*, 15, 137, 1978.

108. Needleman, P., Wyche, A., and Raz, A., Platelet and blood vessel arachidonate metabolism and interactions, *J. Clin. Invest.*, 63, 345, 1979.

109. Needleman, P., Prostacyclin in blood vessel-platelet interactions: perspectives and questions, *Nature (London)*, 279, 14, 1979.

110. Moncada, S. and Vane, J. R., Arachidonic acid metabolites and the interactions between platelets and blood-vessel walls, *N. Engl. J. Med.*, 300, 1142, 1979.

111. Wilson, J. W., Pulmonary disease and the microcirculation, in *The Microcirculation in Clinical Medicine*, Wells, R., Ed., Academic Press, New York, 1973, 169.

112. Cross, C. E. and Hyde, R. W., Treatment of pulmonary edema, in *Lung Water and Solute Exchange*, Staub, N. C., Ed., Marcel Dekker, New York, 1978, 471.

113. Johnson, K. J., Chapman, W. E., and Ward, P. A., Immunopathology of the lung: a review, *Am. J. Pathol.*, 95, 795, 1979.

114. Goldstein, I., Polymorphonuclear leukocyte lysosomes and immune tissue injury, *Prog. Allergy*, 20, 301, 1976.

115. Becker, C. G. and Harpel, P. C., α-Macroglobulin on human vascular endothelium, *J. Exp. Med.*, 144, 1, 1976.

116. Sacks, T., Moldow, C. F., Craddock, P. R., Bowers, T. K., and Jacob, H. S., Oxygen radicals mediate endothelial cell damage by complement-stimulated granulocytes, *J. Clin. Invest.*, 61, 1161, 1978.

117. Sacks, T., Moldow, C. F., Craddock, P. R., Bowers, T. K., and Jacob, H. S., Endothelial damage provoked by toxic radicals released from complement-triggered granulocytes, in *The Red Cell*, Brewer, G. J., Ed., Alan R. Liss, New York, 1978, 719.

118. Anderson, R. R., Holliday, R. L., Driedger, A. A., Lefcoe, M., Redi, B., and Sibbald, W. J., Documentation of pulmonary capillary permeability in the adult respiratory distress syndrome accompanying human sepsis, *Am. Rev. Respir. Dis.*, 119, 869, 1979.

119. Fein, A., Crossman, R. F., Jones, J. G., Overland, E., Pitts, L., Murray, J. F., and Staub, N. C., The value of edema fluid protein measurement in patients with pulmonary edema, *Am. J. Med.*, 67, 32, 1979.

120. Beesley, J. E., Pearson, J. D., Carleton, J. S., Hutchings, A., and Gordon, J. L., Interaction of leukocytes with vascular cells in culture, *J. Cell. Sci.*, 33, 85, 1978.

121. Moore, A., Jaffe, E. A., Becker, C. G., and Nachman, R. L., Myosin in cultured human endothelial cells, *Br. J. Haematol.*, 35, 71, 1979.

122. Simionescu, M. and Simionescu, N., Isolation and characterization of endothelial cells from the heart microvasculature, *Microvasc. Res.*, 16, 426, 1978.

123. Herbst, T. J., Raichle, M. E., and Ferrendelli, J. A., Beta-adrenergic regulation of adenosine 3',5' — microvessels, *Science*, 204, 330, 1979.

124. Ryan, U. S., Clements, E., Habliston, D., and Ryan, J. W., Isolation and culture of pulmonary artery endothelial cells, *Tissue and Cell*, 10, 535, 1978.

125. Habliston, D. L., Whitaker, C., Hart, M. A., Ryan, U. S., and Ryan, J. W., Isolation and culture of endothelial cells from the lungs of small animals, *Am. Rev. Respir. Dis.*, 119, 853, 1979.

126. Fishman, A. P. and Hecht, H. H., Eds., *The Pulmonary Circulation and Interstitial Space*, University of Chicago Press, 1969, 432.

127. Hance, A. J. and Crystal, R. G., The connective tissue of lung, *Am. Rev. Respir. Dis.*, 112, 657, 1975.

127a. Kefalides, N. A., Alper, R., and Clark, C. C., Biochemistry and metabolism of basement membranes, *Int. Rev. Cytol.*, 61, 167, 1979.

128. Huang, T. W., Composite epithelial and endothelial basal laminas in human lungs, *Am. J. Pathol.*, 93, 681, 1978.

129. Kapanci, Y., Assimacopoulos, A., Irle, C., Zwahlen, A., and Gabbiani, G., Contractile interstitial cells in pulmonary alveolar septa: a possible regulator of ventilation/perfusion ratio? Ultrastructural, immunofluorescence, and in vitro studies, *J. Cell Biol.*, 60, 375, 1974.

130. Kapanci, Y., Costabella, P. M., and Gabbiani, G., Location and function of contractile interstitial cells of the lungs, in *Lung Cells in Disease*, Bouhuys, A., Ed., Elsevier, North Holland Press, Amsterdam, 1976, 69.

131. Bartels, H., Freeze-fracture demonstration of communicating junctions between interstitial cells of the pulmonary interalveolar septa, *Am. J. Anat.*, 155, 125, 1979.

132. Lauweryns, J. M. and Baert, J. H., Alveolar clearance and the role of the pulmonary lymphatics, *Am. Rev. Respir. Dis.*, 115, 625, 1977.

133. Wayland, H. and Silberberg, A., Blood to lymph transport, *Microvasc. Res.*, 15, 367, 1978.

134. Wangensteen, O. D., Wittmers, L. E., Jr., and Johnson, J. A., Permeability of the mammalian blood-gas barrier and its components, *Am. J. Physiol.*, 216, 719, 1969.

135. Taylor, A. E. and Gaar, K. A., Jr., Estimation of equivalent pore radii of pulmonary capillary and alveolar membranes, *Am. J. Physiol.*, 218, 1133, 1970.

136. Drake, R., Gaar, K. A., and Taylor, A. E., Estimation of the filtration coefficient of pulmonary exchange vessels, *Am. J. Physiol.*, 234, H266, 1978.

137. Brody, A. R., Kelleher, P. C., and Craighead, J. E., A mechanism of exudation through intact alveolar epithelial cells in the lungs of cytomegalovirus-infected mice, *Lab. Invest.*, 39, 281, 1978.

138. Egan, E. A., Nelson, R. M., and Gessner, I. H., Solute permeability of the alveolar epithelium in acute hemodynamic pulmonary edema in dogs, *Am. J. Physiol.*, 233, H80, 1977.

139. Gardiner, T. H., Quantitative changes in permeability of rat lung epithelium in lung edema, *J. Appl. Physiol. Respir. Environ. Exercise Physiol.*, 44, 576, 1978.

140. Nadel, J. A. and Davis, B., Autonomic regulation of mucus secretion and ion transport in airways, in *Asthma: Physiology, Immunopharmacology and Treatment*, Lichtenstein, L. M. and Austin, K. F., Eds., Academic Press, New York, 1977, 197.

141. Bignon, J., Jaurand, M. C., Pinchon, M. C., Sapin, C., and Warnet, J. M., Immunoelectron microscopic and immunochemical demonstrations of serum proteins in the alveolar lining material of the rat lung, *Am. Rev. Respir. Dis.*, 111, 109, 1976.

142. Gee, M. H. and Staub, N. C., Role of bulk fluid in protein permeability of the dog lung alveolar membrane, *J. Appl. Physiol.*, 42, 144, 1977.

143. Richardson, J., Bouchard, T., and Ferguson, C. C., Uptake and transport of exogenous proteins by respiratory epithelium, *Lab. Invest.*, 35, 307, 1976.

144. Braley, J. F., Dawson, C. A., Moore, V. L., and Cozzini, B. O., Absorption of inhaled antigen into the circulation of isolated lungs from normal and immunized rabbits, *J. Clin. Invest.*, 38, 1240, 1978.

145. Jones, J. G., Berry, M., Hulands, G. H., and Crawley, J. C. W., The time course and degree of change in alveolocapillary membrane permeability induced by aspiration of hydrochloric acid and hypotonic saline, *Am. Rev. Respir. Dis.*, 118, 1007, 1978.

146. Chopra, S. K., Taplin, G. V., Tashkin, D. P., and Elan, D., Lung clearance of soluble radioaerosols in scleroderma, *Thorax*, 34, 63, 1979.

147. Gorin, A. B. and Stewart, P. A., Differential permeability of endothelial and epithelial barriers to albumin flux measured in lungs of sheep, *J. Appl. Physiol.*, 47, 1315, 1979.

148. Ryan, S. F., Barrett, C. R., Lavietes, M. H., Bell, A. L., and Rochester, D. F., Volume-pressure and morphometric observations after acute alveolar injury in the dog from N-Nitroso-N-Methylurethane, *Am. Rev. Respir. Dis.*, 118, 735, 1978.

149. Smith, P. and Heath, D., Paraquat, *CRC Crit. Rev. Toxicol.*, 4, 411, 1976.

150. Picciano, P. and Rosenbaum, R. M., The type I alveolar lining cells of the mammalian lung. I. Isolation and enrichment from dissociated adult rabbit lung, *Am. J. Pathol.*, 90, 99, 1978.

151. Rosenbaum, R. M. and Picciano, P., The type I alveolar lining cells of the mammalian lung. II. *In vitro* identification via the cell surface and ultrastructure of isolated cells from adult rabbit lung, *Am. J. Pathol.*, 90, 123, 1978.

152. Mason, R., Williams, M., Greenleaf, R., and Clements, J., Isolation and properties of type II alveolar cells from rat lung, *Am. Rev. Respir. Dis.*, 115, 1015, 1977.

153. Mason, R. J., Dobbs, L. G., Greenleaf, R. D., and Williams, M. C., Alveolar type II cells, *Fed. Proc. Fed. Am. Soc. Exp. Biol.*, 36, 2697, 1977.

154. Simon, L. M., Robin, E. D., Raffin, T., Theodore, J., and Douglas, W. H., Bioenergetic pattern of isolated type II pneumocytes in air and during hypoxia, *J. Clin. Invest.*, 61, 1232, 1978.

155. Michelson, A. M., McCord, J. M., and Fridovich, I., Eds., *Superoxide and Superoxide Dismutases*, Academic Press, New York, 1977.

156. McCord, J. M. and Fridovich, I., The biology and pathology of oxygen radicals, *Ann. Intern. Med.*, 89, 122, 1978.

157. Clark, J. M. and Lambertson, C. J., Pulmonary oxygen toxicity: a review, *Pharmacol. Rev.*, 23, 37, 1971.

158. Balentine, J. D., Experimental pathology of oxygen toxicity, in *Oxygen and Physiological Function*, Jobsin, F. F., Ed., Professional Information Library, Dallas, 1977, 311.

159. Frank, L. and Massaro, D., The lung and oxygen toxicity, *Arch. Int. Med.*, 139, 347, 1979.

160. **Chow, C. K. and Tappel, A. L.**, An enzymatic protective mechanism against lipid peroxidation damage to lungs of ozone exposed rats, *Lipids,* 7, 518, 1972.
161. **Crapo, J. D. and Tierney, D. F.**, Superoxide dismutase and pulmonary oxygen toxicity, *Am. J. Physiol.,* 226, 1401, 1974.
162. **Kimball, R. E., Reddy, K., Pierce, T. H., Schwartz, L. W., Mustafa, M. G., and Cross, C. E.**, Oxygen toxicity: augmentation of antioxidant defense mechanisms in rat lung, *Am. J. Physiol.,* 230, 1425, 1976.
163. **Anderson, W. R., Tan, W. C., Takatori, T., and Privett, O. S.**, Toxic effects of hydroperoxide injections on rat lung, *Arch. Pathol. Lab. Med.,* 100, 154, 1976.
164. **Cohen, G. and Cederbraum, A. I.**, Chemical evidence for production of hydroxyl radicals during microsomal electron transfer, *Science,* 204, 66, 1979.
165. **Kameda, K., Ono, T., and Imai, Y.**, Participation of superoxide, hydrogen peroxide and hydroxyl radicals in NADPH-cytochrome P-450 reductase-catalyzed peroxidation of methyl linolenate, *Biochim. Biophys. Acta,* 572, 77, 1979.
166. **Shu, H., Talcott, R. E., Rice, S. A., and Wei, E. T.**, Lipid peroxidation and paraquat toxicity, *Biochem. Pharmacol.,* 28, 327, 1979.
167. **Sasame, H. A. and Boyd, M. R.**, Superoxide and hydrogen peroxide production and NADPH oxidation stimulated by nitrofurantoin in lung microsomes: possible implications for toxicity, *Life Sci.,* 24, 1091, 1979.
168. **Babior, B. M.**, Oxygen-dependent microbial killing by phagocytes, *N. Engl. J. Med.,* 298, 659, 1978.
169. **Johnston, R. B., Jr. and Lehmeyer, J. E.**, The involvement of oxygen metabolites from phagocytic cells in bactericidal activity and inflammation, in *Superoxide and Superoxide Dismutases,* Michelson, A. M., McCord, J. M., and Fridovich, I., Eds., Academic Press, New York, 1977, 291.
170. **Badwey, J. A., Curnette, J. T., and Karnovsky, M. L.**, The enzyme of granulocytes that produces superoxide and peroxide: an elusive pimpernel, *N. Engl. J. Med.,* 300, 1157, 1979.
171. **Sharma, S. C., Mukhtar, H., Sharma, S. K., and Murt, C. R. K.**, Lipid peroxide formation in experimental inflammation, *Biochem. Pharmacol.,* 21, 1210, 1972.
172. **Salin, M. L. and McCord, J. M.**, Free radicals in leukocyte metabolism and inflammation, in *Superoxide and Superoxide Dismutases,* Michelson, A. M., McCord, J. M., and Fridovich, I., Eds., Academic Press, New York, 1977, 257.
173. **Johnston, R. B., Jr., Godzik, C. A., and Cohn, Z. A.**, Increased superoxide anion production by immunologically activated and chemically elicited macrophages, *J. Exp. Med.,* 148, 115, 1978.
174. **Schnyder, J. and Baggiolini, M.**, Role of phagocytosis in the activation of macrophages, *J. Exp. Med.,* 148, 1449, 1978.
175. **Drath, D. B., Karnovsky, M. L., and Huber, G. L.**, Hydroxyl radical formation in phagocytic cells of the rat, *J. Appl. Physiol. Respir. Environ. Exercise Physiol.,* 46, 136, 1979.
176. **Nathan, C. F., Brukner, L. H., Silverstein, S. C., and Cohn, Z. A.**, Extracellular cytolysis by activated macrophages and granulocytes. I. Pharmacologic triggering of effector cells and the release of hydrogen peroxide, *J. Exp. Med.,* 149, 84, 1979.
177. **Nathan, C. F., Silverstein, S. C., Brukner, L. H., and Cohn, Z. A.**, Extracellular cytolysis by activated macrophages and granulocytes. II. Hydrogen peroxide as a mediator of cytotoxicity, *J. Exp. Med.,* 149, 100, 1979.
178. **Craddock, P. R., Fehr, J., Dalmasso, A. P., Brigham, K. L., and Jacob, H. S.**, Hemodialysis leukopenia, *J. Clin. Invest.,* 59, 879, 1977.
179. **Goldstein, I. M.**, Polymorphonuclear leukocyte lysosomes and immune tissue injury, *Prog. Allergy,* 20, 301, 1976.
180. **Ryan, G. B. and Majno, G.**, Acute inflammation, *Am. J. Pathol.,* 86, 185, 1977.
181. **Segal, A. W. and Meshulan, T.**, Production of superoxide by neutrophils: a reappraisal, *FEBS Lett.,* 100, 27, 1979.
182. **Lehmeyer, J. E. and Johnston, R. B., Jr.**, Effect of anti-inflammatory drugs and agents that elevate intracellular cyclic AMP on the release of toxic oxygen metabolites by phagocytes: studies in a model of tissue-bound IgG, *Clin. Immun. Immunopathol.,* 9, 482, 1978.
183. **Carp, H. and Janoff, A.**, In vitro suppression of serum elastase-inhibitory capacity by reactive oxygen species generated by phagocytosing polymorphonuclear leukocytes, *J. Clin. Invest.,* 63, 793, 1979.
184. **Cohen, A. B.**, The effects *in vivo* and *in vitro* of oxidative damage to purified α_1-Antitypsin and to the enzyme-inhibiting activity of plasma, *Am. Rev. Respir. Dis.,* 119, 953, 1979.
185. **Olmori, H., Komoriya, K., Azuma, A., Kurozumi, S., and Oto, Y. H.**, Xanthine oxidase-induced histamine release from isolated rat peritoneal mast cells: involvement of hydrogen peroxide, *Biochem. Pharmacol.,* 28, 333, 1979.
186. **Rister, M. and Baehner, R. L.**, Effect of hyperoxia on superoxide anion and hydrogen peroxide production of polymorphonuclear leucocytes and alveolar macrophages, *Br. J. Haematol.,* 36, 241, 1977.

187. Marcus, A. J., Silk, S. T., Safier, L. B., and Ullman, H. L., Superoxide production and recuding activity in human platelets, *J. Clin. Invest.*, 59, 149, 1977.

188. Pratt, P. C., Vollmer, R. T., Shelburne, J. D., and Crapo, J. D., Pulmonary morphology in a multihospital collaborative extracorporeal membrane oxygenation project, *Am. J. Pathol.*, 95, 191, 1979.

189. Myrvold, H. E. and Lewis, D. H., Platelets, fibrinogen, and pulmonary haemodynamics in early experimental septic shock, *Circ. Shock*, 4, 201, 1977.

190. Sandritter, W., Mittermayer, C., Riede, U. N., Freudenberg, N., and Grimm, H., Shock lung syndrome (a general review), *Pathol. Res. Pract.*, 162, 7, 1978.

191. Malik, A. B. and van der Zee, H., Lung vascular permeability following progressive pulmonary embolization, *J. Appl. Physiol. Respir. Environ. Exercise Physiol.*, 45, 590, 1978.

192. Costabella, P. M., Lindquist, Y. K., Kapanci, Y., and Saldeen, T., Increased vascular permeability in the delayed microembolism syndrome, *Microvasc. Res.*, 15, 275, 1978.

192a. Malik, A. B., Lee, B. C., Zee, H., and Johnson, A., The role of fibrin in the genesis of pulmonary edema after embolization in dogs, *Circ. Res.*, 45, 120, 1979.

192b. Binder, A. S., Kageler, W., Perel, A., Flick, M. R., and Staub, N. C., Effect of platelet depletion on lung vascular permeability after microemboli in sheep, *J. Appl. Physiol. Respir. Environ. Exercise Physiol.*, 48, 414, 1980.

193. Ohkuda, K., Nakahara, K., Weidner, W. J., Binder, A., and Staub, N. C., Lung fluid exchange after uneven pulmonary artery obstruction in sheep, *Circ. Res.*, 43, 152, 1978.

194. Craddock, P. R., Hammerschmidt, D. E., Moldow, C. F., Yamada, O., and Jacob, H. S., Granulocyte aggregation as a manifestation of membrane interactions with complement: possible role in leukocyte margination, microvascular occlusion, and endothelial damage, *Semin. Hematol.*, 16, 140, 1979.

195. Flick, M. R., Perel, A., Kageler, W., and Staub, N. C., White blood cells contribute to increased lung vascular permeability after microemboli, *Fed. Proc. Fed. Am. Soc. Exp. Biol.*, 38, 1265, 1979.

195a. Jacob, H. S., Craddock, P. R., Hammerschmidt, D. E., and Moldow, C. F., Complement induced granulocyte aggregation: an unsuspected mechanism of disease, *N. Engl. J. Med.*, 302, 789, 1980.

196. van der Brenk, H. A. S., Kelly, H., and Stone, M. G., Innate and drug-induced resistance to acute lung damage caused in rats by α-naphthyl thiourea (ANTU) and related compounds, *Br. J. Exp. Pathol.*, 57, 621, 1976.

197. Said, S. I., Environmental injury of the lung: role of humoral mediators, *Fed. Proc. Fed. Am. Soc. Exp. Biol.*, 37, 2504, 1978.

198. Gardiner, T. H. and Goodman, F. R., Effect of pulmonary edema on drug transport and binding in rat lung, *Am. J. Physiol.*, 232, C132, 1977.

199. Gardiner, T. H. and McAnalley, B. H., Effect of lung edema on the pulmonary absorption of drugs, *Life Sci.*, 23, 1827, 1978.

200. Malik, A. B., Pulmonary vascular response to increase in intracranial pressure: role of sympathetic mechanisms, *J. Appl. Phys.*, 42, 335, 1977.

201. Bowers, R. E., McKeen, C. R., Park, B. E., and Brigham, K. L., Increased pulmonary vascular permeability follows intracranial hypertension in sheep, *Am. Rev. Respir. Dis.*, 119, 637, 1979.

202. Anderson, R. W. and DeVries, W. C., Transvascular fluid and protein dynamics in the lung following hemorrhagic shock, *J. Surg. Res.*, 20, 281, 1976.

203. Bus, J. S., Aust, S. D., and Gibson, J. E., Paraquat toxicity: proposed mechanism of action involving lipid peroxidation, *Environ. Health Perspect.*, 16, 139, 1976.

204. Talcott, R. E., Shu, H., and Wei, E. T., Dissociation of microsomal oxygen reduction and lipid peroxidation with the electron acceptors paraquat and menadione, *Biochem. Pharmacol.*, 28, 665, 1978.

205. Steffen, C. and Netter, K. J., On the mechanism of paraquat action on microsomal oxygen reduction and its relation to lipid peroxidation, *Toxicol. Appl. Pharmacol.*, 47, 593, 1979.

206. Rotman, H. H., Lavelle, T. F., Jr., Dimcheff, D. G., VandenBelt, R. J., and Weg, J. G., Long-term physiologic consequences of the adult respiratory distress syndrome, *Chest*, 72, 190, 1977.

207. Lakshminarayan, S. and Hudson, L. D., Pulmonary function following the adult respiratory distress syndrome, *Chest*, 74, 489, 1978.

208. Zapol, W. M., Trelstad, R. L., Coffey, J. W., Tsai, I., and Salvador, R. A., Pulmonary fibrosis in severe acute respiratory failure, *Am. Rev. Respir. Dis.*, 119, 547, 1979.

209. Ullrich, R. L. and Casarett, G. W., Interrelationship between the early inflammatory response and subsequent fibrosis after radiation exposure, *Radiat. Res.*, 72, 107, 1977.

210. Greenberg, G. B. and Hunt, T. K., The proliferative response *in vitro* of vascular endothelial and smooth muschle cells exposed to wound fluids and macrophages, *J. Cell. Physiol.*, 97, 353, 1978.

211. Fulmer, J. D., Roberts, W. C., Von Gal, E. R., and Crystal, R. G., Morphologic-physiologic correlates of the severity of fibrosis and degree of cellularity in idiopathic pulmonary fibrosis, *J. Clin. Invest.*, 63, 665, 1979.

212. McCullough, B., Schneider, S., Greene, N. D., and Johanson, W. G., Jr., Bleomycin-induced lung injury in baboons: alteration of cells and immunoglobulins recoverable by bronchoalveolar lavage, *Lung*, 155, 337, 1978.

213. Henderson, R. F., Rebar, A. H., Denicola, D. B., and Henderson, T. R., The use of pulmonary lavage fluid for detecting acute pulmonary injury in toxicological screening programs, *Fed. Proc. Fed. Am. Soc. Exp. Biol.*, 38, 582, 1979.

214. Thrall, R. S., McCormick, J. R., Jack, R. M., McReynolds, R. A., and Ward, P. A., Bleomycin-induced pulmonary fibrosis in the rat: inhibition by indomethacin, *Am. J. Pathol.*, 95, 117, 1979.

215. Last, J. A. and Cross, C. E., unpublished observations, 1978.

216. Last, J. A. and Cross, C. E., unpublished data, 1979.

217. Lenfant, C., Ed., *Lung Biology in Health and Disease,* Vol. 1, Marcel Dekker, New York, 1976.

Chapter 7

MUCUS PRODUCTION AND THE CILIARY ESCALATOR

Jerold A. Last

TABLE OF CONTENTS

I. INTRODUCTION

Surprisingly little is known with certainty about tracheobronchial mucus. Most of our knowledge of this substance comes from either of two types of indirect studies. Most of the chemical studies of tracheobronchial mucus have been performed on sputum collected from individuals afflicted with chronic hyperproducing diseases. Sputum may be an unsatisfactory fluid in which to study tracheobronchial mucus, in that it is almost impossible to distinguish mucus per se from those components that arise from contaminating saliva, serum transudates and exudates, and other fluids not directly related to tracheobronchial mucus. Details of the structure and sequence of the mucus glycoproteins are obtained mostly by analogy with mucus glycoproteins obtained from more abundant sources than the tracheobronchial tree. Most of the detailed studies of glycoprotein structure have been performed on serum glycoproteins such as fetuin; on gastric mucosal glycoproteins, some of which are produced in copious quantities by tumors; and on salivary glycoproteins, especially from sheep and cattle. Since so much of our knowledge of the composition of tracheobronchial glycoproteins and mucus is indirect, there have been very few studies directly addressing themselves through experimental work to studies of the effects of toxic lung damage on the tracheobronchial mucus per se.

We are on somewhat firmer ground when ciliostasis in tracheobronchial tissue, in vivo or in vitro, is the end point studied to reflect toxic lung damage. Due to the relative ease of performing such assays in vitro, and due to the elegant techniques that have been worked out to study clearance in vivo, this has historically been, and presently is, a well-studied area.

It is the purpose of this chapter to review studies on mucus production and ciliary function in experimental models of toxic lung damage. An attempt will be made to cite or discuss examples of many of the techniques that have been applied to these assays. It is probably impossible to cover all of the agents that affect these processes; therefore, no attempt will be made to do so. The tabulated data are intended to survey the various techniques used and several toxic agents and drugs studied to serve as an entry point to the literature, especially the more recently published studies. These tables are not intended to be comprehensive, and there was no deliberate selection of which studies to cite other than our desire to include a representative cross section. Finally, a brief discussion of our personal bias as to appropriate directions for future work in this area will be included.

Several recent reviews of aspects of this topic should be noted. Neuronal[1] and pharmacological[2-5,121] control of mucus secretion and/or tracheobronchial clearance, the effects of air pollutants and cigarettes on clearance rates[6] and on neuronal responses,[7] and histological evaluation of the respiratory mucus membrane[8] have all been discussed by authoritative sources. Clinical implications of mucociliary dysfunction with regard to bronchial asthma have also been recently reviewed.[118,120]

II. MUCUS

A. Composition

Little or nothing is known about the composition of tracheobronchial mucus from direct analyses of this material. Rather, most of our dogma about this substance comes from extrapolations of data obtained from ovarian cyst mucus, from salivary gland mucus, from gastrointestinal tract mucus, and from sputum. Sputum, for example, is rich in water (about 95%), and in Na^+ and Cl^- ions, with lesser amounts of K^+, Ca^{++}, amino acids, low-molecular-weight carbohydrates, high-molecular-weight glycoproteins (acidic and neutral), lysozyme, lactoferrin, immunoglobulins A and G, albumin, transferrin, α_1-antitrypsin, various other globulins, fibrinogen, and ceruloplasmin. Whether this multiplicity of components arises from tracheobronchial mucus per se or from serum transudates and/or exudates (or from other nonmucus sources) is not known with certainty.[9] Similar complexity of fluid composition exists when tracheo-bronchial lavage fluids are analyzed,[10,11] or when the material collected onto screens inserted into the large airways is sampled.[12]

On the other hand, the mucus produced by various glands and epithelial cells of the body is a fluid of much simpler composition. Usually, the typical mucus fluid consists of about 90 to 95% water, isotonic levels of Na^+, Ca^{++}, and Cl^- ions, and the high-molecular-weight glycoproteins that are characteristic of these substances. The serum proteins enumerated above are usually absent, or when present are recognized to be contaminating impurities. The typical glycoprotein is very large, generally about 0.5 to several million daltons, and is very high in relative content of sugars (as high as 80% by weight). For the tracheobronchial mucus glycoproteins, the characteristic sugars present in oligosaccharide side chains are fucose, galactose, N-acetylgalactosamine, and N-acetylglucosamine. Sialic acid residues, which can be present, are found at the nonreducing ends of oligosaccharide chains. Galactose residues may or may not be sulfated, presumably at the 6-position (as galactose-6-sulfate).[13] On the basis of their separation by ion-exchange chromatographic and/or by electrophoretic techniques, these glycoproteins have been classified as neutral and acidic, with the acidic group further broken down into sulphomucins and sialomucins.[11] The same nomenclature has also been used by histologists,[8] based on differential staining properties of putative glycoproteins with periodic acid-Schiff stain and alcian blue stain at various pH values, and based on staining properties of tissue sections before and after treatment with neuraminidase to remove terminal sialic acid residues. We know of no evidence that proves that the biochemically defined neutral, sialo-, and sulfomucins are the same substances as the histologically defined glycoproteins of the same names. Reports of mannose being present in mucus glycoproteins[14] have not been confirmed by more recent studies; the reported mannose content presumably arose by contamination of these substances with serum components. Specific blood group antigens and virus hem-agglutination assays have also been used to characterize partially purified glycoproteins prepared from tracheobronchial mucus or sputum.[9] Virus hemagglutination by certain viruses with a glycoprotein preparation is apparently caused by these glycoproteins containing terminal sialic acid residues and thus may be used as a probe for structure; similarly, blood group specificity is conferred by the presence of specific sugar residues in specific linkages at the end of the oligosaccharide side chains. For example, terminal N-acetylgalactosamine residues in β-linkage confer blood group-A antigenic specific-ity, while type B individuals have galactose residues at these same terminal positions. Glycoproteins from type AB individuals contain both terminal galactose and N-acetyl-galactosamine residues; while glycoproteins from type O subjects contain neither. Thus, information about the presence or absence of specific sugar residues at the ter-mini of the oligosaccharide side chains may be obtained from a knowledge of the blood group specificity, which is readily determined by serological techniques. Glycoproteins containing blood group activity in sputum are apparently found only in the (biochem-ically defined) neutral fraction.[15]

B. Structure

Conventional dogma, based upon the two-fluid model of Lucas and Douglas,[16] sug-gests that tracheobronchial mucus exists as two layers, a lower sol and an upper gel. The upper layer, a viscoelastic gel, contains primarily mucus glycoproteins and their counter-ions. The lower serous layer, through which the cilia beat, is assumed to be an aqueous isotonic salt solution. The mucus gel is thus visualized as floating on the sol layer, along which it is propelled by the beating of the cilia, probably by direct contact of the tips of the cilia with the underside of the gel. While essentially all investigators in this field would accept this model, it is pertinent to point out that it is a model, and that such a structure for tracheobronchial mucus has never actually been proven. In addition, there are controversies concerning various details within this model. For example, while the majority point of view is presumably that such a mucus layer is continuous along the epithelial surface,[17,18] others have argued[19,20] that a discontinuous layer, with "islands" of mucus floating on a serous "sea", better describes the normal state. It is also not clear whether various serum constituents found in association with mucus glycoproteins in sputum[9,21] are normal constituents of the mucus layer or whether they arise from artifactual associations (through disulfide bonding, see below) during isolation and purification of glycoproteins and sputum.

Tracheobronchial mucus glycoproteins themselves are highly branched proteins with oligosaccharide side chains, usually attached by ester linkages to either serine or threonine residues. They contain relatively large quantities of sugars, up to 80% by weight.[9,21] The very high molecular weights observed for these glycoproteins, of the order of several millions,[21] is presumably due to the attachment of protein subunits via disulfide bridges between cysteine residues on different protein chains.[21] This view is consistent with the known ability of mercaptoethanol and other sulfhydryl reducing agents to disperse and dissolve mucus glycoproteins[22] as well as with the fact that reduction and alkylation with iodoacetic acid renders mucus irreversibly soluble.[9] Thus, the structure of tracheobronchial mucus is currently visualized as a two-phase system, sol and gel, with the gel consisting of glycoproteins of very high sugar content (hence, very hygroscopic) that are extensively cross-linked via disulfide bonds to give very high molecular weights to these molecules. As a result of this high molecular weight, coupled with the limited flexibility conferred on the chains by the frequent occurrence of oligosaccharide side chains along the protein backbone, these glycoproteins give rise to extremely viscous solutions at relatively low concentrations of dissolved solute.

C. Rheology

As with many other aspects of the study of tracheobronchial mucus structure, the major problems in this field are (1) obtaining adequate quantities of material for study, (2) obtaining mucus free of contaminating saliva and/or materials from cellular and bacterial degradation (especially DNA) when sputum is used as the starting material, and (3) extrapolation of data from studies of sputum obtained from diseased humans (e.g., chronic bronchitis, bronchorrhea) or studies of mucus from animal sources (e.g., bovine cervical mucus) to a definition of the properties of normal human tracheobronchial mucus. In addition, possible organ-specific, as well as species-specific, properties of mucus must be considered. Also of importance is the chemical structure of the constituent glycoproteins; for example, whether or not the glycoprotein contains terminal sialic acid residues on its constituent oligosaccharide side chains is thought to be an important determinant of mucus viscosity. It should be pointed out that much of our knowledge of the biochemistry and viscosity of mucus glycoproteins come from studies of submaxillary and of gastric mucus, which are easy to obtain. These sources of mucus are convenient to use, but their constituent glycoproteins are more soluble and contain much simpler oligosaccharide side chains than those of tracheobronchial mucus; hence, much of what we know of the detailed structure of mucus may not be directly relevant to respiratory tract mucus. Finally, since the mucus glycoproteins are high-molecular-weight polyelectrolytes, their rheological properties and behavior in solution will depend upon their concentration and upon the pH and ionic strength of the solvent, a factor of obvious importance in the interpretation of in vitro studies.

The viscoelastic properties of tracheal mucus are thought to be determined exclusively by the high-molecular-weight glycoprotein fraction.[22] Native tracheal mucus is insoluble, except when severe mucolytic agents such as mercaptoethanol are used. Such agents irreversibly destroy the fibrillar structure of mucus, with concomitant loss of its elastic properties. Tracheal mucus can be solubilized in 6M urea, which may then be removed by dialysis. After lyophilization, the mucus gel can be reconstituted to standardized conditions of pH, concentration, and ionic strength for further study. Sodium thiocyanate has also been recommended as a solubilizing agent for mucus that allows its dispersion with retention of its elasticity properties.[24] The picture of tracheal mucus that has emerged from studies of such in vitro solubilized materials is that of a typical mucus, a substance showing viscoelasticity; that is, the properties of viscosity (the ability to dissipate stored energy or energy transmitted to it by external forces) and of elasticity (the ability to store energy).

Why are these considerations of importance to toxicology? One parameter that can be quantitated when humans or experimental animals are exposed to potential pneumotoxins is the tracheobronchial clearance rate, the rate at which foreign particulate substances are cleared from the respiratory epithelial surfaces (as will be discussed in detail below). The measured clearance rate is almost invariably decreased by pneumotoxins. Such decreased tracheobronchial clearance rates can be caused, in principle, by any (or all) of the following: (1) increased mucus viscosity, (2) decreased mucus production, (3) decreased rate of ciliary beating, (4) decreased numbers of cilia per unit area of surface, and/or (5) increased mucus (hyper) secretion, such that mucus-producing glands and ducts or small airways may be blocked. Obviously, these factors may be interrelated under some circumstances; for example, increased mucus viscosity may cause a decreased ciliary beat frequency. Differentiation of these mechanisms may be fundamental in assessing the long-term consequences of exposure to a pneumotoxin, predicting effects of pneumotoxin mixtures, etc. It is not known whether mucus rheology can be modulated in vivo to accommodate differences in the driving force caused by differences in cilia density and/or beat frequency. It is usually assumed that the depth of the putative serous layer is rigidly controlled so as to allow only the tips of the cilia to make contact with the floating gel layer. If the amount of serous fluid varied or was affected by a pneumotoxin, the cilia would either not make proper contact with the glycoprotein gel or would be forced to beat through the viscous gel layer, a process that would dissipate a much greater amount of energy and, perhaps, completely prevent mucociliary clearance. Conversely, it is not known whether ciliary beat frequency can be modulated to accommodate putative changes in mucus viscosity that might be caused by exposure to a toxic agent. Also highly relevant in this context is the unresolved question of whether cilia must propel a continuous mucus blanket or isolated islands of mucus. Clearly, equivalent changes in the physical properties of the mucus layer will exert a more profound effect on the organism if the blanket is continuous than if intermittant "blobs" must be propelled, especially if the gel were solidified, in which case intermittent "blobs" could be propelled upwards as if they were a series of rafts.[25]

A very interesting series of experiments on the effect of chronic SO_2 inhalation on the rheological properties of canine tracheal pouch mucus has been reported.[22] The striking findings in this study were a decrease in the viscoelastic properties of the tracheal mucus during exposure of two dogs to 550 ppm of SO_2 for 2 hr, twice a week, for 80 to 90 weeks. The greatest decrease correlated with decreased levels of high-molecular-weight glycoproteins (relative to low-molecular-weight proteins, presumably arising from serum exudates and/or transudates) in the collected mucus. Since only relative ratios were determined, the potential role of inflammation on the denominator (low-molecular-weight proteins) term must be considered. Since these changes were observed in mucus collected from tracheal pouches, which were not contiguous with the functional respiratory airways, the role of neural or circulatory mediators in eliciting changes in tracheal mucus viscoelasticity was suggested.[22]

More recent studies by this group[26] have been performed on normal dogs with tracheal pouches in an attempt to correlate changes in mucus viscoelastic properties with mucociliary clearance rate. These workers conclude that as the elastic modulus increases about 10-fold, the clearance rate is halved. These findings suggest either that the methods used are too crude to detect subtle relationships between clearance rate and elasticity (certainly possible, if not probable) or that changes in mucus viscosity are not used in vivo for fine tuning the tracheobronchial mucociliary clearance rate.

D. Effects of Toxic Substances on Mucus Secretion

Reid[27] has stated that "mucus hypersecretion is an accepted inflammatory response from a mucus secreting surface". Even cursory examination of Table 1 indicates that one standardized response to pneumotoxin exposure is an increased mucus secretion rate. Examples of agents eliciting this response in Table 1 include NH_3 vapor, SO_2, ozone, chromate, and H_2SO_4 aerosol. If we assume that mucus hypersecretion is a cause of decreased mucociliary clearance rate and/or decreased mucus flow rate (these terms are operationally identical), then this response is shown to essentially all of the listed insults to the lung. In addition, the mucus-secreting surface, in this case the respiratory epithelium, seems to be able to modulate (increase) the number of mucus-producing cells it contains upon chronic exposure to such irritant fumes as SO_2 and cigarette smoke. Depilation of cilia is another stereotyped result to inhalation of acidogenic gases such as NO_2 and SO_2. It is not known whether these observed responses (loss of cilia, goblet cell hypertrophy, mucus hypersecretion) of the respiratory tract epithelium are ultimately harmful to the organism. Few, if any, studies have systematically explored the effects of long-term recovery from such insults, so it is not known whether such observed changes are reversible or irreversible. It is also not known whether the ubiquity of these observed responses to noxious substances denotes identical underlying mechanisms, identical prognoses as to harm to the organism, and/or identical prognoses as to recovery or return to the original state (which may not be synonymous). One speculation is that irreversible spread of mucus-secreting cells into smaller bronchi and/or bronchioles may cause continued secretion of mucus in an inappropriate area, leading to chronic airway obstruction analogous to that seen in chronic bronchitis.

E. Mucus Secretory Mechanisms

Mucus is secreted in the tracheobronchial tree both by surface epithelial cells ("goblet cells", others?) and by submucosal glands of the trachea and large bronchi. The submucosal glands, which contain both mucus and serous cells, are under parasympathetic cholinergic nervous control.[28] Thus, either parasympathetic nerve stimulation or parasympathomimetic drugs such as acetylcholine, pilocarpine, and methacholine cause an increase in the volume and glycoprotein content of mucus secreted (Table 2). These effects can be blocked by an acetylcholine antagonist such as atropine. Less is understood about the regulation of secretion by the surface epithelial cells. Apparently, direct contact of mechanical or chemical irritants with the mucosal surface is a stimulus for secretion. The role, if any, of cholinergic or adrenergic stimulation in stimulating mammalian epithelial cells to secrete mucus or fluid is not clear,[28] even though it is known that in geese (which do not have submucosal glands) goblet cells do respond to cholinergic stimuli.[29] Increases in mucus transport rates are elicited by catecholamines, acetylcholine, and nicotine; decreases are elicited by cholinergic antagonists α- and β-receptor blockers, and some tranquilizers.[28] It is not clear whether these changes are due to effects on mucus secretion, on ciliary beat frequency, or on both processes. Some of these effects are also summarized in Table 2.

Table 1

EFFECTS ON VARIOUS SUBSTANCES ON THE TRACHEAL MUCOCILIARY ESCALATOR

Agent	Level	Duration	Species tested	Affect on mucociliary apparatus observed	Technique(s) used for evaluation	Ref.
NH_3	102 ppm	12 Weeks	Rats	Damage to tracheal mucosa; no effect on rate of ciliary beating	Microscopic visualization; histopathology	52
NH_3 plus carbon (< 3 μm)	119 ppm 3.4 mg/m^3	12 Weeks	Rats	Severe damage to tracheal mucosa; decreased rate of ciliary beating		52
NO_2	6 ppm	6 Weeks	Rats	Decreased mucociliary transport rate	Direct observation	57
NO_2	17 ppm	3 Weeks	Rats	Loss of cilia from bronchial epithelium	Histopathology	45
SO_2	650 ppm	19-74 Days	Hamsters	Loss of tracheal cilia, tracheal hypersecretion	Histopathology	55
SO_2	9-11 ppm	> 3 Days	Mice	Loss of cilia	Histopathology	56
SO_2	10 ppm	10 Weeks	Rats	Decreased mucus flow rate and ciliary velocity	Direct observation	35
SO_2	1 ppm	12 Months	Dogs	Decreased tracheal mucus velocity	Teflon® disc movement	54
SO_2	74-239 ppm	45 Minutes	Rabbits	Decreased tracheal ciliary velocity	Direct observation	53
SO_2 plus carbon	74-239 ppm 2.5-3 mg/m^3	45 Minutes	Rabbits	Decreased tracheal ciliary velocity	Direct observation	53
Ozonized gasoline vapor	1-3 ppm	24-48 Days	Rabbits	Ciliostasis	Direct observation	58
Aerosol hair spray	—	20 Seconds	Humans	Tracheal mucus velocity decreased	Radioopaque discs followed by X-ray	43
Freon propellant for hair spray	—	20 Seconds	Humans	No effect		43
Cigarette smoke	—	Minutes	Cats	Slowing of mucus flow and slowing of ciliary beat frequency	Rate of transport of marker substance on mucus layer	59, 60

Table 1 (continued)
EFFECTS ON VARIOUS SUBSTANCES ON THE TRACHEAL MUCOCILIARY ESCALATOR

Agent	Level	Duration	Species tested	Affect on mucociliary apparatus observed	Technique(s) used for evaluation	Ref.
Formaldehyde, acetaldehyde, formic acid, benzene, NH_3, NO_2, Acetylene, dimethyl ether, hydrocyanic acid	—	0.5 Min	Cats	Slowing of mucociliary transport velocity. No effect on ciliary beat frequency	Direct observation of cilia beating	59, 60
NH_4Cl	3 mg Aerosol	0.5 Min	Cats	Decreased mucus flow rate	Rate of transport of marker spores	60
Cigarette smoke	Several puffs	Minutes	Rabbits	Decreased mucus flow rate	Rate of transport of marker particles	61
Isoprene	—	—	Cats	Decreased mucus flow rate	Rate of transport of marker particles	59, 60, 62
Various anesthetics enflurane, NO-halothane, NO-morphine	0.6—2.4 MAC	15 Min	Dogs	Decreased mucociliary transport rate	Tracheal mucociliary flow rate by radioactive tracer	63
Chlorpromazine prochlorperazine	100—200 $\mu g/ml$	15—20 Min	Rats	Decreased ciliary beat frequency	Microscopic observation of tracheal rings in culture by stroboscopy	64
Oxygen	10%, 40%, 100%	20 Min	Cats	Decreased mucociliary transport rate	Particle transport rate by direct observation	65
Cigarette smoke	4-6 Puffs	12-Sec exposures	Chicken	Decreased mucociliary transport rate	Microscopic observation of movement of tracer particles	66
Cigarette smoke	25 Cigarettes per day	24 Days	Rats	Changes in tracheal epithelial cells	Morphological techniques	67, 68
SO_2	400 ppm	⩽ 6 Weeks	Rats	Changes in mucus-producing cells	Histopathological observation	68, 69
NH_3 vapor	0.1-0.3 mol%	3 Minutes	Cats	Increased mucus secretion rate	Flushing of mucus from tracheal lumen	70

Agent	Concentration	Duration	Species	Effect	Method	Ref.
Carbon particles	4-40 mg/mℓ	1 Hour	Hamsters, pigs, guinea pigs	Changes in tracheal mucosal cells	Morphological techniques	71
SO_2	500-600 ppm	4-5 Months	Dogs	Changes in tracheal and bronchial epithelial cells	Morphological techniques	72
SO_2	600-700 ppm	10 Days	Rats	Increased numbers of bronchial goblet cells	Histological evaluation	73
Ozone	0.8 ppm	1-90 Days	Rats	Changes in rate of mucus glycoprotein secretion	Secretion rate of labeled glycoproteins by tracheal explants	74
Ozone and/or H_2SO_4 aerosol	0.5 ppm (O_3) and/or 1 mg/m³ (H_2SO_4)	3-14 Days	Rats	Changes in rate of glycoprotein secretion	Secretion rate of labeled glycoproteins by tracheal explants	75
Sodium chromate	0.04-2.16 mM	1 Day	Rats	Changes in rate of glycoprotein secretion	Secretion rate of labeled glycoproteins by tracheal explants	76, 77
Calcium chromate	10 mg/mℓ	20 Minutes	Rats	Ciliostasis	Phase microscopy	50
SO_2	800 ppm	2 Hours	Rats	Loss of ciliated epithelial cells	Microscopy	78
H_2SO_4 aerosol	15 mg/m³	4 Hours	Mice	Decreased tracheobronchial clearance rate	Clearance of labeled streptococci	79
Acrolein	5% aerosol	5 Minutes	Guinea pigs	Loss of ciliated epithelial cells	Microscopy	80
H_2SO_4 aerosol	100 µg/m³	1-26 Weeks	Donkeys	Changes in tracheobronchial clearance rates	Migration rate of radioactive particles	81
Ozone	1.2 ppm	4 Hours	Rats	Decreased tracheobronchial clearance rates	Clearance of labeled latex spheres	106
Local anesthetics	≤ 1% (w/v)	Minutes	Ferrets	Ciliostasis, some damage	Observation of ciliary beating	114
Thiopental, halothane	40 mg/kg, 1.2 MAC	2 Hours	Dogs	Decreased mucociliary clearance rate	Tantalum bronchography	115
X-irradiation	mCi levels	Minutes	Sheep	Increased mucociliary clearance rate	Teflon® disc movement	116
Tobacco smoke	—	30 Days	Rats	Increased number of tracheal gland cells	Morphometry	117
Atropine, ipritropium bromide	—	Minutes	Dogs	Decreased mucociliary clearance rate	Migration rate of radioactive particles	119
Lidocaine	4% topical	15-45 Minutes	Humans	None	Teflon® disc movement	122

Table 1 (continued)

EFFECTS ON VARIOUS SUBSTANCES ON THE TRACHEAL MUCOCILIARY ESCALATOR

Agent	Level	Duration	Species tested	Affect on mucociliary apparatus observed	Technique(s) used for evaluation	Ref.
X-irradiation	mCi levels	Minutes	Dogs	Increased mucociliary clearance rate?	Teflon® disc vs. X-ray camera movement	123
Trichloroethylene	—	—	Rabbits	Ciliostasis	Direct observation	124

Table 2
EFFECTS OF PHARMACOLOGICAL AGENTS ON MUCOCILIARY TRANSPORT

Drug	Ref.	Animal	Effect	Remarks	Assay
Atropine	44	Dog	Decreased clearance rate, increased viscoelasticity	Surprisingly, no effect on volume (did not dehydrate despite popular dogma)	Clearance of labeled α-emitter, volume by tracheal pouch
Terbutaline	44	Dog	Increased secretion volume	—	—
N-acetylcysteine	44	Dog	Increased clearance rate	—	—
Serotonin	82	Cat	Increased mucus flow rate	Potentiation by Ca++ ion	Particle transport time over tracheae
5-Hydroxytryptophan	82	Cat	Increased mucus flow rate	—	Tracheal ciliary activity, extent & vigor
Lidocaine, cocaine	83	Chicken	Ciliostasis in vitro	No long-term effects in vivo (3 days)	Transport of labeled Teflon® particles
Bethanecol	84	Humans	Increased rate of tracheobronchial clearance	Cholinergic stimulation	
Acetylcholine, pilocarpine	85	Rats	Increased ciliary beat frequency	Sympathomimetic drugs	Direct observation or high-speed cinematography
Ammonium chloride, potassium iodide	85	Rats	Increased ciliary beat frequency	"Mucolytic agents"	
N-acetylcysteine	85	Rats	Decreased ciliary beat frequency	Reduced mucus viscoelasticity	
Aminophylline	86	Dogs	Increased mucus flow rate	α-Adrenergic agonist	Transport of labeled Teflon® discs
Epinephrine, ephedrine, isoproterenol, noradrenalin	87	Cats, rats	Increased ciliary beat frequency	Adrenergic agents, catecholamines	High-speed cinematography
Methacholine	97	Humans	Increased mucus secretion rate	Drug in tissue culture medium; antagonized by atropine	Discharge of labeled mucus
Pilocarpine	98	Cats	Increased mucus secretion rate	Drugs & precursors administered in vivo	Discharge of labeled mucus to tracheal lumen
Histamine, prostaglandins	99	Cats, geese	Increased mucus secretion rate	Drugs & precursors administered in vivo	Discharge of labeled mucus to tracheal lumen
Acetylcholine, lignocaine	100	Geese	Increased mucus secretion rate	Drugs & precursors administered in vivo	Discharge of labeled mucus to tracheal lumen
Methacholine	12	Dogs	Increased mucus secretion rate	Administered subcutaneously; blocked by atropine	Weight of mucus trapped on tracheal screen

Table 2 (continued)
EFFECTS OF PHARMACOLOGICAL AGENTS ON MUCOCILIARY TRANSPORT

Drug	Ref.	Animal	Effect	Remarks	Assay
NA 872, NAB 365	102	Rats, cats, hamsters	Increased ciliary beat frequency	Adrenergic drugs	High-speed cinematography
Methacholine, physostigmine	103	Human	Increased activity of mucus glands	Parasympathomimetic agents	Histological techniques
Ephedrine	104	Rat	Decreased ciliary beat frequency	Sympathomimetic agent	Observation
Atropine	105	Rabbit	Decreased ciliary beat frequency	Parasympathomimetic blocker	Observation
Physostigmine	105	Rabbit	Increased mucus transport rate	Parasympathomimetic agent	Direct observation
S-Carboxymethyl cysteine	107	Human	None	Putative mucolytic agent	Tracheal mucus velocity by radioactive tracer
Phenylephrine, oxymetazoline, acetylcysteine	88	Chicken	Cessation of ciliary beating	Nasal decongestants used as proprietary drugs	Microscopic observation
Isoproterenol, epinephrine	89	Humans	Increased clearance rate	Adrenergic agents administered as aerosols	Clearance of Fe_2O_3 particles, α-emitter
Atropine	89	Humans	Decreased clearance rate	Administered orally	Clearance of Fe_2O_3 particles, α-emitter
Acetylouabain	90	Cats	Increased mucus flow rate	Administered intravenously	Direct observation
Isoprenaline, pilocarpine	91, 101	Rats	Increased size and number of mucus-producing cells	Injected repetitively subcutaneously	Histological observation
Pilocarpine	92	Cats	Increased ciliary beat and increased mucus volume	Drug given in culture fluid bath	Direct observation
Isoprenaline	93	Pigs	Increased size and number of goblet cells	Injected intramuscularly	Histological observation
Acetylcholine, pilocarpine, carbachol	94	Humans	Increased mucus secretion rate	Drugs added to bath for tissue culture	Autoradiography
Atropine, hyoscine	94	Humans	Decreased mucus secretion rate	Drugs added to tissue culture medium	Autoradiography
Acetylcholine	95	Dogs	Increased mucus secretion rate	Drugs added to tissue culture medium; antagonized by atropine	Discharge of labeled mucus into medium

Kallidin, other kininogenic polypeptides	96	Dogs	Increased mucus secretion rate	Drug in tissue culture medium	Discharge of labeled mucus
Phenylephrine, terbutaline	108	Cats	Increased mucus secretion	In vitro assay	Discharge of labeled mucus to tracheal lumen
Bethanechol, isoprenaline, methoxamine	109	Cats	Increased mucus secretion	In vitro assay	Release of mucus droplets by glands
Isoproterenol, salbutamol	110	Rats	Increased number of secretory cells, changes in glycoprotein types	Drugs given systemically	Morphological techniques
Cholinergic and α-adrenergic agents	111	Cats	Increased submucosal gland secretory rate	In vitro assay	Discharge of mucus by single glands
α-Adrenergic agents	112	Cats	Increased secretion of [^{35}S] glycoproteins by tracheal glands	In vitro assay	Discharge of labeled mucus by single gland
Atropine	113	Dogs	Increased tracheal clearance rate	—	Tracheal mucus velocity by radioactive tracer

III. CILIARY ESCALATOR

A. The Ciliary Escalator

The clearance of foreign substances up the mucociliary escalator is a function both of the ciliary action (length and density of cilia per unit area, beat frequency of cilia) and of the viscosity of the fluid traveling on the escalator. It is not at all simple to separate these components when evaluating the effects of toxic agents on ciliary activity. An additional complicating factor is that to be propelled by ciliary action there must exist an optimal viscosity for the tracheobronchial fluid: if the fluid is too viscous it resists being propelled by ciliary beating, while if it is too fluid the cilia beat through the fluid rather than pushing it forward.[30,31] These same considerations of viscosity, coupled with the elastic properties of mucus and the fluidity of aqueous solutions, represent the major theoretical basis for the familiar two-layer[3,16] model of serous and mucus fluids overlaying the respiratory tract cilia. Such a model proposes that the extended cilia beat forward through a nonviscous aqueous sol layer, with only their tips in contact with the mucus gel layer, which is thus propelled forward. On the return stroke, the curved cilia beat backward through the sol layer, imparting no movement to the gel layer. In this model, the cilia themselves can directly affect the transport of mucus up the ciliary escalator in only one way, that is by variations in their beat frequency.

Where are the cilia that drive the ciliary escalator? For the purposes of this chapter we will not deal with the nose at all, even though it plays a very important role in the removal of particulate components from inhaled air streams. The entire topic of the structure and function of the nasal defenses has recently been reviewed in detail.[32] It is pertinent to point out, however, that rodents such as rats are obligate nose breathers, and that studies of the effects of inhaled toxic substances, especially those that contain particulate components, must take the nasal defenses into consideration when rats are used as the experimental animal. Thus, the cilia of interest in this chapter are those of the trachea, of the bronchi, and of the small airways.

What is known about the respiratory tract cilia in rats? There are about 200 cilia per cell, which are about 5 μm long, about 0.25 μm in diameter, and beat at a frequency of about 20 to 22 strokes per second[30] at the tracheal level. Cilia beat at successively lower frequencies as airways become smaller; beat frequency has been estimated[33] to be about 7 Hz in rat peripheral airways. This level of ciliary activity is sufficient to propel mucus at velocities estimated to be about 0.4 mm per minute in small bronchioles,[34] about 11.5 mm/min in the lobar bronchus,[34] and about 13 mm/min in the rat trachea in vivo.[35] These values are complicated by questions of whether the mucus blanket is continuous or whether it occurs in patches or islands (see the discussion of this question in Section II B of this chapter). There are reported species variations in ciliary beat frequency and in mucus transport rates[3] that may be related to this question if the observed differences are indeed real. The biochemical basis of ciliary beating and the structure of the cilia are discussed below.

B. Mechanisms of Ciliary Beating

Cilia consist of three working parts: the shaft, the basal body, and the roots. The shaft contains protein fibrils running parallel to its long axis called the axoneme. These fibrils, also known as microtubules, appear as characteristic structures with two central fibrils surrounded by an outer ring of nine more complex microtubules consisting of one complete and one incomplete fibril (axonemes have, in fact, been called "9 + 2" bundles because of their structure). Other structures associated with the shaft include pairs of arms ("dynein") projecting from one microtubule toward the next at frequent intervals along the microtubule, connections between peripheral pairs of microtubules called "nexins" that are arrayed like rungs on a ladder, and connections occurring at regular intervals between the peripheral and central fibrils called "spokes" or "radial links". Central microtubules contain additional projecting "rods" at regular intervals that may serve as connections to the radial links.

As the ciliary shaft enters the cell itself the resulting structure is called the basal body. The peripheral nine fibers continue throughout the length of the basal body to eventually terminate at its roots. As the peripheral microtubules cross the plane of the cell surface they are enriched by the addition of a third incomplete fibril. These triple fibrillar structures are twisted about their axes and interconnected by thin filaments, which also connect these structures to the cell membrane. A pattern of "hub and spokes" is often seen. The central fibrils of the ciliary shaft teminate near the plane of the cell surface, often embedded in a dense granule.

The main anchoring of the axoneme occurs at the ciliary roots, where it is attached to the basal body by a set of "root fibers". Often these fibers are striated aggregates of filaments or are microtubular.

The biochemical basis of ciliary function is strikingly similar to that of muscle.[30] The microtubule protein, which constitutes the structural component of the long axis of the axoneme, is an approximately 120,000 dalton molecule called tubulin. Tubulin as isolated usually contains guanosine triphosphate (GTP) and guanosine diphosphate (GDP), about one molecule of each per tubulin dimer (i.e., per unit of 120,000 daltons). The analogy with actin is obvious, albeit the primary structures of tubulin and of actin are different. Similarly, dynein may be considered as analogous to myosin in some respects, even though it is a very different protein structurally. Dynein and myosin both possess adenosine triphosphatase (ATPase) activity, but the dynein ATPase requires only Mg^{++} for activity and is more specific for ATP than is myosin ATPase, which also requires Ca^{++} as a cofactor. Dynein is a large protein, molecular weight about 540,000 (again analogous to myosin in size), which appears to catalyze the hydrolysis of ATP necessary to generate the energy required to allow ciliary beating. No convincing candidate has as yet been found to serve the functional role of troponin in muscle, but a 150,000 dalton protein has been identified as the "nexin" connecting links of the axoneme. Also in common with the known mechanisms of muscle contraction, it is assumed that ciliary beating is the consequence of sliding of peripheral microtubule filaments with respect to one another. Thus, it is assumed that the length of the ciliary microtubules remains constant throughout a stroke, but that sliding of the filaments, which are anchored together in the basal body, causes a cilium to bend in one direction for the effective stroke and the opposite direction for the recovery stroke. Dynein arms are assumed to bind and hydrolyze ATP and, as a consequence, undergo cyclic changes of shape. These changes are transduced into relative movement of microtubule filaments with respect to one another, the sliding referred to above.

Ciliary dysfunction in humans has thus far been linked to an absence of dynein arms (Kartagener's syndrome)[36] or to an absence of radial links.[37]

C. Measurements of Ciliary Beat Frequency

Beat frequency may be measured in vivo or in vitro, by any of several methods.[3,38] Direct observation of the flicker caused by varying reflection from the moving cilia of a light beam parallel to the visual axis is the classical method for this measurement. This method is simple, but is grossly inaccurate and severely underestimates the true frequency; the technique is still, however, of great value in toxicological studies where large changes in beat frequency or actual arrest of beating may be observed. Alternatively, ciliary beat frequency may be quantitated by determining the synchronous frequency under a microscope with a calibrated stroboscopic lamp. The accuracy of this method is limited by a large (subjective) experimental error in frequency matching and by variations in flicker frequency among adjacent areas of the epithelial surface. Photographic methods, using high-speed cinematography to freeze motion, have been used.[39] These methods generally require such high intensity of illumination to allow photography rapid enough to freeze the motion of rapidly beating cilia in mammalian respiratory tissue that there is enough heat produced to damage the tissue epithelium itself. Flicker frequency may also be determined electronically with precision, but this technique is only useful in vitro as respiratory and other extraneous motions interfere in vivo with the measurement of voltage changes by which flicker frequency is ascertained. In vivo measurements are usually performed on anesthetized animals with surgically exposed tracheae or with tracheostomies. Careful control of temperature and humidity are critical (as is also true for in vitro preparations). In vitro measurements are usually done on extirpated frog palates, isolated tracheae, or tracheal rings in tissue culture.

D. Measurements of Mucus Transport Velocity

The simplest method for such measurements is by direct observation of the rate of transport of a particle along the epithelium under low-power magnification.[38] Other methods include X-ray or gamma scintillation camera measurements of clearance of radio-opaque substances such as $BaSO_4$ or of isotopically labeled gamma-ray emitters,[40-42] cinematography or videotape measurement of clearance of Teflon® discs,[43] measurement of rate of movement of isotopically labeled tracer substances between two well-collimated fixed detectors,[44] and use of magnetic flux detectors or scintillation cameras to trace the clearance of tagged particles (usually with Fe^{++} or ^{99}Tc, respectively) through the tracheobronchial tree. Mucus transport rates measured for tracheae in vivo have been reported to range from about 13 to 22 mm/min (chicks and rats through cats and frogs, respectively), while values in vitro have been reported as about 21 to 36 mm/min for rats and monkeys or cats and dogs, respectively. These values may in fact all be the same within experimental error.[3]

E. Effects of Toxic Substances on Ciliary Movement

Exposure to high levels of SO_2[45] and to enormous levels of NH_3 and NO_2 causes ciliostasis in vitro. Formaldehyde vapor is a rapid ciliostatic agent.[45] Cigarette smoke is also ciliotoxic.[3] Exposure to ozone and other oxidant pollutants in vivo can cause sloughing of cilia from large and small airways.[46] H_2SO_4 aerosol, administered in vivo at 900 $\mu g/m^3$, decreased the ciliary beat frequency of hamster tracheal rings evaluated in vitro.[47] A large number of trace-metal ions are ciliotoxic as evaluated by tissue culture techniques. For example,[48] Ni^{++} decreases ciliary beat frequency of hamster tracheal rings at levels below 1 $\mu g/m\ell$ (about 10 μM). Complete ciliostasis was observed in this study at 65 $\mu g/m\ell$. When $NiCl_2$ was administered to hamsters in vivo as an aerosol of 100 $\mu g/m^3$ for 2 hr, similar depressions of ciliary beat frequency were observed with freshly excised tracheae. These same authors[49] have also demonstrated that the ciliary beat frequency of hamster tracheal rings in vitro is depressed by concentrations of $CdCl_2$ as low as 6 μM, with correlative in vivo data obtained with aerosols of 50 $\mu g/m^3$ of $CdCl_2$. Similarly, chromate (CrO_4^{-2}) ion damages ciliated cells at levels of 10 $\mu g/m\ell$ (50 μM) and above and is ciliostatic at levels of 10 mg/mℓ and above in vitro.[50]

F. Mechanisms of Ciliotoxicity

It is tempting to speculate on general mechanisms whereby classes of toxic substances might interfere with ciliary function based upon our knowledge of normal beating of cilia. For example, heavy metals such as chromium, cadmium, and nickel might interfere with dynein ATPase by acting as antagonists of the essential Mg^{++} ion required as a cofactor for this reaction. In this (speculative) case, we could then distinguish between effects on ciliary beating and effects on mucus viscosity as a mechanism of action of these toxic substances.

Many agents that affect mucociliary clearance rates (Table 1) do so presumably by directly affecting the viscosity of the mucus layer. In this category would probably fit ammonium chloride (and other "expectorants"), as well as short-term acute exposure to vapors of water-soluble compounds such as ammonia, formic acid, formaldehyde, acetaldehyde, hydrocyanic acid, and possibly sulfur dioxide. As mentioned previously, agents that directly dilute the mucus layer by hydration, or that lower its viscosity by dissociation of bonds holding together high-molecular-weight substances responsible for such viscosity, would presumably decrease the mucus flow rate.

It is almost certain that many toxic agents acutely affect the mucociliary escalator indirectly by triggering the release of mediators[1,5] or of neurogenic stimuli, which in turn exert the observed effects. The secretory response of epithelial (goblet) cells to irritants[27] may be an example of such an indirect mechanism. Goblet cell or gland hyperplasia and spread to lower airways, a chronic response to irritant pollutants such as tobacco smoke or SO_2 (see Table 1), may also be brought about, at least in part, by mediator substances released by affected cells. The role of, for example, histamine in such processes remains to be explored in detail. We do not know whether such rearrangements of mucus secreting cells affect the proximal cilia nearby. Little is known about the short- or long-term implications of removal of cilia upon exposure to a pneumotoxic gas as evaluated morphologically[46] on the mucociliary escalator in vivo, nor even by what mechanisms the cilia are removed. Can they regenerate? Is there a reversible and/or an irreversible level of removal?

IV. CONCLUSIONS

As has been pointed out at several places within this chapter, we do not presently have the tools with which to distinguish between changes in mucociliary transport rate caused by changes in mucus (viscosity, level of hydration, amount) from those caused by changes in the cilia (beat frequency, number, depth of the putative serous layer in which they are immersed). Even though such changes need not be mutually exclusive, the ability to understand and predict the types of interactions that might occur between pollutants does require that we understand such mechanistic bases of interactions of substances with the mucociliary escalator. Another area requiring intense study, for which we may indeed presently possess the appropriate methodology, is the question of whether we can resolve direct effects of toxic agents on the mucociliary escalator components from indirect effects caused by the release of adrenergic or cholinergic effectors and/or other mediator substances by cells in response to such pneumotoxins. Further correlation of results from in vitro and in vivo exposure systems should provide insights into the answers to these questions. In addition, in vitro preparations are reaching a level of sophistication wherein neuronal and direct responses can be dissociated from each other[1,51] to allow these questions to be asked.

The level of basic knowledge of several of the component processes of mucociliary transport, especially in normal healthy individuals, is too deficient in many areas to allow us to understand the cellular and molecular basis of pathophysiology. Among questions needing answers in this context are: can mucus composition and/or quantity be modulated in vivo to (deliberately) change the viscosity of mucus? What are the relative roles of neutral, "sulpho-", and "sialo"-mucins in determining the physical and biological properties of mucus? What are the relative roles of epithelial secretory cells and submucosal glands in producing the different kinds and amounts of mucus glycoproteins in health and in response to pneumotoxins? What is the exact structure of the mucus layer? Can this structure be altered to the benefit or detriment of the organism? Are the changes in mucus transport rate measured after exposure to noxious substances good or bad responses from the point of view of the affected animal? Are there definable limits to such responses that allow them to be reversible or irreversible? Can respiratory tract cilia, once damaged, be regenerated by a given epithelial cell, or must this cell be replaced to restore the ciliary layer to its preinsult quality? Can the organism (deliberately) modulate its ciliary beat frequency?

Other questions of the type proposed above will undoubtedly occur to the thoughtful reader. It is in the nature of the assays that have been routinely applied in this field over the last 20 years that they raise more questions than they answer for those concerned with the mechanistic bases of the observed effects. While screening of substances for their ability to affect ciliary beat frequency or mucus transport rate in vitro will remain an important tool in the armamentarium of toxicologists, such assays are not themselves able to provide the mechanistic insights required to understand a rational basis for therapeutic intervention, for evaluation of interactions of toxic substances, and for the rational setting of air quality criteria for public health and safety.

REFERENCES

1. Widdicombe, J. G., Control of secretion of tracheobronchial mucus, *Br. Med. Bull.,* 34, 57, 1978.
2. Parke, D. V., Pharmacology of mucus, *Br. Med. Bull.,* 34, 89, 1978.
3. Asmundsson, J. and Kilburn, K. H., Mechanisms of respiratory tract clearance, in *Sputum: Fundamentals and Clinical Pathology,* Dulfano, M. J., Ed., Charles C Thomas, Springfield, 1973, 107.
4. Boyd, E. M., Pharmacological agents and respiratory tract fluid, in *Sputum: Fundamentals and Clinical Pathology,* Dulfano, M. J., Ed., Charles C Thomas, Springfield, Ill., 1973, 544.
5. Keal, E. E., Physiological and pharmacological control of airways secretions, in *Respiratory Defense Mechanisms,* Part I, Brain, J. D., Proctor, D. F., and Reid, L. M., Eds., Marcel Dekker, New York, 1977, 357.
6. Hee, J. and Guillerm, R., La fonction muco-ciliare et ses modifications sous l'influence de certaines agressions, *Bull. Eur. Physiopathol. Resp.,* 13, 11, 1977.
7. Alarie, Y., Sensory irritation by airborne chemicals, *CRC Crit. Rev. Toxicol.,* 2, 299, 1973.
8. Jeffery, P. K. and Reid, L. M., The respiratory mucus membrane, in *Respiratory Defense Mechanisms,* Part I, Brain, J. D., Proctor, D. F., and Reid, L. M., Eds., Marcel Dekker, New York, 1977, 193.
9. Boat, T. F. and Matthews, L. W., Chemical composition of human tracheobronchial secretions, in *Sputum: Fundamentals and Clinical Pathology,* Dulfano, M. J., Ed., Charles C Thomas, Springfield, Ill., 1973, 243.
10. Yeager, H., Jr., Tracheobronchial secretions, *Am. J. Med.,* 50, 493, 1971.
11. Roussel, P., Degand, P., Lamblin, G., Laine, A., and Lafitte, J. J., Biochemical definition of human tracheobronchial mucus, *Lung,* 154, 241, 1978.
12. Reasor, M. J., Cohen, D., Proctor, D. F., and Rubin, R. J., Tracheobronchial secretions collected from intact dogs. II. Effects of cholinomimetic stimulation, *J. Appl. Physiol. Respir. Environ. Exercise Physiol.,* 45, 190, 1978.
13. Roussel, P., Lamblin, G., Degand, P., Walker-Nasir, E., and Jeanloz, R. W., Heterogeneity of the carbohydrate chains of sulfated bronchial glycoproteins isolated from a patient suffering from cystic fibrosis, *J. Biol. Chem.,* 250, 2114, 1975.
14. Ellis, D. B., Synthesis and secretion of respiratory tract mucus by tracheal explants, *Mod. Probl. Pediatr.,* 19, 110, 1977.
15. Gallagher, J. T. and Corfeld, A. P., Mucin-type glycoproteins — new perspectives on their structure and synthesis, *Trends Biochem. Sci.,* 8, 38, 1978.
16. Lucas, A. M. and Douglas, L. C., Principles underlying ciliary activity in the respiratory tract. II. A comparison of nasal clearance in man, monkey, and other mammals, *Arch. Otolaryngol.,* 20, 518, 1934.

17. Kilburn, K. H., A hypothesis for pulmonary clearance and its implications, *Am. Rev. Respir. Dis.*, 98, 449, 1967.
18. Sturgess, J. M., The mucous lining of major bronchi in the rabbit lung, *Am. Rev. Respir. Dis.*, 115, 819, 1977.
19. Van As, A., Pulmonary airway clearance mechanisms: a reappraisal, *Am. Rev. Respir. Dis.*, 115, 721, 1977.
20. Lopez-Vidriero, M. T., Das, I., and Reid, L. M., Airway secretion: source, biochemical, and rheological properties, in *Respiratory Defense Mechanisms,* Part I, Brain, J. D., Proctor, D. F., and Reid, L. M., Ed., Marcel Dekker, New York, 1977, 289.
21. Roberts, G. P., Isolation and characterization of glycoproteins from sputum, *Eur. J. Biochem.*, 50, 265, 1974.
22. Litt, M., Khan, M. A., Chakrin, L. W., Sosnowski, G., and Wardell, J. R., Jr., Effect of chronic sulfur dioxide inhalation on rheological properties of tracheal mucus, *Biorheology*, 13, 107, 1976.
23. Litt, M., Khan, M. A., and Wolf, D. P., Mucus rheology: relation to structure and function, *Biorheology,* 13, 37, 1976.
24. Khan, M. A., Wolf, D. P., and Litt, M., Effect of mucolytic agents on the rheological properties of tracheal mucus, *Biochim. Biophys. Acta,* 444, 369, 1976.
25. Litt, M., Mucus rheology and mucociliary clearance, *Mod. Probl. Pediat.,* 19, 175, 1977.
26. Giordano, A. M., Holsclaw, D., and Litt, M., Mucus rheology and mucociliary clearance: normal physiologic state, *Am. Rev. Respir. Dis.,* 118, 245, 1978.
27. Reid, L., Bronchial mucus production in health and disease, in *The Lung,* Liebow, A. A. and Smith, D., Eds., Williams & Wilkins, Baltimore, 1968, 87.
28. Widdicombe, J. G., Defensive mechanisms of the respiratory system, in *Respiratory Physiology II,* Vol. 14, Widdicombe, J. G., Ed., University Park Press, Baltimore, 1977, 291.
29. Phipps, R. J. Physiological control of airway mucus secretion, *Eur. J. Res. Dis.,* 61, 33, 1981.
30. Sleigh, M. A., The nature and action of respiratory tract cilia, in *Respiratory Defense Mechanisms,* Part I, Brain, J. D., Proctor, D. F., and Reid, L. M., Eds., Marcel Dekker, New York, 1977, 247.
31. Chen, T. M. and Dulfano, M. J., Mucus viscoelasticity and mucociliary transport rate, *J. Lab. Clin. Med.,* 91, 423, 1978.
32. Bang, B. G. and Bang, F. B., Nasal mucociliary systems, in *Respiratory Defense Mechanisms,* Part I, Brain, J. D., Proctor, D. F., and Reid, L. M., Eds., Marcel Dekker, New York, 1977, 405.
33. Iravani, J., Flimmerbewegung in den intrapulmonalen Luftwegen der Ratte, *Pflugers Arch.,* 297, 221, 1967.
34. Iravani, J. and Van As, A., Mucus transport in the tracheobronchial tree of normal and bronchitic rats, *J. Pathol.,* 106, 81, 1972.
35. Dalhamn, T., Mucus flow and ciliary activity in the trachea of healthy rats and rats exposed to respiratory irritant gases, *Acta Physiol. Scand.,* 36(Suppl. 123), 1, 1956.
36. Afzelius, B. A., A human syndrome caused by immotile cilia, *Science,* 193, 317, 1976.
37. Sturgess, J. M., Chao, J., Wong, J., Aspin, N., and Turner, J. A. P., Cilia with defective radial spokes. A cause of human respiratory disease, *N. Engl. J. Med.,* 300, 53, 1979.
38. Rylander, R., Current techniques to measure alterations in the ciliary activity of intact respiratory epithelium, *Am. Rev. Respir. Dis.,* 93, 67, 1966.
39. Cheung, A. T. W. and Jahn, T. L., High speed cinematographic studies on rabbit tracheal (ciliated) epithelia: determination of the beat pattern of tracheal cilia, *Pediatr. Res.,* 10, 140, 1976.
40. Yeates, D. B., Sturgess, J. M., Kahn, S. R., Levison, H., and Aspin, N., Mucociliary transport in trachea of patients with cystic fibrosis, *Arch. Dis. Child.,* 51, 28, 1976.
41. Wong, J. W., Keens, T. G., Wannamaker, E. M., Crozier, D. N., Levison, H., and Aspin, N., Effects of gravity on tracheal mucus transport rates in normal subjects and in patients with cystic fibrosis, *Pediatrics,* 60, 146, 1977.
42. Albert, R. E., Lipmann, M., Peterson, H. T., Berger, J., Sanborn, K., and Bohning, D., Bronchial deposition and clearance of aerosols, *Arch. Int. Med.,* 131, 115, 1973.
43. Friedman, M., Dougherty, R., Nelson, S. R., White, R. P., Sackner, M. A., and Wanner, A., Acute effects of an aerosol hair spray on tracheal mucociliary transport, *Am. Rev. Respir. Dis.,* 116, 281, 1977.
44. Giordano, A., Holsclaw, D., and Litt, M., Effects of various drugs on canine tracheal mucociliary transport, *Ann. Otol.,* 87, 484, 1978.
45. Dalhamn, T. and Sjoholm, J., Studies on SO_2, NO_2, and NH_3: effect on ciliary activity in rabbit trachea of single *in vitro* exposure and resorption in rabbit nasal cavity, *Acta Physiol. Scand.,* 58, 287, 1963.
46. Mellick, P. W., Dungworth, D. C., Schwartz, L. W., and Tyler, W. S., Short term morphological effects of high ambient levels of ozone on lungs of rhesus monkeys, *Lab. Invest.,* 36, 82, 1977.

47. Grose, E. C., Miller, F. J., and Gardner, D. E., The effects of ozone and sulfuric acid on ciliary activity of syrian hamsters, *Am. Rev. Respir. Dis.*, 117, 237, 1978.

48. Adalis D., Gardner, D. E., and Miller, F. J., Cytotoxic effects of nickel on ciliated epithelium, *Am. Rev. Respir. Dis.*, 118, 347, 1978.

49. Adalis, D., Gardner, D. E., Miller, F. J., and Coffin, D. L., Toxic effects of cadmium on ciliary activity using a tracheal ring model system, *Environ. Res.*, 13, 111, 1977.

50. Mass, M. J. and Lane, B. P., Effect of chromates on ciliated cells of rat tracheal epithelium, *Arch. Environ. Health*, 31, 96, 1976.

51. Nadel, J. A. and Davis, B., Regulation of Na⁺ and Cl⁻ transport and mucous gland secretion in airway epithelium, in *Respiratory Tract Mucus*, Ciba Foundation Symposium #54, Elsevier-North Holland, Amsterdam, 1978, 142.

52. Dalhamn, T. and Reid, L., Ciliary activity and histologic observations in the trachea after exposure to ammonia and carbon particles, in *Inhaled Particles and Vapours*, Vol. 2, Davies, C. N., Ed., Pergamon Press, New York, 1967, 299.

53. Dalhamn, T. and Strandberg, L., Acute effects of sulfur dioxide on the rate of ciliary beat in the trachea of the rabbit (*in vivo* and *in vitro*) with studies on the absorption capacity of the nasal cavity, *Int. J. Air Water Pollut.*, 4, 154, 1967.

54. Hirsch, J. A., Swenson, E. W., and Wanner, A., Tracheal mucus transport in beagles after long-term exposure to 1 ppm sulfur dioxide, *Arch. Environ. Health*, 30, 249, 1975.

55. Goldring, I. P., Greenberg, L., Park, S., and Ratner, I. M., Pulmonary effects of sulfur dioxide exposure in the Syrian hamster, *Arch. Environ. Health*, 21, 32, 1970.

56. Giddens, W. E., Jr. and Fairchild, G. A., Effects of sulfur dioxide on the nasal mucosa of mice, *Arch. Environ. Health*, 25, 166, 1972.

57. Giordano, A. M. and Morrow, P. E., Chronic low-level nitrogen dioxide exposure and mucociliary clearance, *Arch. Environ. Health*, 25, 443, 1972.

58. Kotin, P., Falk, H. L., and McCammon, C. J., The experimental induction of pulmonary tumors and changes in the respiratory epithelium in C57B1 mice following their exposure to an atmosphere of ozonized gasoline, *Cancer*, 11, 473, 1958.

59. Carson, S., Goldhamer, R., and Weinberg, M. S., Characterization of physical, chemical, and biological properties of mucus in the intact animal, *Ann. N.Y. Acad. Sci.*, 130, 935, 1966.

60. Carson, S., Goldhamer, R., and Carpenter, R., Responses of ciliated epithelium to irritants, *Am. Rev. Respir. Dis.*, 93, 86, 1966.

61. Kensler, C. J. and Batista, S. P., Chemical and physical factors affecting mammalian ciliary activity, *Am. Rev. Respir. Dis.*, 93, 93, 1966.

62. Weissbecker, L., Creamer, R. M., and Carpenter, R. D., Cigarette smoke and tracheal mucus transport rate, *Am. Rev. Respir. Dis.*, 104, 182, 1971.

63. Forbes, A. R. and Hornigan, R. W., Mucociliary flow in the trachea during anesthesia with enflurane, ether, nitrous oxide, and morphine, *Anesthesiology*, 46, 319, 1977.

64. Adler, K. B. and Fand, I., Cilioinhibitory effect of phenothiazines *in vitro* and its antagonism by Ca⁺⁺, *Arch. Int. Pharmacodyn.*, 227, 309, 1977.

65. Laurenzi, G. A., Yin, S., and Guarneri, J. J., Adverse effect of oxygen on tracheal mucus flow, *N. Engl. J. Med.*, 279, 333, 1968.

66. Battista, S. P. and Kensler, C. J., Mucus production and ciliary transport activity, *Arch. Environ. Health*, 20, 326, 1970.

67. Jones, R., Bolduc, P., and Reid, L., Protection of rat bronchial epithelium against tobacco smoke, *Br. Med. J.*, 2, 142, 1972.

68. Reid, L., Evaluation of model systems for study of airway epithelium, cilia, and mucus, *Arch. Int. Med.*, 126, 428, 1970.

69. Lamb, D. and Reid, L., Mitotic rates, goblet cell increase, and histochemical changes in mucus in rat bronchial epithelium during exposure to SO₂, *J. Pathol. Bacteriol.*, 96, 97, 1968.

70. Phipps, R. J. and Richardson, P. S., The effects of irritation at various levels of the airway upon tracheal mucus secretion in the cat, *J. Physiol.*, 261, 563, 1976.

71. Mossman, B. T., Adler, K. B., and Craighead, J. E., Interaction of carbon particles with tracheal epithelium in organ culture, *Environ. Res.*, 16, 110, 1978.

72. Spicer, S. S., Chakrin, L. W., and Wardell, J. R., Jr., Effect of chronic sulfur dioxide inhalation on the carbohydrate histochemistry and histology of the canine respiratory tract, *Am. Rev. Respir. Dis.*, 110, 13, 1974.

73. Knauss, H. J., Robinson, W. E., Medici, T. C., and Chodosh, S., Cell vs. noncell airway temporal response in rats exposed to sulfur dioxide, *Arch. Environ. Health*, 31, 241, 1976.

74. Last, J. A., Jennings, M. D., Schwartz, L. W., and Cross, C. E., Glycoprotein secretion by tracheal explants cultured from rats exposed to ozone, *Am. Rev. Respir. Dis.*, 116, 695, 1977.

75. Last, J. A. and Cross, C. E., A new model for health effects of air pollutants: evidence for synergistic effects of mixtures of ozone and sulfuric acid aerosols on rat lungs, *J. Lab. Clin. Med.*, 91, 328, 1978.

76. Last, J. A., Jennings, M. D., and Moore, P. F., Chromate inhibition of metabolism by rat tracheal explants, *Lab. Invest.*, 37, 276, 1977.

77. Last, J. A., Raabe, O. G., Moore, P. F., and Tarkington, B. K., Chromate inhibition of metabolism by rat tracheal explants. II. In vivo exposures, *Toxicol. Appl. Pharmacol.*, 47, 313, 1979.

78. Wells, A. B. and Lamerton, L. F., Regenerative response of rat tracheal epithelium after acute exposure to tobacco smoke: a quantitative study, *J. Natl. Canc. Inst.*, 55, 887, 1975.

79. Fairchild, G. A., Stultz, S., and Coffin, D. L., Sulfuric acid effect on the deposition of radioactive aerosol in the respiratory tract of guinea pigs, *Am. Ind. Hyg. Assoc. J.*, 36, 584, 1975.

80. Dahlgren, S. E., Dalen, H., and Dalhamn, T., Ultrastructural observations on chemically induced inflammation in guinea pig trachea, *Virchows Arch. Abt. B. Zellpathol.*, 11, 211, 1972.

81. Schlesinger, R. B., Lipmann, M., and Albert, R. E., Effects of chronic inhalation of sulfuric acid upon mucociliary clearance from the lungs of donkeys, *Am. Ind. Hyg. Conf. Abstr.*, 76, 1978.

82. Dadaian, J. H., Yin, S., and Laurenzi, G. A., Studies of mucus flow in the mammalian respiratory tract. II. The effects of serotonin and related compounds on respiratory tract mucus flow, *Am. Rev. Respir. Dis.*, 103, 808, 1971.

83. Dudley, J. P. and Cherry, J. D., Effect of topical anesthetics on ciliary activity of chicken embryo tracheal organ cultures, *Ann. Otol.*, 87, 533, 1978.

84. Camner, P., Strandberg, K., and Philipson, K., Increased mucociliary transport by cholinergic stimulation, *Arch. Environ. Health*, 29, 220, 1975.

85. Melville, G. N. and Iravani, J., Factors affecting ciliary beat frequency in the intrapulmonary airways of rats, *Can. J. Physiol. Pharmacol.*, 53, 1122, 1975.

86. Serafini, S. M., Wanner, A., and Michaelson, E. D., Mucociliary transport in central and intermediate size airways: effects of aminophyllin, *Bull. Eur. Physiopathol. Respir.*, 12, 415, 1976.

87. Melville, G. N., Horstmann, G., and Iravani, J., Adrenergic compounds and the respiratory tract, *Respiration*, 33, 261, 1976.

88. Dudley, J. P. and Cherry, J. D., The effect of mucolytic agents and topical decongestants on the ciliary activity of chicken tracheal organ cultures, *Pediatr. Res.*, 11, 904, 1977.

89. Foster, W. M., Bergofsky, E. H., Bohning, D. E., Lippmann, M., and Albert, R. E., Effect of adrenergic agents and their mode of action on mucociliary clearance in man, *J. Appl. Physiol.*, 41, 146, 1976.

90. Laurenzi, G. A. and Yin, S., Studies of mucus flow in the mammalian respiratory tract, *Am. Rev. Respir. Dis.*, 103, 800, 1971.

91. Sturgess, J. and Reid, L., The effect of isoprenaline and pilocarpine on (a) bronchial mucus-secreting tissue and (b) pancreas, salivary glands, heart, thymus, liver, and spleen, *Br. J. Exp. Pathol.*, 54, 388, 1973.

92. Horstmann, G., Iravani, J., Melville, G. N., and Ulmer, W. T., Physiological and electron-microscopic investigations of the trachea after pilocarpine, *Pneumonologie*, 152, 105, 1975.

93. Baskerville, A., The development and persistence of bronchial gland hypertrophy and goblet-cell hyperplasia in the pig after injection of isoprenaline, *J. Pathol.*, 119, 35, 1976.

94. Strugess, J. and Reid, L., An organ culture study of the effect of drugs on the secretory activity of the human bronchial submucosal gland, *Clin. Sci.*, 43, 533, 1972.

95. Chakrin, L. W., Baker, A. P., Christian, P., and Wardell, J. R., Jr., Effect of cholinergic stimulation on the release of macromolecules by canine trachea *in vitro*, *Am. Rev. Respir. Dis.*, 108, 69, 1973.

96. Baker, A. P., Hillegass, L. M., Holden, D. A., and Smith, W. J., Effect of kallidin, substance P, and other basic polypeptides on the production of respiratory macromolecules, *Am. Rev. Respir. Dis.*, 115, 811, 1977.

97. Boat, J. F. and Kleinerman, J. I., Human respiratory tract secretions. II. Effect of cholinergic and adrenergic agents on *in vitro* release of protein and mucous glycoprotein, *Chest*, 67, 32S, 1975.

98. Gallagher, J. T., Kent, P. W., Phipps, R., and Richardson, P., Influence of pilocarpine and ammonia vapour on the secretion and structure of cat tracheal mucins: differentiation of goblet and submucosal gland secretions, *Adv. Exp. Med. Biol.*, 89, 91, 1977.

99. Phipps, R. J. and Richardson, P. S., The nervous and pharmacological control of tracheal mucus secretion in the goose, *Proc. Physiol. Soc.*, 116P, 1976.

100. Phipps, R. and Richardson, P., The role of pharmacological mediators and irritants in the secretion of mucins from the trachea, *Adv. Exp. Med. Biol.*, 89, 515, 1977.

101. Bolduc, P. and Reid, L., The effect of isoprenaline and pilocarpine on mitotic index and goblet cell number in rat respiratory epithelium, *Br. J. Exp. Pathol.*, 59, 311, 1978.

102. Iravani, J. and Melville, G. N., Mucociliary activity in the respiratory tract as influenced by prostaglandin E-l, *Respiration*, 32, 305, 1975.

103. Coles, S., Regulation of the secretory cycles of mucous and serous cells in the human bronchial gland, *Adv. Exp. Med. Biol.*, 89, 155, 1977.

104. Scudi, J. V., Kimura, E. T., and Reinhard, J. F., Study of drug action on mammalian ciliated epithelium, *J. Pharmacol. Exp. Ther.*, 102, 132, 1951.

105. Kordik, P., Bülbring, E., and Burn, J. H., Ciliary movement and acetylcholine, *Br. J. Pharmacol.*, 7, 67, 1952.

106. Frager, N. B., Phalen, R. F., and Kenoyer, J. L., Adaptation to ozone in reference to mucociliary clearance, *Arch. Environ. Health*, 37, 51, 1979.

107. Goodman, R. M., Yergin, B. M., and Sackner, M. A., Effects of S-carboxymethylcysteine on tracheal mucus velocity, *Chest*, 74(6), 615, 1978.

108. Davis, B., Phipps, R. J., and Nadel, J. A., A new method for studying tracheal secretion *in vitro:* effect of adrenergic agonists in cats, *Chest*, 75(2), 224, 1979.

109. Quinton, P. M., Composition and control of secretions from tracheal bronchial submucosal glands, *Nature (London)*, 279, 551, 1979.

110. Jones, R. and Reid, L., β-Agonists and secretory cell number and intracellular glycoprotein in airway epithelium: the effect of isoproterenol and salbutamol, *Am. Rev. Respir. Dis.*, 121, 407, 1979.

111. Ueki, I., German, V. F., and Nadel, J. A., Micropipette measurement of airway submucosal gland secretion. Autonomic effects, *Am. Rev. Respir. Dis.*, 121, 351, 1980.

112. Phipps, R. J., Nadel, J. A., and Davis, B., Effect of alpha-adrenergic stimulation on mucus secretion and on ion transport in cat trachea *in vitro*, *Am. Rev. Respir. Dis.*, 121, 359, 1980.

113. Chopra, S. K., Effect of atropine on mucociliary transport velocity in anesthetized dogs, *Am. Rev. Respir. Dis.*, 118, 367, 1978.

114. Manawadu, B. R., Mostow, S. R., and LaForce, F. M., Local anesthetics and tracheal ring ciliary activity, *Anesth. Analg.*, 57, 448, 1978.

115. Forbes, A. R. and Gamsu, G., Depression of lung mucociliary clearance by thiopental and halothane, *Anesth. Analg.*, 58, 387, 1979.

116. Ahmed, T., Januszkiewicz, A. J., Landa, J. F., Brown, A., Chapman, G. A., Kenny, P. J., Finn, R. D., Bondick, J., and Sackner, M. A., Effect of local radioactivity on tracheal mucous velocity of sheep, *Am. Rev. Respir. Dis.*, 120, 567, 1979.

117. Hayashi, M., Sornberger, G. C., and Huber, G. L., Morphometric analyses of tracheal gland secretion and hypertrophy in male and female rats after experimental exposure to tobacco smoke, *Am. Rev. Respir. Dis.*, 119, 67, 1979.

118. Wanner, A., The role of mucociliary dysfunction in bronchial asthma, *Am. J. Med.*, 67, 477, 1979.

119. Sackner, M. A., Chapman, G. A., and Dougherty, R. D., Effect of nebulized ipratropium bromide and atropine sulfate on tracheal mucus velocity and lung mechanics in anesthetized dogs, *Respiration*, 34, 181, 1977.

120. Wanner, A., Clinical aspects of mucociliary transport, *Am. Rev. Respir. Dis.*, 116, 73, 1977.

121. Nadel, J. A., Control of mucus secretion and ion transport in airways, *Ann. Rev. Physiol.*, 41, 369, 1979.

122. Friedman, M., Scott, F. D., Poole, D. O., Dougherty, R., Chapman, G. A., Watson, H., and Sackner, M. A., A new roentgenographic method for estimating mucus velocity in airways, *Am. Rev. Respir. Dis.*, 115, 67, 1977.

123. Wolff, R. K. and Muggenburg, B. A., Comparison of two methods of measuring tracheal mucous velocity in anesthetized beagle dogs, *Am. Rev. Respir. Dis.*, 120, 137, 1979.

124. Tomenius, L., Effect of trichloroethylene on cilia activity in rabbit trachea, *Acta Pharmacol. Toxicol.*, 44, 65, 1979.

Index

INDEX

A

Abnormalitis of connective tissue, II: 162
Abnormal levels of inhibitors, II: 36
Accumulation
    of basic amines, I: 172—175
    of foreign compounds, I: 169—177
    of nutrophil, II: 41
    of phagocyte, I: 235
    steady-state, I: 170, 171
Acetaldehyde, I: 254, 263
C-Acetate, II: 105
Acetylcholine, I: 257, 258; II: 74, 78—79
Acetylcysteine, I: 258
N-Acetylcysteine, I: 257
Acetylene, I: 254
Acetylouabain, I: 258
Acid phosphatase, I: 135; II: 38
Acrolein, I: 255; II: 43, 44
ACTH, see Adrenocorticotropic hormone
Actin, I: 135
Activated macrophages, II: 21, 22
Activated mediators, II: 70, 89
Activated oxygen, II: 86, 106
Activated phagocytes, I: 231, 235
Activity median aerodynamic diameter (AMAD)
    of particles, I: 33
Activity median diameter (AMD) of particles, I:
    31
Activity median diffusive diameter (AMDD) of
    particles, I: 33
Acute bronchitis, II: 46—47
Acute pancreatitis, II: 78
Adenosine diphosphate (ADP), II: 76
Adenosine triphosphate (ATP), II: 71, 105
ADH, see Antidiuretic hormone
ADP, see Adenosine diphosphate
α-Adrenergic blocking agents, I: 259
β-Adrenergic blocking agents, I: 170
Adrenergic effectors, I: 263
β-Adrenergic system, II: 130
Adrenocorticotropic hormone (ACTH), II: 67,
    69, 80
Adult respiratory distress syndrome (ARDS), II:
    77
Adventitia, see Tunica adventitia
Aerodynamic diameter of particles, I: 32, 33,
    49—51, 59
Aerodynamic properties of particles, I: 31—33,
    41
Aerodynamic separation, I: 49
Aerodynamic size of particles, I: 41
Aerosol hair spray, I: 253
Aerosols, I: 254, 255
    coagulation rate for, I: 33
    defined, I: 29
    dispersion characteristics of, I: 33—34
    hydrolytic, I: 64
    monodisperse, I: 47, 50, 53, 56
    polydisperse, I: 53, 56

    properties of, I: 29—35
Aflatoxin B_1, II: 92
AHH, see Aryl hydrocarbon hydroxylase
Air-blood barrier, I: 79, 93, 97, 123, 151, 220
Airflow, I: 41—47
    patterns of in airway, I: 65
    resistance in, I: 4
Air pollution, I: 59, 248; II: 14, 15, 164
Air tissue-lymph interface, I: 146
Airway branching, I: 4
    angles of, I: 4, 5, 38, 39
    irregularity in, I: 5
    patterns in, I: 39
Airways, I: 213, 223, 260
    airflow patterns in, I: 65
    branching in, see Airway branching
    cell death and renewal in, I: 189—218
    epithelium of, I: 6—10
    geometry of, I: 4, 35—41
    models of, I: 40—41
    morphometry of, I: 4—5, 35—40, 50, 51
    organization of, I: 6—11
    resistance in, II: 162, 171
Albumin distribution volume, I: 222
Alkalosis, II: 74—75, 89—91
Alkylation products, II: 95
Allergic bronchopulmonary aspergillosis, II:
    50—51
Aluminum silicate, II: 13
Alveolar air spaces, I: 123, 139, 147, 150, 151,
    236; II: 4, 7, 10, 42, 52, 191
Alveolar atrophy, II: 173
Alveolar basement membranes, II: 4
Alveolar bronchiolization, I: 207
Alveolar capillaries, I: 78, 81, 93, 97, 127, 150,
    151, 190, 231; II: 49
Alveolar-capillary membrane, see also Air-blood
    barrier, I: 220, 231
Alveolar cells, I: 207
    morphometry of, I: 204
Alveolar clearance, I: 59—61
Alveolar deposition, I: 51
Alveolar ducts, I: 38, 91, 131; II: 11, 12, 47, 67,
    76, 174, 175, 178
Alveolar edema, I: 220, 232; II: 11, 42
Alveolar epithelial cells, I: 174, 176; II: 99
    permeability of, I: 229
    Type I, I: 16; II: 48, 105
    Type II, I: 16; II: 48, 105
Alveolar epithelium, II: 191—196, 228, 230—233;
    II: 4, 49, 177, 178, 194
Alveolar flooding, see also Pulmonary edema, I:
    222, 223
Alveolar forces, I: 228
Alveolar hemorrhage, II: 96
Alveolar hypoxia, II: 77
Alveolar interstitium, II: 125, 128
Alveolar lymphatic vessels, I: 127
Alveolar macrophage collagenase, II: 35
Alveolar macrophages, I: 190, 209, 211, 223;